Amste[illegible]

"*Amsterdam Ascendant* is a rich, compelling work of historical fiction that follows the lives and relationships of lovers, traders, soldiers, immigrants, shipbuilders, and other fascinating individuals in the late 1500s. Several themes related to the book's history are smoothly integrated throughout the story, making it easy to lose track of time and become immersed in its historical world. This book is a must-read for everyone interested in the history of Europe, particularly Amsterdam." ***—Manhattan Book Review***

"A well-researched historical novel with a very human core . . . The story proper opens dramatically with Maarten van der Voort and the Sea Beggars, essentially privateers, capturing a Spanish warship, which sets the tone for the next several years of back-and-forth fighting . . . The principal characters, each drawn with distinct personalities, include Maarten, the adopted son of saintly old Papa Hasbrouk, Maarten's wife Betje, and their two sons, Nicolaas and Dirck . . . Considering the many plot threads that could easily have become tangled, such as those following Dirck's social cluelessness, Nicolaas' womanizing, and Betje's endless fretting, Richards is to be congratulated for keeping each strand in place, all requiring just the right amount of our attention. Richards is a competent and earnest writer, not given to lyricism. But her love for the time and place is palpable, and this well-told tale leaves the reader eager for further chapters." ***—Kirkus Reviews***

". . . inviting and rich in its actions and details . . . The vivid 'you are here' feel of the story brings the times to life . . . the competing visions and experiences of a variety of characters create an especially realistic tone as events unfold . . . Richards employs an evocative, descriptive voice that brings these times and families to life . . . *Amsterdam Ascendant*'s ability to capture an engrossing, changing social and political landscape in the 1500s makes it a top recommendation for libraries and readers who look to be immersed in the times and the people . . ." ***—Midwest Book Review***

Amsterdam Ascendant

A novel of rebellion, faith, and daring enterprise that launch a Golden Age

JUDITH W. RICHARDS

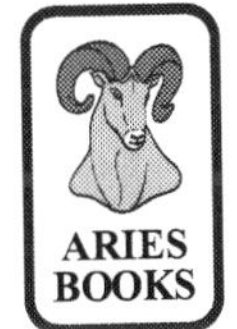

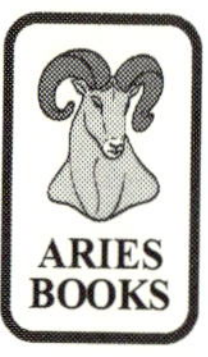

ARIES BOOKS – Fiction

Washington, D.C.

www.AriesBooks.com

This book is a work of fiction. The characters are products of the author's imagination or are used fictitiously, and any resemblance to a real person is entirely coincidental. The portrayals of well-known historical personages, however, are based on recorded history.

Library of Congress Cataloging-in-Publication Data

Richards, Judith W.

Aries Books first edition, 2023, Washington, D.C.

Title: Amsterdam Ascendant. Subtitle: A novel of rebellion, faith, and daring enterprise that launch a Golden Age

Main categories: Historical novel | Amsterdam | 1500s | Action adventure | Family saga.

ISBN 978-0-9845410-8-9 (paper)

ISBN 978-0-9845410-9-6 (ebook)

for David

My husband, author D. Manning Richards,
who offered invaluable critiques and
support along the way.

Table of Contents

Author's Note to the Reader

This story is fictional, but the history is true. In case you are not fully familiar with the time period of the novel, I offer Background History below to help set the stage. Following that is a Language section, which explains my choices of Dutch vs. English words.

At the back of the book is additional information. *Fact or Fiction?* sorts out real people and events from invented ones. *Acknowledgements and Principal Sources* lists reference books you may want to read to learn more about specific subjects covered in the story. If you are curious about what motivated me, an American real estate developer, to write this novel, you will find the answer in *About the Author.* For those who like to share their reading experiences, there is a *Book Club Discussion Guide.* Lastly, I hope the *Epilogue* will whet your appetite for my next two books that will carry the Van der Voort saga into Amsterdam's 1600s Golden Age and to exotic destinations around the world.

BACKGROUND HISTORY

When the story starts in 1572, Amsterdam is a small Catholic-dominated trading city that is best known for a miracle that occurred in 1345, which made it an important pilgrimage destination. The miracle involved a Holy Communion host that was vomited up by a dying man and would not burn when tossed into a fire and instead levitated above the flames. Though Amsterdam is the largest city in the northern part of the Netherlands, it is nowhere near as wealthy or grand as Antwerp and Brussels in the south. There is nothing about Amsterdam in 1572 to suggest it would become an economic powerhouse by the end of the century.

The Netherlands is owned by Spain and consists of present-day

Netherlands, Belgium, Luxemburg, and parts of France. It is a watery world because land reclamation is not yet underway on a large scale. The estuaries of the major rivers—Rhine, Maas, Waal, and Scheldt—are vast and untamed. The Zuider Zee too is sprawling, and between it and Amsterdam is a sluggish river, the Ij. Amsterdam is separated from Haarlem by a lake, which has since been drained. Dikes provide crucial protection against the sea, the same as today.

The Netherlands has been at war for four years with its mighty ruler, King Philip II of Spain, who is intent on purging Protestant heretics from his realm. Prior to the rebellion, cities and provinces in concert with a small aristocracy enjoyed a degree of self-governance, including making their own laws and having a say on taxes. So when the king introduced a new ten-percent tax without their consent, marched troops into the Netherlands, and imposed a brutal Inquisition, both Catholic and Protestant Netherlanders objected. They were rebuffed and many were forced to flee, including Prince William of Orange, who became the leader of the revolt and whose House of Orange is the monarchy of the Netherlands today. In exile, Prince William recruited an army and issued letters of marque to exiled sea captains, known as the Sea Beggars, authorizing them to attack and capture Spanish ships.

During the period of this novel, 1572 to 1597, Amsterdam is shaped by religious strife, war, seafaring enterprise, immigrants, business-friendly civic leadership, and innovations in shipbuilding and mapmaking. All are woven into the story.

LANGUAGE

The written language of the 1500s is an old form of Dutch with formal and flowery phraseology. I make no attempt to mimic it in dialogue and instead use direct, casual, and friendly discourse, which is in keeping with my perception of Amsterdam's merchant class at that time: competitive, pragmatic, and loving of family. For ease of reading by my primary readership, Americans, I limit the use of Dutch words to *ja* (yes) and *nee* (no), pronounced "ya" and "nay," and *speculaas koekjes* (spice cookies), pronounced "spaykool-ahs kookyuhs." For ease of recognition, place names are spelled in English, such as Netherlands for Dutch *Nederland*, Brill for the town *Den Briel*, and Gdansk for *Dantzig*, and some geographic references are simplified. For example, Italy refers to the Italian peninsula and Italian as their language, even though a unified Italy with a single language does not exist at the time. Similarly, Calvinism is used in place of the less familiar proper name Reformed Church. I realize my choices may rankle Netherlanders and apologize in advance.

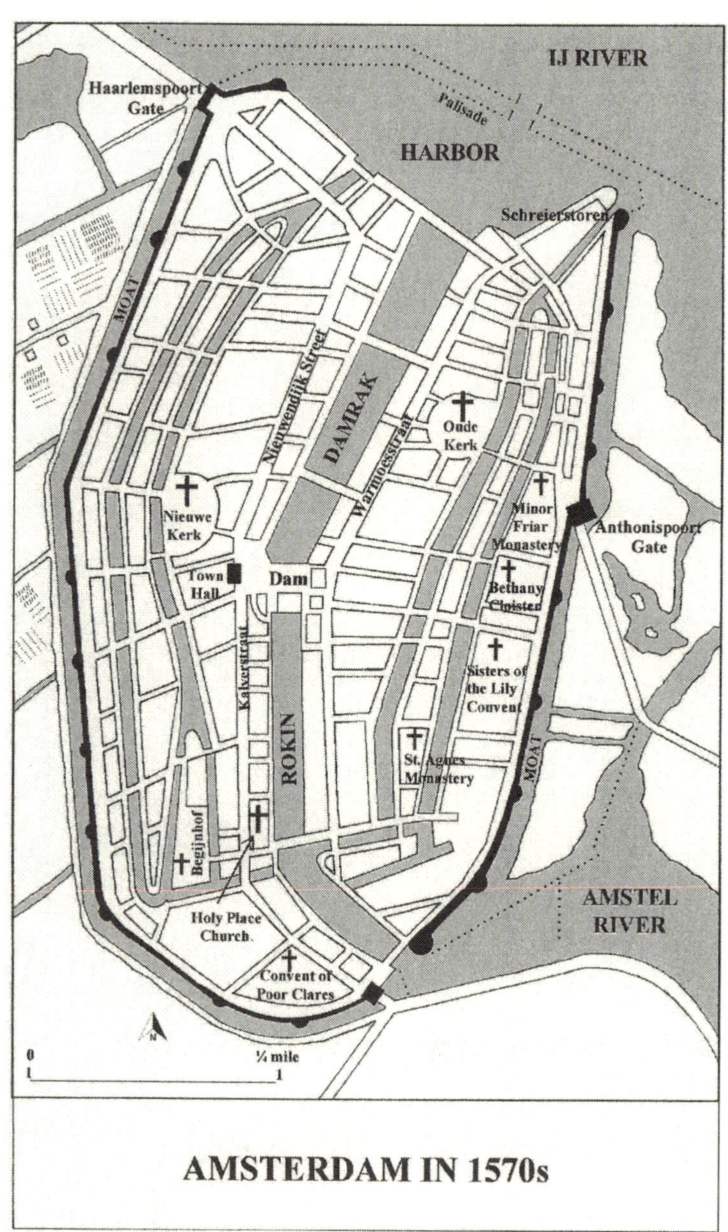

AMSTERDAM IN 1570s

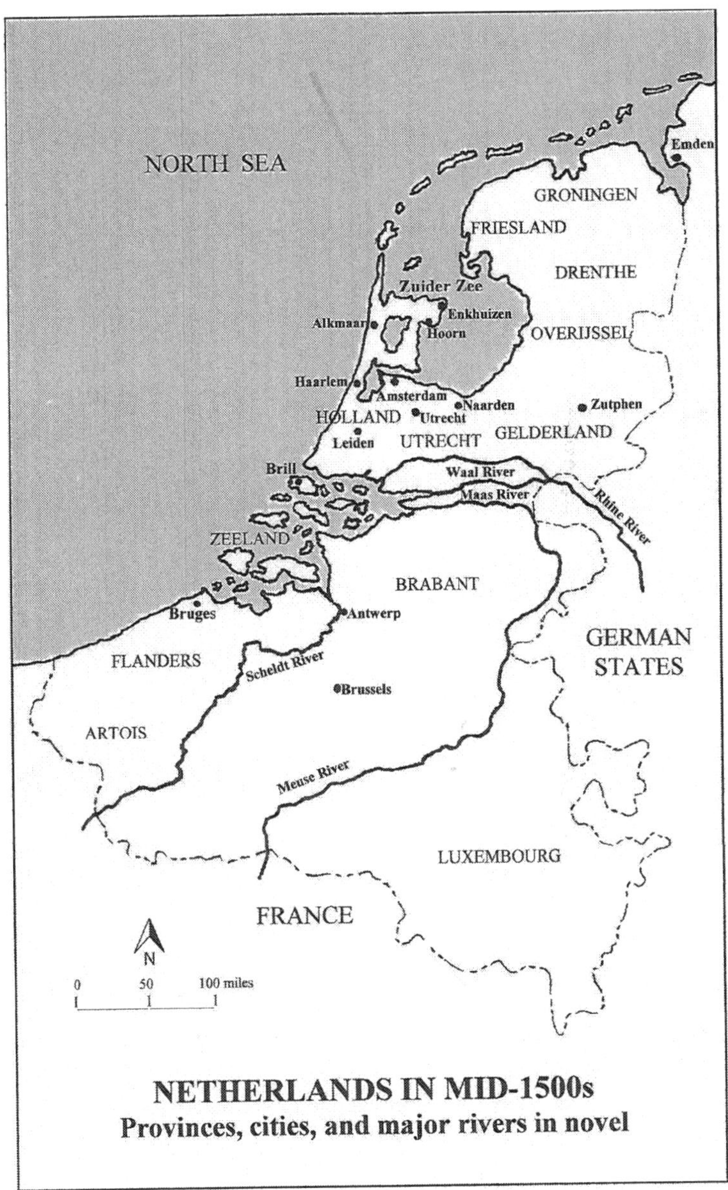

NETHERLANDS IN MID-1500s
Provinces, cities, and major rivers in novel

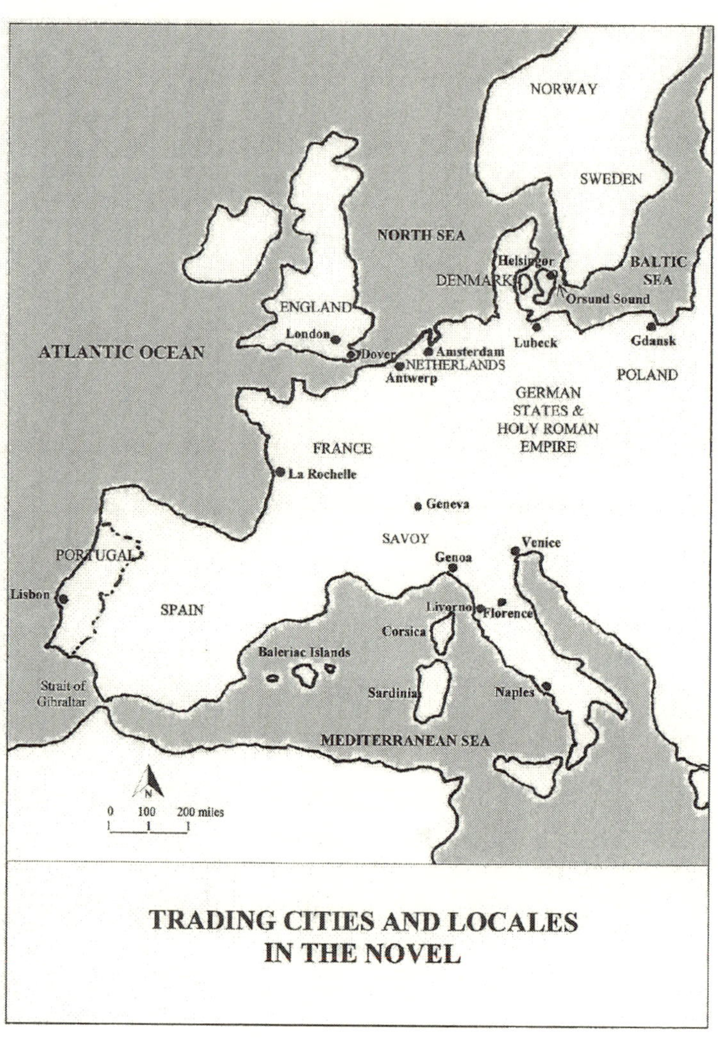

TRADING CITIES AND LOCALES IN THE NOVEL

Family Tree

Principal Fictional Characters in 1572

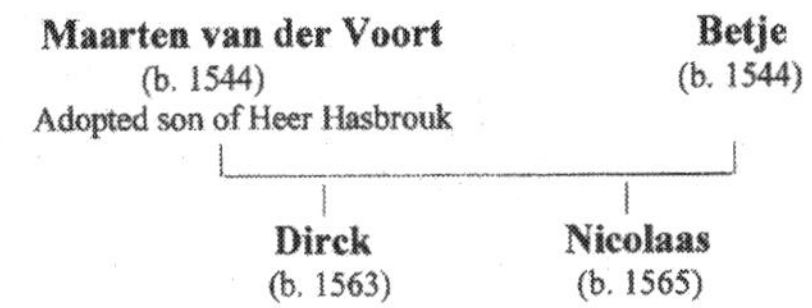

Heer Hasbrouk
(b. 1516)
Adoptive father of Maarten
married to Jaane (b. 1534, d. 1562)

Catrijn
(b. 1562)
Godchild of Maarten and Betje

Margaretha Hasbrouk
(b. 1516)
Twin sister of Heer Hasbrouk
Member of the Beguines

Pieter
(b. 1547)
Brother-in-law of Maarten and brother of Betje

Rijp Dekker
(b. 1543)
Petty criminal and Maarten's nemesis

Note: The purpose of this brief Family Tree is to help the reader establish relationships among principal characters at the start of the novel. Subsequent events in their lives—marriages, children, and dates of deaths—are excluded to avoid unduly disclosing the story.

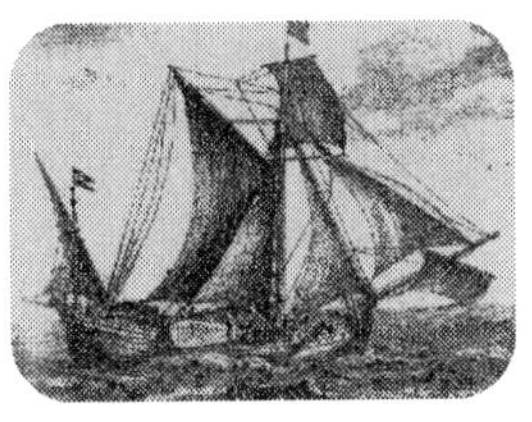

CHAPTER 1

The Sea Beggars—1572

Dutch sea captain Maarten van der Voort stood on the deck of his merchant ship, the *Dirck*, and watched his men, looking ghostlike in the dense fog, go over the side and into the waiting longboat. It was a cold March night and three in the morning, yet sweat beaded on his brow, for he knew he was taking a calculated risk with their lives. They were going to attack a Spanish ship before it attacked them.

Earlier that night, his most trusted sentry had awakened him after hearing something in the distance that sounded like water gently lapping against a ship's hull. Though no other sentry had heard it, to be cautious Maarten sent the man out in the longboat, tethered by a lengthy line to the *Dirck*, to drift silently and reconnoiter. Upon returning, the sentry reported seeing the vague outline of a ship, which appeared to be Spanish because it was larger and had a higher stern than a typical Dutch vessel. The ship was utterly quiet, with no movement on deck. No other ships were in sight.

After weighing the options, Maarten had decided the only choice was to strike first and use the element of surprise to his advantage. With luck, the ship would indeed be alone, having been separated from its convoy by the same storms that had scattered his own fleet, the notorious Dutch Sea Beggars.

Maarten went below to rouse the men, cautioned them to be as quiet as possible, and explained the imminent threat and need to act before the fog lifted. The men listened intently and without alarm, as Maarten had expected. He knew them well, for they had been together for four years since leaving Amsterdam in 1568 to flee the Spanish Inquisition and join the Dutch revolt against Spain.

He also laid out the risks. "We've taken many a ship with our fleet over the years, but make no mistake, this time is different. We're in unknown waters. And we're on our own." Maarten looked each man in the eye to make sure he understood.

"If we're successful," he continued, "we *alone* will reap the rewards."

The men nodded, understanding the profit potential. Maarten possessed a letter of marque from the leader of the Dutch revolt, Prince William of Orange, which allowed him to seize enemy ships and sell them as so-called prizes of war. The proceeds were theirs to keep, except for the ten percent to be given to Prince William to help fund the ongoing rebellion.

"If any man has a question, or objects to the assault—speak now," Maarten said. Hearing none, he prepared them for battle, saying in a quiet voice: "Our cause is just. You are brave, and I know I can count on you." He raised his fist. "To God! To Prince William!"

The men repeated the vow in equally low voices and thrust their clenched hands into the air. All knelt, and Maarten led them in a Calvinist prayer.

On deck, he observed the oarsmen wrapping rags around the oar supports to muffle sound, while the men slipped over the side and into the longboat. The last man to go down the ladder was his brother-in-law Pieter, and he scrutinized his face to see whether he was letting his superstitious imagination get away from him. If he was, the men would see. Fear was contagious.

Pieter feigned a confident look, but was worried, not only about the possibility of other Spanish ships being nearby, but also the reported lack of noise and movement on the ship. Are the crew dead? From some horrifying disease? Is the ship cursed?

Maarten saluted the two men staying aboard the *Dirck* and

then prepared to descend. After pushing a lock of damp blond hair back under his beret and giving a final tug to the belt securing his knife and sword, he stepped onto the rope ladder. Though burly and taller than the average Dutchman, he nimbly climbed down and took his seat at the bow of the longboat.

The eyes of his eighteen men followed him, looking for the slightest sign of doubt on their captain's face.

Maarten returned their stares with a look of determination and confidence and gave the command to start rowing. His finger went to his lips: silence. The oarsmen pulled as noiselessly as possible, and the sentry pointed the way.

The men squinted into the thick mist, searching ... searching for the elusive ship. The sentry was the first to spot its hazy image.

Maarten signaled to lay up oars. The longboat drifted soundlessly, and the ship grew more distinct. It was indeed Spanish. Seeing that it was not too much bigger than the *Dirck*, Maarten thought: Good, this should be a fairly equal fight, man-for-man.

He let the longboat drift to the ship's anchor line, and the boatswain grabbed hold of it. Maarten stood, got a boost from a sailor, and hoisted himself up the rough rope. One by one, his men followed. The boatswain remained behind to prevent the longboat from bumping noisily against the enemy hull and to signal if another ship showed up.

At the top, Maarten gripped his feet on the fretwork, grasped the gunwale, and peered over. No movement ... no sentries in sight. He climbed over and squatted. His eyes narrowed and surveyed the deck. Why no sentries? He inched forward. Next to the capstan, he saw a slumped man and another near the hatch. The stupid sentries are asleep! Maarten tiptoed toward the capstan with knife in hand, while his first mate crept to the hatch. Behind them, more Dutchmen came over the gunwale.

Maarten sank his knife into the slumbering sentry's neck. The man moaned, and Maarten muffled the sound with his hand. The sentry slumped against the capstan, dead.

The first mate stumbled, waking the sentry next to the hatch, and had to lunge to stab him. A groan escaped as he died. The first mate crouched next to the hatch with his knife poised, and crew members joined him.

From below deck, footfalls. The hatch opened with a creak. A Spaniard peeked out. "Fernando?"

The first mate stabbed him with quick jabs. The man fell inside, and the hatch slammed shut.

Maarten hurried to the forecastle door, sword raised. His crew assumed positions behind him. Below deck, men shouted in Spanish.

An officer burst through the door. Maarten rammed his sword into him and pushed the crumpled body aside. A hefty deckhand emerged wielding a long dagger. He dodged Maarten's sword and smashed into him, sending them both tumbling. The man landed on top, banged Maarten's hand onto the deck until he released the sword, and then raised his own dagger. Maarten twisted to get out of its reach and thrust his hand into the deckhand's face, his fingers gouging into the eyes.

"*Aargh*." The man jerked back his head but Maarten's fingers only dug deeper. His dagger started slashing wildly, and Maarten threw up an arm to shield himself. The blade grazed his forearm, and another swipe hit his upper arm. Suddenly the man bolted straight up; his body twitched twice and collapsed onto Maarten, knocking the wind out of him. Maarten's first mate knelt down and with great effort shoved the body off. After yanking his pike out of the man's back, the first mate pivoted to face the next foe, while Maarten caught his breath.

On his feet again, Maarten retrieved his sword in time to swing at a Spaniard emerging from the forecastle, felling him. Seeing a man atop Pieter, Maarten charged, knocking him over and then finishing him off with a hit of his sword. He pulled Pieter to his feet.

Maarten paused to assess the melee. Nearby, one of his men was strangling a flailing Spaniard. Next to the mast, another was under attack, and Pieter was slipping and sliding across the bloody deck to aid him.

A figure appeared in the doorway at the stern of the ship, and

Maarten's eyes fixed on him. His haughty demeanor and impeccable clothes told Maarten he was the captain and an aristocrat.

The Spanish commander needed little time to size up the situation. Many of his men lay dead, others were struggling for their lives, and those coming up from below were being cut down before even entering the fray. The assailants clearly were Dutchmen—big, fair-skinned and ferocious—who would rather die for their heretical religion than give up. Why battle on? he thought. The ship belongs to the king, nothing to lose your life over. His eyes rested on Maarten, and intuition told him that this was their captain, despite his being dressed similarly to his crew, a common practice of Dutch sea captains.

Maarten strode toward him, daring the captain to fight man-to-man.

The Spanish captain assumed an erect pose and put one hand into the air. With dignity and formality, he reversed the hilt of his sword and presented it to Maarten. "*Me rindo. Tú ganas.*" I surrender. You win.

Maarten stood motionless, his eyes boring into the captain's and body straining against the urge to strike him down.

To his men, the Spanish captain ordered, "*HOMBRES! ALTO! ENTREGUEN SUS ARMAS!*" Men! Stop! Hand over your weapons!

Maarten called out, "MEN! SEA BEGGARS! STOP! THEY'RE SURRENDERING!"

The combatants froze. Warily they eyed their captains ... and each other.

"*ENTREGUEN SUS ARMAS!*" the captain repeated. Hand over your weapons!

"TAKE THEIR WEAPONS!" Maarten ordered.

The Spanish captain was still offering his sword.

Maarten snatched it contemptuously and glared back, as if to say: You coward, you didn't even put up a fight!

The Spanish captain crossed himself and kissed the gold crucifix hanging from a necklace.

In Maarten's adrenaline-pumped state, *that* was an insult. How dare you flaunt your Catholicism—in front of *me*, a Calvinist Sea Beggar! I ought to run you through. Maarten swung his sword up to the captain's throat. He hesitated, and the sword hung there, just touching the Adam's apple. He glanced at his first mate, whose hate-filled expression was saying: Go ahead, kill the lousy papist! Maarten's eyes flitted to his brother-in-law Pieter, whose message was clear: Don't kill him. You're not a murderer. Maarten's gaze returned to the cowardly captain.

Dutchmen and Spaniards fell silent, watching.

With a deft flick of his sword, Maarten popped the captain's gold chain. It and the cross went flying and landed on the deck next to Pieter's foot with a clink.

"THROW THE BASTARD INTO HIS BOAT!" Maarten barked, waving a hand toward the vessel lashed to the deck. "HIS MEN TOO. THEN CUT THEM ADRIFT."

Amid the fog and carnage, an eerie calm set in as Maarten put his men to work. The first mate and a team of sailors herded the Spaniards toward the bow of the ship, a second group collected their weapons and piled them at the stern, and Pieter's crew unlashed and lowered the longboat into the water. Meanwhile, Maarten did a quick scan of the surrounding sea for enemy vessels. Seeing none, he focused on treating the six wounded Dutchmen.

Once the Spanish longboat was full, it rode deep in the water and tipped precariously until the Spaniards redistributed themselves. Maarten saluted the captain and gave the order to cut them loose. Without oars or sail, the boat bobbed and drifted into the fog and out of sight.

Maarten gathered his men to pray over their two dead comrades and commit their bodies to the sea. Afterward, he congratulated each and every man for the hard-earned victory, and together they recited the Sea Beggars' motto, "Help thyself and God will help thee," followed by three exuberant hurrahs.

Maarten remained on the Spanish ship along with brother-in-law Pieter and half the men. The first mate took the others back to the *Dirck*, and a line was attached to the two ships to keep them from drifting apart.

At daybreak, neither the Spanish longboat nor any other ship was visible in the thinning fog. Maarten ordered the sails raised, and the two ships set sail southwestward on a light wind. The destination was England, where sympathetic Protestant Queen Elizabeth allowed Dutch Sea Beggars to provision in safety and where an active market existed for selling captured ships. En route, Maarten hoped to meet up with the rest of his fleet.

Once the ships were on a steady course, Maarten relaxed and pulled out the bottle of sherry and elegant crystal goblet he had taken from the Spanish captain's richly appointed cabin. While pouring himself a heaping glassful, he marveled at how differently Spanish and Dutch sea captains lived. He himself had no cache of fine wines and crystal, or fancy accommodations. In fact, he shared his austere cabin with Pieter, the first mate, *and* the steering rudder. Every Dutch captain lived similarly, even noblemen fleet commanders.

Maarten glanced around his captured ship, admiring its well-designed rigging ... freshly washed deck ... all in excellent condition. I wish I could keep her, he lamented, but she's too rich for my purse. At least she'll fetch a nice sum to tide me over for a while. His eyes shifted to his own *Dirck*: the single-masted, seventy-foot vessel he had purchased used in Amsterdam before the revolt started. The last four years on the run haven't been kind to her, he concluded. Those makeshift repairs the boatswain made after the last battle won't hold much longer ... and those patched sails *must* be replaced. That's where a good bit of the money will go.

Maarten gave a squeeze to the beggar's purse hanging from his neck, taking comfort in the symbol of the Sea Beggars that had sustained him through many a hardship. He had first donned the purse when leaving Amsterdam to escape the Inquisition sent by Spanish King Philip II to eradicate heretics, such as him. Protestants from all walks of life had been forced to leave their hometowns, and some dissenting Catholics as well. Like Pieter, many had never been to sea, and none had been to war.

The Sea Beggars' moniker had originated when Dutch lower-ranking nobles were spurned as "mere beggars" for asking King

Philip to reconsider his decisions to send an Inquisition and troops into the Netherlands, replace local officials with his own men, and impose a ten-percent tax without local concurrence. In defiance, they put on beggar purses and clothes—and then fled. High-level nobility too had been forced to escape, and some lost their lives. Catholic Count Egmont was beheaded and became the hero of the revolt, and Prince William of Orange emerged as its leader. Despite Prince William having been a protégé of King Philip's own father, he was forced into exile and from his German estate raised a Beggar army and issued letters of marque to the Sea Beggars.

By the time Pieter came on deck after having completed his inventory of the ship's contents, the fog had burned off. He paused to enjoy the warmth of the sun and took out the Saint Nicolaas medal given to him by his sister Betje, Maarten's wife. Thoughts of his big sister and of Saint Nicolaas, Amsterdam's patron saint, always centered him, especially at times like this when memories of last night's bloodshed still lingered. Though he was a sturdy fellow and as capable as the next man of fighting, his gentle and compassionate nature prevented him ever becoming inured to killing another human being. With a sigh, Pieter returned to the task at hand and gave a final once-over to his inventory.

He looked for Maarten and spotted him at the bow, contemplative and clutching his beggar purse. Again, Pieter was struck by the uncanny resemblance between Maarten and his adoptive father, Papa Hasbrouk. Both were big men with broad faces, thoughtful eyes, and easy smiles, but aside from the physical similarities, they were very different. Papa was calm and impressively erudite; Maarten was anything but. Yet, Pieter had to admit that Maarten had acquired some of Papa's traits during their four years at war. He was now less hotheaded, more disciplined, and on occasion even used quotes from Papa's favorite books when needing to buoy up the crew.

Pieter stepped forward after Maarten let go of his beggar's purse. "I'm done with my inventory, Maarten."

Maarten accepted the list, passed the goblet to Pieter to finish, and started reading.

Pieter savored the sherry and beamed when Maarten's head began nodding in approval, which reconfirmed his value as a meticulous and accurate record-keeper. Those skills along with his scrupulous honesty had made him a sought-after bookkeeper in Amsterdam and purser aboard the *Dirck*. Like everyone else on the ship, though, he also had other jobs, including helping with the mainsail, scrubbing the deck when his turn came up, and being a combatant when required. The role he was most proud of, however, was being Maarten's moral compass, though Maarten would probably never perceive or acknowledge his work in that regard. Maarten was a good and honorable man, but sometimes his moral fiber was tested by the burdens of being captain and making difficult decisions, which was when Pieter stepped in to give a nudge in the right direction.

Maarten handed the inventory back to Pieter, and an involuntary burp came out, almost directly into his face. Pieter pulled back and waved the noxious odor away. Both chuckled.

"Good work, Pieter," Maarten said and slapped him on the back.

When Dover came into view, Maarten climbed up to the top of the mast and with sea gulls circling overhead surveyed the harbor. There were twenty-three Sea Beggar ships by his count, easily identified by the colorful patterns painted on their hulls and brazen ten-coin flags, which signified hatred of King Philip's ten-percent tax. The rest of the ships were mostly English, with a few French ones sprinkled in. Importantly, he saw no captured Spanish ships, which meant his prize would command a high price. On occasion, Sea Beggars had brought as many as ten prizes at once to Dover, causing prices to be depressed for weeks as they were sold off.

The *Dirck* and the prize set anchor among the Sea Beggar ships, and captains shouted congratulations to Maarten. Soon the crews were gathering at the gunwales, yelling questions back and forth about the taking of the Spanish ship and the best pubs to visit in the boisterous little town of Dover. Meanwhile, Maarten and Pieter went ashore to find buyers.

By late afternoon, Maarten had secured two firm offers for his prize and expected a higher third one from a successful privateer, whose business was buying slaves from Portuguese suppliers in Africa and selling them in Spain's American colonies. He was in the final stages of assembling a new fleet with money from well-heeled and powerful backers and was reportedly eager to get underway, so Maarten guessed he would make an attractive offer to seal the deal quickly.

While Maarten waited for the privateer's offer, he invited fellow Sea Beggar captains onto his prize to look around and sample wines from her hold.

The Sea Beggars' commander arrived late and was wearing his trademark uniform, a priest's vestment, this time a gold-threaded purple velvet robe from a recent raid on a monastery. Under normal circumstances his appearance was bizarre with his wild eyes and unruly long hair and beard, which he vowed never to cut until he avenged King Philip's murder of his relative Count Egmont. This evening, though, the commander looked even more menacing. His face was contorted with rage, as he stalked across the deck toward Maarten.

Pieter took a step back, for he detested the unpredictable, ruthless, and cruel commander and believed his unreasonable hatred of Catholic clergy gave the Sea Beggars a bad name. Although Maarten found the commander to be volatile and merciless, he preferred to focus on his good qualities: fearlessness and brilliance as a leader.

"Maarten," the commander said, "sell your prize right away—before word gets out that Queen Elizabeth is expelling us from England."

Gasps all around.

Maarten nodded he understood. "Why is she forcing us out?"

"Ja, why?" others queried.

"Because she's *gutless,*" the commander snarled, spittle flying. In case they could not deduce what had happened, he explained it in simple terms. "His Royal High-*ass* threatened her—of course!" referring to Spain's King Philip II.

Pieter was not surprised that the queen of a backwater country like England would sacrifice the Sea Beggars' cause, after being threatened by the most powerful king in the world.

"Weak, *sniveling* royals like Elizabeth," the commander raged on, "don't have the *guts* to stand up for their principles!" He looked at Maarten. "Get the best price you can, before your buyers hear about it and you lose all bargaining power." To the other captains he added, "Get ready to sail on the next high tide and favorable wind. *Gutless* Elizabeth is sending her agents to ensure we leave right away."

The commander swiftly departed. The captains gulped down their remaining wine and thanked Maarten, and grumbled as they went over the side. Maarten was watching them climb down the ship's ladder when he noticed the privateer sitting in his longboat.

The privateer waited for the last Sea Beggar captain to be rowed away, before coming aboard. He stated his offer—it was substantially higher than the other two—and he and Maarten shook hands on the deal.

The privateer's men plunked a strongbox on the deck. While his purser observed, Pieter began counting the coins, starting with gold Spanish ducats. Half way through, he came upon a suspicious looking coin that felt too soft to be solid gold. He bit down on it and checked its weight on his balance scale. "Lead," Pieter declared, meaning there was gold on the outside but lead inside. He passed the ducat to Maarten and gulped hard, aware that Maarten had punched the last guy who tried to pass off a fake coin.

Maarten bit the ducat. Fuming, he thrust it into the privateer's face. "What's *this*?"

The privateer took the ducat, tested it, and glared at his purser. "*You know I don't do business like this!*" With a vicious kick, he sent the man sprawling. "*Get him out of my sight!*" Returning to Maarten, he pulled a replacement ducat from his money pouch. "Take this. I'm sorry."

Maarten snatched the coin, frowned, and put it between his teeth. With a nod of approval, he handed it to Pieter.

Pieter resumed counting. After the gold ducats, he went on to English gold sovereigns and lastly the silver: some Antwerp groats, but mostly thalers from Bohemia. Relieved that the privateer had not tried to sneak in any copper coins, so low in value to be essentially useless, Pieter sat back on his haunches. "It's all there, Maarten. All good."

Calmer now, Maarten put out his hand to shake. "She's yours, captain. Good luck on your venture."

Maarten and his men returned to the *Dirck,* and the strongbox was placed on the deck. With the crew gathered close, Pieter divided the coins into neat stacks, each representing one man's share. He also created piles for provisions and the required ten percent for Prince William of Orange. Done, he sat back and smiled broadly at the men. They cheered, and Maarten poured a round of drinks. Congratulations and backslapping went around.

When the commander gave the signal to put to sea, there had been too little time for Maarten to fully provision the *Dirck,* or for the crew to seek out the pleasures of Dover.

As the Sea Beggar fleet sailed out of the harbor, the sun was shining and not a cloud was to be seen. Maarten van der Voort should have been a happy man, but he was not. The future worried him. Queen Elizabeth, a coward in his opinion, had put the Sea Beggars in an extremely precarious situation. In these parts, the fleet had only one other friendly port, La Rochelle in France, which was controlled by Huguenots (French Calvinists). The only other port open to them was Emden, their base in the far north beyond the Zuider Zee in Germany.

The Sea Beggar cause itself also troubled Maarten. When leaving his home in 1568, he had been full of indignation and self-righteousness, and fleeing ahead of the Inquisition was the smart thing to do to save his ship from possible confiscation. He had expected to return home soon, because any rational king would realize he was losing good tax-paying merchants and quickly capitulate to their demands.

Now four years on, had King Philip II yielded? No, Maarten had to admit. What had the Sea Beggars accomplished, aside from marauding Catholic monasteries and harassing Spanish ships? Had they figured out how to trade in hostile realms to support themselves and the rebel cause? No. Had they won over any converts to their cause? No. Had they won any battles or gained any strategic advantage for Prince William of Orange? No. Was the Prince winning any battles on land? No. Maarten was coming to the sad conclusion that the last four years had been pretty much a huge waste of time.

At this point, all he wanted to do was go home and make an honest living again. Nothing more. Back there, he could take care of his family, try to sort out how things had ever come to this, and possibly regain some of his youthful exuberance, for right now he was feeling much older than his twenty-eight years. Of course, going home was impossible, so he did the next best thing. He closed his eyes and summoned a comforting image of his family and the home he left behind in Amsterdam.

In his mind, his adoptive father Papa Hasbrouk was in his cozy little house engaged in lively conversation with his twin sister, Aunt Margaretha. Catrijn, Papa's daughter and Maarten's goddaughter, was falling asleep on her father's lap with a book in her hands.

At his own home, Maarten envisioned his wife Betje looking voluptuous, silhouetted against the warm glow of the hearth. She was stirring a pot of Maarten's favorite stew. The boys were wrestling on the floor, with Nicolaas trying in vain to get the upper hand on older brother Dirck.

A pang of guilt crept into Maarten's reverie about the mountain of debt he owed on his house and the *Dirck*. He ignored it, and the idyllic vision of home resumed. Never did he suspect that life in Amsterdam might be far different in reality.

~

In Amsterdam, nine-year-old Dirck van der Voort saw his former home ahead as he rounded the corner with brother Nicolaas and Catrijn Hasbrouk. It still angered him that the Inquisition had kicked him out of his house, along with his mother and Nicolaas, nearly four years ago.

"Stay here," Dirck said and headed toward the house.

Catrijn knew not to ask questions when Dirck had that determined look on his face, so she grabbed seven-year-old Nicolaas's hand and tugged him next to her.

At the front door, Dirck fumbled through his multilayered clothes—two stockings, long shirt, two quilted doublets, and leather jerkin—and succeeded in pulling out his penis. After grinning back at Catrijn and Nicolaas, he proceeded to unload on the threshold. Steam rose.

Catrijn's hand flew to her mouth—a ten-year-old young lady isn't supposed to laugh at such crudeness!

Feeling Catrijn's grip relax, Nicolaas yanked his hand loose and made a dash for the house. Dirck was finished with the threshold and working on the front door when Nicolaas showed up and began digging into his clothes.

The door opened, and a man stepped onto the wet stoop. "Fuck!" His big hand came down and seized Dirck by the arm.

"RUN!" Dirck yelled and pushed his brother back.

Nicolaas fell backward and was crawling away, when Catrijn arrived and dragged him to his feet. Together they sprinted away.

"You son of a whore!" The man was shaking Dirck. "Fuckin' little brat!"

Dirck let his body go limp and twisted to break the man's hold. The well-worn threads of his sleeve began to tear, and he squirmed harder until the sleeve ripped from the jerkin. In the instant that the man's fingers loosened to get a firmer grasp, Dirck broke free and ran as fast as he could.

"*Fuckin' brat!*"

Dirck stopped and with a wicked grin faced the man, who was angry as can be and shaking his fist. Dirck retrieved his penis again. As the trickle started, he let out an exaggerated laugh and defiantly pumped his fist into the air.

"*Next time I see you, I'll break that little dick off!*"

All the way home, the three repeated the profanities and laughed uncontrollably. They quieted down when Catrijn opened the front door, peeked inside, and confirmed that neither her father nor the boys' mother was in the front room. Nicolaas scampered in, and Dirck followed closely behind Catrijn, trying to hide his torn sleeve.

"There you are, finally," Betje van der Voort said, as she came out of the kitchen wiping her hands on her apron. She noticed the sleeve right away. "What have you been up to, Dirck?" Scowling, she waved him into the kitchen and told him to remove his jerkin.

Still excited, Nicolaas blurted out, "Dirck was—"

"Dirck had to," Catrijn interrupted, "uh, fight a boy who tried to steal this." She held out the cheese they had been sent to buy.

Betje van der Voort examined the cheese, declared it to be "paltry" and grumbled about the high cost of food.

"Ja, it's fuckin—"

"Nicolaas!" Betje's head whipped around. "What did you say?"

"He said *pfaltry*, Mother," Dirck clarified. "He meant to say *paltry*, but his tongue got tangled." Dirck flashed a malevolent look at his brother.

Betje did not believe a word of it, but did not have time to get to the bottom of the torn sleeve or the swearing.

"I know you've been up to something," Betje warned, "but I have work to do. I'll deal with you later. Now shoo, go sit down."

Considering themselves lucky to have gotten off so easily, the kids hurried to the seat next to the window.

Betje went to the linen cabinet for a needle, thread, and some solace. It was the place where important possessions were stored under lock and key and was the heart of every woman's household and womanhood. This cabinet had belonged to Catrijn's deceased mother, and Heer Hasbrouk had given the key to Betje as a welcoming gesture on the day she and the boys moved in with him and Catrijn. That day, Betje had lost everything to the Inquisition: the Van der Voort home, its contents, and Betje's own linen cabinet. Maarten had been convicted of heresy in absentia and his property seized as punishment for being a self-proclaimed Protestant who advocated for a Calvinist church in Amsterdam.

Betje found the needle and thread and sat down to sew.

The front door opened, and Hasbrouk came in. "Betje, I'm home."

She called back a greeting and turned her attention to preparing the evening meal.

Hasbrouk kissed Catrijn on the forehead, patted Dirck's shoulder, tousled Nicolaas's hair, and noticed they were unusually subdued. He regarded it as a blessing, for quiet moments were a rarity in the front room, which served as his office, his and Catrijn's bedroom, and the family sitting room. He took the opportunity to do some reading.

Catrijn and Dirck traded smirks, still reveling in their escapade. Nicolaas whispered alternately "dick" and "fuckin" to muffled giggles. Soon, Nicolaas was fully engaged in his usual incessant chatter, which eventually wore on fifty-six-year-old Hasbrouk.

"Nicolaas, you must remember that *moderation* in all things is a virtue, including talking. Don't you want to be like your father? He never chatters. Always thinks first, then speaks if he has something worthwhile to say." Hasbrouk knew that wasn't entirely true, because Maarten in his youthful exuberance had frequently spoken indiscreetly and excessively about the mistreatment of Calvinists.

"Ja, I want to be like father." Nicolaas's legs went into motion, swinging back and forth. "When's Father coming home? Oh ja, he can't." Frowning, he declared, "I *hate* the Spanish."

"We only hate them," Catrijn said, "because they hated us first. Right, Papa?"

"We shouldn't hate them in any case. They *don't* hate us. They *envy* us," Hasbrouk said, trying as usual to turn the discussion into a learning opportunity. "We Netherlanders are heirs to the proud and independent Batavians who resisted the Romans and as a result won special privileges and freedoms. Remember? Tacitus wrote of them." Hasbrouk reached over and retrieved a volume from the shelf. "I shall read to you from Tacitus about the Batavians to refresh your memories."

Hasbrouk began reading aloud, translating from Latin to Dutch as he went. The passage did not describe the facts in simple enough terms, and he went on to a second one, and a third. Seeing the kids' eyes glaze over, he closed the book and in summary said:

"So you see, the Batavians were impossible to defeat. Consequently, the Romans had to stop fighting them and instead treat them with respect. The Romans granted the Batavians special privileges that were honored and enhanced over the centuries by successive rulers, including the Hapsburgs and Holy Roman Emperor Charles V. Ah, Charles V, he was a good man. He was of noble birth, the son of King Ferdinand and Queen Isabella, yet he was one of us ... spoke our language, and was well loved by us Netherlanders. It was a shame when he abdicated in 1555 and gave the Netherlands to his son King Philip. Did I ever tell you that I once saw Philip? He was a cold and distant man."

By now the boys' minds were elsewhere, and only Catrijn was eager to continue.

"Shall we work on Latin?" Hasbrouk said and opened Tacitus again.

"Nee, I'd rather speak French," Catrijn said. "*Maman* spoke French."

Not again! Dirck complained to himself, for he knew this was going to be the start of another lengthy discussion about Catrijn's dead mother and Antwerp. He moved over to the desk where his father had sat as an apprentice. Nicolaas followed, took out the wooden boat their father had carved for them, and sailed it across to his brother.

"Ja, Catrijn," Hasbrouk said a bit wistfully. "Your mother, my beloved Jaane, spoke French, Latin and Greek. And a little Italian too."

Of course, Catrijn already knew that, but these reaffirming truths were her only link to a mother she never knew, because her mother Jaane had died giving birth to her. Hasbrouk had met Jaane in Antwerp while doing business with her father. Despite their growing affection for each other, he never proposed marriage, owing to their significant age difference. He ultimately did so at the urging of Jaane's father from his deathbed, who feared that his daughter, the last of his line of Antwerpers, was going to be alone. Jaane moved to Amsterdam with her new husband, and the couple had two blissful years together before death took her away.

Father and daughter proceeded to recite French phrases that Jaane had found particularly poetic.

With a contented smile, Catrijn rested her cheek on her hand. "Tell me again about Antwerp, Papa. What was it like?"

Hasbrouk again described the magnificent cathedral, elegant homes, warehouses brimming with exotic goods, and well-dressed people everywhere.

"I wish I was a bird," Catrijn said dreamily. "I'd fly away ... reach up and touch the clouds ... and then zoom straight to Antwer—"

"Before you go!" Betje called from the kitchen, "come set the table."

The trance broken, Catrijn ignored Dirck's snicker and trudged into the kitchen to lay down the table cloth and put out wooden and pewter plates, knives, beer mugs and a salt shaker, and lastly fill the mustard dish.

Just before supper, Hasbrouk's twin sister Margaretha arrived. It was easy to hear her coming because of the clicking of her cane, which she had used since childhood after a boating accident crippled one leg. She lived nearby in the Begijnhof, the compound of the Catholic lay order of the Beguines, and regularly had meals with the family. Because of her simple black robe and stiff white collar, she could be mistaken for a nun, but she was not. Nuns took lifelong vows, while Beguines merely agreed to devote themselves to the service of others and to be chaste. Many Beguines, like Margaretha, purchased homes in the Begijnhof and supported themselves with investments. Margaretha's own money had come from an inheritance from her father, a modestly successful Amsterdam merchant. During her forty years as a Beguine, she specialized in working with orphaned and wayward children, which was how she had met nine-year-old Maarten van der Voort shortly after his arrival in Amsterdam.

As soon as Margaretha came through the door, Hasbrouk rose

and gave his diminutive sister a loving embrace. To anyone observing them, it was obvious they had a strong bond but not that they were twins. Aside from their alert and compassionate blue eyes, they looked nothing alike. He was big-boned, round-faced and ever-jovial, and she, slight and always skeptical. The thing they shared, though, was an unquenchable thirst for knowledge.

The children planted affectionate kisses on Aunt Margaretha's cheeks. Betje greeted her warmly and summoned them all to eat.

Theirs was a meager meal of cheese, salted herring, boiled onions, a lone white carrot, and two eggs that Betje's scrawny hens had reluctantly given up.

After supper the kids helped Betje in the kitchen, and Hasbrouk and his sister sat down in the front room. He opened Tacitus again, and Margaretha pulled out a small book of writings by Saint Francis, whom she admired for his message of love and concern for the common man. She leafed through the pages, looking for an uplifting passage.

Hasbrouk closed his book and leaned back. "Margaretha, it is a rare fortune these days to think what one wants and to say what one thinks," he said, paraphrasing Tacitus. "Have you noticed? You and I never talk about religion anymore."

Margaretha sighed. "Ja." Despite she being a Catholic and he embracing Calvinism, they used to have stimulating conversations that were as much philosophical as religious. Dutch scholar and philosopher Erasmus was often the subject of discussion. Both liked his humanist beliefs that man is by nature peaceful, loving, and a seeker of knowledge, and that religion is a matter for individuals and not governments. They agreed with Erasmus's railing against popes for their never-ending wars, but had differing opinions on his legacy. Margaretha believed he did much to help reform Catholicism, while her brother thought his greatest contribution was to fuel the rise of Protestantism.

"Now, children speak of hatred," Hasbrouk said. "And Betje ... she hardly speaks at all. Never complains about the loss of the house or Maarten's absence, though I can see it weighs heavily on her."

"Hmm, ja." Margaretha closed her book. "Have you had any news of Maarten? Or the Sea Beggars?"

Hasbrouk shook his head no.

"I heard rumors that Prince William has raised a new army and is set to invade the southern provinces again." Margaretha was an ardent supporter of Prince William of Orange and his pursuit of religious tolerance. For King Philip II she had nothing but contempt, believing him to be immoral for waging war and inflicting a cruel Inquisition on fellow Christians.

"And I heard that Prince William *still* hasn't raised enough money for a decent army and won't be invading anywhere, anytime soon."

Both shook their heads in despair, for the rebels had made no progress in the four long years of the revolt.

"I saw Rijp Dekker today," Margaretha commented. "He was selling a gold ring, which I'm certain was stolen. We had words." Her head started turning side to side. "I must say, it pains me even now to see him. He was my *one* great failure."

"You should think on the positive side, Margaretha. Rijp could never be changed; larceny is built into him. But *you* saved Maarten from Rijp's grip."

Margaretha sensed her brother was right, and her spirits lifted. "I can still remember the day I rescued little Maarten. He was a typical homeless orphan, scrawny and scared. The long journey from Alkmaar had exhausted him. Fortunately, he was a good boy and was easily dissuaded from a life of crime."

Hasbrouk recalled the joy on Maarten's face when he had proposed adopting him and the fulfilling father-son relationship that blossomed. A warm feeling came over him, until a vision of Rijp appeared, taunting and threatening Maarten to try to coerce him back into his gang, and Maarten responding with fists.

"I hate to think how Maarten will react," Hasbrouk said, "when he learns that Rijp has taken over his house."

Becalmed, the Sea Beggar ships floated on the North Sea within sight of each other. Days passed. With food supplies running low, Maarten cut rations. When they ran out, he rowed himself to other ships, which had been in Dover long enough to fully provision, and secured enough dried herring and water for a few more days. To occupy the men, he had them scrub the deck, clean their clothes, air their bedding, fish, repair sails, and repaint faded geometric patterns on the *Dirck*'s hull.

The fleet continued drifting on a minimal southwesterly wind, and supplies fell to dire levels. At night, crews lounged on deck amusing themselves with banter, dice, and cards to avoid thinking about their empty stomachs.

Aboard his *Dirck*, Maarten took astrolabe readings. After reconfirming the alignment of the instrument with the North Star and reading the latitude indicated on the rim, he turned to the men nearby.

"If my astrolabe reading is correct, we're at about the same latitude as Antwerp," Maarten said and pointed eastward. "The city should be over there."

Pieter, the first mate, and several other men rose and stared, hoping to sight land or city lights.

"How far away from Antwerp do you think we are, cap'n?"

"Can't tell." Maarten was being honest because he had no way of determining longitude. The method would not be invented for another two hundred years.

Disappointed at seeing nothing, the men sat down, and Maarten joined them.

"Skipper, you ever been to Antwerp?" the first mate asked, saying the word Antwerp reverently, for it was the spiritual center for Calvinists and now surrounded by Spanish troops.

"Nee, but almost feel like I have. My Papa loves Antwerp and tells me it's the biggest, *richest* city in all Netherlands, and beautiful ... with a huge cathedral."

The mention of Papa in conjunction with Antwerp stirred memories for Maarten of his conduct as a teenager when Papa had gone to Antwerp to visit a sick business colleague and had come home with a bride, who was *much* younger than Papa. Maarten tried to purge the recollection from his mind and stretched out on the deck with his hands behind his head. He began counting stars. The memories, nonetheless, crept back in, forcing him to relive them.

I was selfish and resented Jaane from the start, Maarten chastised himself. That's what Aunt Margaretha said, and she was right. But back then, no one understood that life as I'd known it was coming to an end. Before Jaane, Papa and I did everything together, relied on each other. After she came, all that changed. I know I broke Papa's heart when I moved out of the house, but there was no way I could stay. Then I proposed to Betje without giving it much forethought ... I guess I wanted my own family. And stupidly borrowed *all* that money from Uncle Nostrand to buy the house and the *Dirck*, and the revolt started. I never repaid Uncle and hate to imagine what he and Papa must think of me now.

In the morning, Maarten was feeling better. A stiff wind had arisen, and the twenty-four Sea Beggar ships were on a course toward the Netherlands coast.

As the first day of April dawned, Maarten thought he saw land and excitedly told Pieter.

"I hope it's not just a trick on your eyes," Pieter said, skeptical. "After all, this *is* April Fools' Day."

"April Fools' Day? Don't we have enough problems, without worrying about superstitious April Fools' tricks?"

"Sorry."

Maarten stared hopefully at the horizon. A low-lying landmass appeared. A small walled city with a tall church and several graceful spires came into view on the bank of a major estuary. Maarten had never sailed in these parts, but guessed the waterway was the mighty Rhine River, based on their latitude. Having no map of the area, he could not identify the town.

When the ships were nearing shore, the commander gave the signal to drop anchor. From this position, the fleet could keep an eye on sea and land alike. The sea posed relatively little threat because Spanish ships typically traveled in small convoys and were unlikely to attack such a large Sea Beggar fleet. Landward was the real hazard because King Philip II's military leader, the Duke of Alva, was fighting a ground war to control cities, and Spanish troops could be expected anywhere in this region.

While sails were being taken down and anchors set, the commander sent men in rowboats to summon Sea Beggar captains to his ship for a meeting.

The commander and his vice commander, a nobleman from Holland province, were waiting on deck when the captains arrived.

"Vice Commander van Treslong," the commander began, "tells me that the town over there is Brill, in southern Holland."

"My father," Van Treslong explained, "was once an official in Brill, and I know people there."

"The plan," the commander said, "is to send a small number of men to reconnoiter. If it's safe to go ashore, the vice commander will go to negotiate for supplies. Meanwhile, I want you to remain with your ships, arm your men, and stay alert."

Maarten returned to the *Dirck* and observed Brill, while his men brought their weapons on deck. He had a good vantage point, his ship being nearest to shore. The city gate was partway open, and people were rushing to get inside. A ferryboat crossing the estuary docked, and its passengers frantically scurried into the city. The city gate slammed shut.

The ferryman remained in his boat, and Maarten watched him with interest. The man seemed unafraid and sat calmly while studying the fleet. Finally, he rowed himself out.

"*Are you Sea Beggars?*" the ferryman called out.

"*Ja, we are,*" Maarten replied, and other captains confirmed the same.

The vice commander leaned over the gunwale and yelled to the man, "*We badly need provisions. We want to talk with Brill's mayors about acquiring food and water.*"

The ferryman squinted at him. "*Are you Heer van Treslong? Remember me? Pieter ... Pieter Kopplestock?*"

"*Kopplestock ... ja, ja,*" Vice Commander van Treslong said and waved to him. "*Come up. Come up.*"

On board, the vice commander greeted Kopplestock with a firm handshake, and the commander acknowledged him with suspicion.

"People are afraid," Kopplestock said, while trying not to stare at the commander's blood-stained and brilliant-blue priest's vestment. "They guessed you were Sea Beggars and think you'll kill everyone and steal everything, because ... er ... begging your pardon, sirs, they think you're *just* pirates."

The commander laughed uproariously.

Kopplestock's eyes darted nervously between Vice Commander van Treslong and the bizarre-looking commander. "My passengers begged me to go inside Brill with them. Said you'd kill me, but I told them you were Prince William's men. And *his* men wouldn't hurt me because I'm loyal to the prince too."

"You're right," the vice commander said and shook Kopplestock's hand again. "We don't intend to hurt any loyalists."

"Is there a garrison in Brill?" the commander asked.

"Nee. Spanish troops are only here in summer, when the Duke of Alva thinks you Sea Beggars might show up. This time of year? Not usually. And Alva's not apt to come here either, because I heard he's at the French border, expecting an invasion by the armies of Prince William and France."

The commander harrumphed. "We can count on France helping us about as much as we can count on England."

Puzzled by the commander's comment, Kopplestock's eyes shifted to Vice Commander van Treslong. "There're other loyalists in Brill, like me, and lots who hate Alva for billeting troops in their homes. But I'm not sure they'll help you. If they help you and Alva returns, *he'll* kill them. If they don't help you, they think *you'll* kill them."

"We don't want to kill anyone," the vice commander assured him. "We just want food and water."

"Kopplestock," the commander said, "I want you to go to the town fathers and tell them to send envoys to me, so we can discuss our needs." His eyes narrowed. "If they refuse—then they'll find out whether we're pirates, or not!" He burst into a sardonic laugh.

"You can tell them I'm here," Vice Commander van Treslong

said and handed Kopplestock his signet ring. "Show them this. They know they can trust a Van Treslong."

When Brill's envoys arrived in Kopplestock's ferryboat, they nodded acknowledgements to Sea Beggars leaning over the gunwales. Maarten saw optimism in their faces and assumed it reflected the profits expected from selling provisions to so many ships.

The envoys passed by again after meeting with the commander, and Maarten noticed their optimism had vanished. All were frowning, and some appeared fearful.

Soon rowboats came around with new orders from the commander to the Sea Beggar captains.

"*Captain van der Voort!*" the man in the rowboat called out. "*The commander has decided to make Brill our new base and has ordered the mayors to surrender the city to us within two hours. If they don't, we'll take it by force in the name of Prince William of Orange. Make sure your men are ready to fight, if necessary.*"

"*They'll be ready.*" Maarten saluted back. A new base? Good idea.

"I hope they surrender," Pieter said, nervous. "We've never taken a city before." Their fleet had attacked plenty of villages and monasteries, but never a city with a high wall. Arrows raining down and cauldrons of boiling oil were too unnerving to contemplate, so instead Pieter scrutinized Brill and its tall church again. "Do you think Brill is full of Catholics, like Amsterdam?"

"Maybe," Maarten said, "but probably not as fanatical as in Amsterdam. Amsterdam is unique ... has all those monasteries, monks and nuns ... *and* the miracle." The miracle had occurred in 1345 when a dying man was administered his last communion and vomited up the host. The host was tossed into a fire, would not burn, and levitated above the flames. Over the years the phenomenon drew religious orders that built cloisters near the site. It also attracted the devout, making Amsterdam a pilgrimage destination. Even Holy Roman Emperors Maximillian and Charles V had come.

"Amsterdam would fight to the death rather than surrender," Pieter commented.

"Definitely." Maarten glanced again at the unremarkable little city. "But Brill? Who's heard of Brill? Why would anyone fight to the death for it?"

"Hopefully no one."

Maarten studied the low-lying countryside and realized he knew almost nothing about this part of the Netherlands. He was familiar with the north—beyond the great Rhine, Waal and Maas rivers—having lived there his entire life and plied its waters while trading. For fun, he decided to test his knowledge and make a game of naming all those northern provinces. It was the sort of thing Papa liked to do. Maarten started with his own province, Holland, where his hometown Amsterdam and birthplace Alkmaar were. Nearby were Utrecht and Gelderland, though he had never been to either. To the north was Overijssel, and way up north were Friesland and Groningen provinces. Maarten congratulated himself—That was easy!—in spite of having forgotten Drenthe. Returning to Brill and its environs, he tried to envision where the major southern provinces and cities lay.

"Pieter," Maarten said, "if Brill is in the southern end of Holland, then the province of Zeeland must be there." His finger pointed south.

"Ja, must be. Zeeland's just a bunch of islands."

"And south and east of Zeeland is Antwerp ... in Brabant? And Flanders is to the south?"

"Yep, I think so."

"Where are those other southern provinces? Luxembourg, Artois—"

"Artois?" Pieter said. "I believe that's a city ... but I'm not sure. They speak French there, don't they?"

Those mostly French-speaking southern provinces were a blur, and they gave up trying to sort them out. To the common man, the Netherlands was a fairly incomprehensible sprawling and low-lying place, crisscrossed by massive rivers, and home to innumerable towns and cities. It consisted of what would ultimately become the Netherlands, Belgium, Luxembourg and parts of France.

After two hours passed and no one came out of Brill to surrender, the commander sent word to board the longboats. He also ordered some to carry extra masts for use as battering rams and wood for making fires.

Once ashore, the commander and vice commander positioned themselves in front of the city, just beyond range of the city's archers. Behind them, Sea Beggar captains lined up their men. Brill was placid, seemingly unaware or uncaring that a horde of Sea Beggars was massing.

The commander strode among his 600 Sea Beggars, inspecting them and their weapons. He himself carried a sword and had a pistol jammed into his belt, and most of the men were armed with swords, pikes, metal-studded clubs, and bows and arrows. Many proudly shouldered crossbows or long guns known as harquebuses. Several carried only sticks. Satisfied he had assembled a suitably menacing army, the commander turned toward Brill, expecting to see city fathers rushing out with white flags waving.

There was no surrender, nor evidence of resistance, only a few heads popping up here and there along the parapet. The Sea Beggars looked at their leaders.

Suspecting the lack of activity was a ploy to lure them close to the city for a surprise attack, the commander decided to delay advancing his army. Instead, he ordered Vice Commander van Treslong to go to the city gate and demand that Brill surrender. Van Treslong chose Maarten and his men to go with him.

While marching toward the gate, Pieter anxiously scanned the parapet and spied two heads. He poked Maarten. "Maybe those men have boiling oil and will drop it on us when we get closer."

Maarten sniffed the air. "Nee, don't smell fire, or oil. But they could be archers." His eyes searched for a place to take cover. "If they start shooting, run to the gate and lean up against it. Arrows won't reach us there. Agreed?"

"Ja."

Maarten glanced back at the Sea Beggar army and took comfort in seeing the commander moving his archers, crossbowmen, and harquebusiers forward to answer any attack from the parapets. A little cloud of smoke was already forming above their heads from harquebusiers lighting slow-burning wicks for their matchlocks.

At the city gate, the vice commander instructed Maarten to announce their arrival. He and five of his men lined up and in unison struck the butts of their weapons against Brill's front door. BAM. BAM. BAM.

The vice commander hollered, "I AM HEER VAN TRESLONG, VICE COMMANDER OF THE SEA BEGGARS. IN THE NAME OF PRINCE WILLIAM OF ORANGE, I ORDER YOU TO OPEN THE GATE AND SURRENDER BRILL TO ME!"

No response. He repeated the order. Still nothing. "YOU HAVE THIRTY MINUTES TO SURRENDER! IF NOT, WE WILL BREAK DOWN YOUR GATE!" The men marched back to the commander's position, and the battering rams and tinder were readied.

Thirty minutes passed, and no one came out to surrender. The commander divided his army. Half went with the vice commander to assault the rear gate, and the commander advanced on the main gate with the other half, including Maarten and his men. To instill terror in Brill's defenders, the commander directed the men to howl and growl and shake their weapons.

At the main gate, the commander ordered a fire built at the base. When the gate was charred and weakened, burly men rammed a mast into it again and again. The gate crashed in, and Sea Beggars streamed into Brill, yelling and brandishing their weapons. After seeing the streets spookily devoid of people, they fell silent, and the commander took the lead and marched straight ahead.

By the time the column reached Brill's main square, it was obvious the city was nearly empty and no one was going to oppose them. The city was theirs.

One man let out a whoop. Another hollered. Others joined in. Hats flew into the air.

The commander let the men carry on, for they deserved to celebrate for having successfully taken a city in enemy territory, something Prince William of Orange had not yet done.

"*Stupid Alva!*" one man shouted, "*You're at the French border, and we—the mighty Sea Beggars—took your town!*"

Another yelled, "*April fool, Alva!*"

The men roared with laughter, and "*April fool, Alva!*" rippled through the crowd.

"*Alva! We stole Brill!*" Pieter called out, and in a stroke of genius added, "*You lost your bril!*" It was a joke, playing on the name of the city, Brill, and the Dutch word for spectacles, *bril.*

Maarten guffawed and slapped Pieter so hard on the back he flew forward.

The men started chanting, "*April fool, Alva! You lost your bril!*" Even the commander added his voice.

The vice commander entered the town square from the south, and his 300 men joined in. "*April fool, Alva! You lost your bril!*"

The commander saluted and shook his vice commander's hand and then noticed he had captured a well-dressed man.

"SETTLE DOWN!" the commander called out to his Sea Beggars. "QUIET!"

To the captive, he demanded, "Where is everyone? Why is your town empty?"

"The fishermen are at sea. The city fathers and most of the residents, th-they all left after Kopplestock told us you had *5,000* men." He glanced around, skeptical, as if questioning the veracity of Kopplestock's number.

"*5,000 men?*" The commander laughed uproariously, and the 600 raucous Sea Beggars repeated, "*5,000 men!*"

Tiring of the chants, the commander studied the square, and his eyes settled on the church. With renewed excitement he ordered, "FOLLOW ME!" With equal zeal, the Sea Beggars converged on the steepled edifice.

Finding the church door locked and bolted from within, they brought the battering ram forward. After several poundings, the door flew open, and the Sea Beggars went on a rampage, smashing graven images and stained glass windows and collecting everything of value. When a barricaded room was spotted, they demolished the obstruction, bashed in the door, and found thirteen terrified priests huddled within. The priests were dragged out, slapped around, and stripped of their clothes.

With night falling and little time to do much else, the commander ordered the priests locked up in their room and the plunder stacked behind the altar under guard. The next day, the priests would be dealt with and the spoils of war divided among the Sea Beggars.

Maarten gathered his men and, after sending some of them with the first mate to guard the ship, led the rest to find an abandoned house to sleep in. Other captains did the same.

Maarten awoke with the first rays of dawn, hung over from the wine he and the men had found in the cellar. He heard one of the men rise and say, "April fool, Alva!" and slap Pieter's butt as he walked by. "You lost your *bril!*"

Chuckles went around the room.

Maarten lay quietly, dreading to hear Pieter's April Fools' witticism again. It had been hilarious the first time, funny the second, but after six hundred men had repeated it a dozen times each, the silly joke had definitely lost its punch.

Pieter was staring at the wall, thinking. He turned and motioned Maarten to get up and go outdoors with him. In front of the house they sat down on a bench, and Maarten pulled out the bread and cheese he had saved from the previous night. After offering some to Pieter and he declining, Maarten began munching.

"Maarten, I've been thinking about those priests. It's ungodly to kill holy men, even corrupt papists. And I'm not sure they're guilty of anything—we don't even ask." His eyes met Maarten's. "I'm afraid we'll go to hell if we kill them. Some of the crew are worried too. Could you talk to the commander?"

"Are you *crazy,* Pieter? *He* won't listen to me." Maarten looked down at the cheese, took another bite, and hoped Pieter would drop the subject.

"Maybe then Vice Commander van Treslong. He seems to be a reasonable man."

"I don't know," Maarten said, his head turning side to side. Having lost his appetite, he put away the food. Pieter was still staring at him. "Pieter, those priests knew we were coming. They should've left. It's not our fault they didn't."

"Well, maybe they felt obligated to stay with the church and their precious relics or whatever is stored inside. Or they believed they were safer in God's home than outside the city with 5,000 Sea Beggars roaming around. Who knows? But their decision doesn't justify us killing them."

Maarten's brow furrowed. "I suppose you're right." He stood up, made his way down the street, and found the vice commander sitting in front of another house.

Maarten returned to Pieter with a smile on his face.

"Van Treslong is a good man. Said he'd speak to the commander and suggest we hold the priests for ransom, rather than kill them. Van Treslong's such a great strategist. I found out that he was the one who suggested taking Brill as a base."

Pieter was pleased.

"Of course, Van Treslong said the commander will have the final say on the priests. After all, he's in charge."

At noon, the commander made his decision. The thirteen battered priests were marched into the town square and summarily executed.

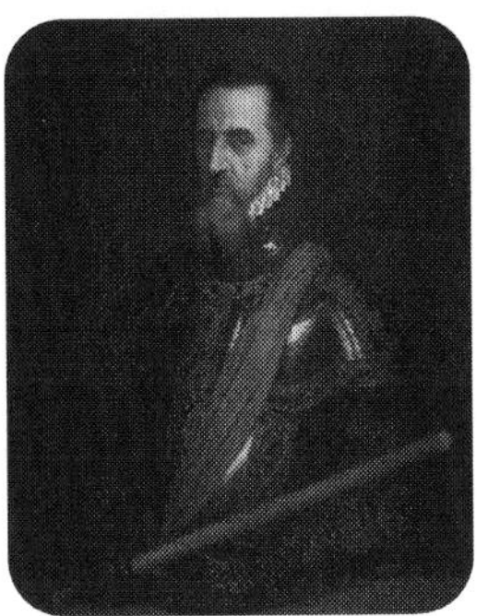

Duke of Alva

CHAPTER 2

Tests of Faith – 1572-1573

In Amsterdam, the Hasbrouk household learned of the Sea Beggars' capture of Brill from Margaretha, who had been told by a visiting bishop from the south. The joke was also relayed, and the kids repeated it endlessly, "April fool, Alva! You lost your *bril*!"

In May, word spread that the Sea Beggars had repulsed an attack on Brill by the Duke of Alva's troops. They fought from Brill's parapets, set fire to Alva's boats in the river, and cut the dikes to flood the land. The Spanish troops fled in confusion and terror.

Positive reports kept trickling in, confirming that the Sea Beggars' victory at Brill had started something. The nearby town of Vlissinger in Zeeland revolted and asked for help from the Sea Beggars, as did Flushing. Emboldened, merchants in Brussels closed their shops rather than pay Alva's contemptible ten-percent tax. Other Sea Beggar fleets seized more cities.

With each bit of news, Hasbrouk took out his yellowed and frayed map of the Netherlands to locate the action, and for the first time Dirck found the map fascinating. No longer was it simply a boring mass of dots identifying places of great beauty or wealth. Now the map represented battles and adventure.

"Is this where Prince William's northern army is?" Dirck asked, pointing to Germany.

"Ja. From there, the army will attempt to free the northern provinces of Gelderland and Overijssel from Spain's control." Hasbrouk put a finger on the border between the Netherlands and France. "And his southern army is here with the French army and the Huguenots preparing to attack Alva."

Betje burst through the front door, excited. "There's going to be a Calvinist service on June 5 at Heer Nostrand's house. I want to go. All these victories—*surely* they're a sign that God's on our side."

Hasbrouk frowned. "That might not be wise, Betje. The Inquisitors will be watching closely on that day." June 5, 1572, was going to be the fourth anniversary of King Philip II's infamous beheading of the Catholic patriot and hero of the revolt, Count Egmont, for daring to ask the king to reconsider his decision to send an Inquisition and troops into the Netherlands.

"Maarten would want his sons and me to go. He shows courage every day. We need to as well."

"Hmm."

On June 5, Betje could not be dissuaded, and Hasbrouk felt obliged to go along in case something went wrong. Not wanting to jeopardize Catrijn, he left her behind with Margaretha. When they reached the opposite side of the canal from Nostrand's home, Hasbrouk stopped and, with Betje and the boys behind him, stepped forward to check for suspicious activity. Seeing none, he led them across the bridge, into the alley, and to Nostrand's side door.

Inside, a beaming Betje warmly greeted Heer Nostrand, his wife and other Calvinists. Hasbrouk and old friend Nostrand shook hands and exchanged concerned looks.

A lay minister officiated, and he began with the Lord's Prayer.

Betje recited with passionate conviction, "Our Lord, who are …"

Dirck mouthed, "Our devil, Duke of Alva, who are from hell, cursed be thy name …"

At the end of the prayer, Hasbrouk patted Dirck's knee and whispered, "I'll be right back."

Dirck figured he was leaving to have a good poop, judging from the way he'd been squirming. His and Betje's eyes followed Hasbrouk to the door.

Outside, Hasbrouk went to the wooden toilet box over the canal. The odor was strong. He knocked on the door.

"Can't a man have a good crap in peace?" came from within.

Hasbrouk hurried to the next box … it was occupied. On to the next, which was free. Before stepping inside, he apprehensively glanced back at Nostrand's house that was almost out of view.

Bored, seven-year-old Nicolaas fidgeted with one of many loose threads on his sleeve. Dirck poked him to stop, and Nicolaas impishly reached over and yanked a thread from Dirck's doublet.

Betje glared at them as if to say, don't you two know bett—

The doorknocker sounded. The room fell silent.

Heer Nostrand let a man in, whom everyone recognized as Sheriff Johann.

The sheriff said, "Joseph took mother and child and fled to Egypt."

The worshipers understood the code words: a raid was imminent and they should flee.

Sheriffs were required to raid these illegal worship services and arrest the heretics, but Johann lacked the stomach for such heartless work.

The sheriff swiftly departed, and Heer Nostrand directed everyone to the side door. "This way." One by one they slipped out, with Nostrand serving as lookout. Betje held back.

"You must go, Betje. You'll be all right, but you *must* go now."

"We can't leave without Heer Hasbrouk."

"He's probably waiting outside for you. If he returns after you've gone, he'll be safe. I'll sit down with him, pour a drink, and talk business—there's nothing illegal about that."

Betje's heart was beating wildly as she scurried down the alley with the boys. At the corner, she stopped, peeked around it, and was alarmed to see the Van Trapp family detained by two men. She knew from experience that the men were collecting incriminating evidence for the Inquisition, because such men had built the case against Maarten in advance of his trial for heresy.

Dirck craned his neck to see around his mother. She stepped back—"Oops!"—and almost fell over him. Both froze. Dirck tugged her hand and inclined his head toward the opposite side of the canal, to suggest: We should race across the bridge.

She agreed and stuck her head out again. The Van Trapps were still being questioned. Betje dashed into the street with her kids—

"*Halt, madam!*" one of the men yelled and started toward her.

Betje kept moving, hoping to outrun him, but Nicolaas had stumbled and she was already dragging him. Heavenly Lord, please help me!

The man caught up with her. "Did you just come from *that* house?" he said, pointing.

Betje's mind raced. Should I confess? Don't look at him, she told herself. Maybe he'll go away.

He did not.

Betje made the sign of the cross.

"Are you a Catholic?" the man asked skeptically.

Don't make me say no, Betje was pleading over and over again in her mind. Don't make me say no.

The man's piercing eyes shifted to the juveniles.

"Of c—" Nicolaas felt a knuckle crunching squeeze to his hand as he was about to say: Of course we're not!

"Madam." The man reminded her he was waiting and getting impatient.

Betje nodded imperceptibly.

"Catholic?" the man repeated.

The movement of her head was slightly more visible.

"Be on your way."

Without looking up, Betje walked off with a tight grip on the boys' hands.

Dirck glanced back. "I don't see Heer Hasbrouk."

Upon reaching home, Betje's hand was shaking so badly she could barely unlock the door. While pushing the children inside, she scanned the room and thought: Good, no one's home. No explanations needed. She closed the door, leaned up against it, shut her eyes, and tried to regain composure. Sensing someone was watching, she opened her eyes. Both sons were staring at her, and Nicolaas was on the verge of tears.

Dirck would not allow himself to cry, believing he was the man of the house until his father returned, but was perplexed. What is a man supposed to do in this situation? he wondered. I'm not even sure what happened. Why is Mother so upset? After all, we did get away from that man. Hmm, what did she do on the bridge? Did Mother indicate she was a Catholic? It all happened so fast.

Betje peered into Dirck's questioning eyes. He disapproves of what I did, she surmised, and is disappointed with me. He's too young to know I had no choice. "Adults must make choices, Dirck." What a stupid thing to say! There's no excuse for what I did. It's immoral and unforgiveable. What kind of person denies her own religion—especially in front of her children?

The door handle clinked, and in walked an anxious Hasbrouk. His face lit up on seeing them.

"I'm so relieved you're safe," he said, while wrapping his arms around the youngsters and giving a squeeze. "I was worried when I saw the Van Trapps talking to a man, and you and the boys walking away from another." He went on to explain his absence.

Betje said nothing, and the kids' eyes shifted anxiously between her and Heer Hasbrouk.

"Is something wrong?"

"Nee, nothing," Betje said in an unsteady voice. "God was on *our* side today." She grimaced. Why did I say that? The Lord will never be on my side again.

During the summer of 1572, Prince William of Orange held meetings with Sea Beggar delegates and leaders of towns in Zeeland and Holland that had come over to his side. All agreed to reconstitute the Zeeland and Holland provincial governments and restore Prince William to his rightful place as their governor. They would no longer recognize the authority of the governor appointed by King Philip or pay taxes to him. For his part, the Prince promised religious freedom and to use their taxes to protect them and fund his army.

Prince William then focused on the invasion of southern Netherlands that he was planning in concert with the Huguenot-led French army. On August 24, however, the assault was abruptly called off after French Catholics unexpectedly began slaughtering Huguenots by the thousands, which became known as the Saint Bartholomew's Day massacre.

With no more threat of attack from France, the Duke of Alva set his massive army in motion northward, intent on retaking every town in Zeeland, Holland, and the other northern provinces allied with Prince William. In the process, he would deprive the prince of any hoped for tax revenues.

Ahead of Alva's advancing troops, Prince William's army retreated northward and the Sea Beggars withdrew from Brill.

As the Sea Beggar fleet got underway, Maarten and Pieter turned for one last glimpse of the city.

"It was inevitable that we'd lose Brill," Maarten commented, resigned. "We were lucky to repulse Alva the first time. The next time, he'll send a bigger army and artillery. Those old city walls would never withstand heavy bombardment for very long."

"I know." Pieter sighed in despair, not because the Sea Beggars were abandoning Brill, but for himself. In the four years at war, he had become pragmatic, and that worried him. In the past, he would have grieved for those poor people left behind in Brill, who were going to face Alva's wrath when he returned. Now he understood that life was just a never-ending cycle of ups and downs. Those townspeople who had helped the Sea Beggars would rotate out of Brill, and those who had fled from the Beggars would return. Some were going to lose their lives, and others were going to survive. Life just goes on, and somehow those who survive adjust. What upset Pieter most was the banality of all the suffering and injustice. Worse yet, he was becoming inured to it all.

"You know something, Pieter?" Maarten said. "This is going to work out fine for us. In the north, more and more towns are coming over to Prince William. Some will be on the Zuider Zee, and from those friendly ports we'll liberate Amsterdam."

"We'll have a good head start on Alva, so we should reach Amsterdam before he does," Pieter said, hopeful now. "Crossing those wide rivers with such a big army is going to slow him down."

"Ja, and by the time he gets to Amsterdam, we'll be waiting for him."

Both men chuckled at the ridiculousness of the idea. Then again, was it really completely beyond the realm of possibilities? After all, they had taken Brill easily and held it. Why not Amsterdam?

"We're going home, methinks," Maarten said and clapped his arm around Pieter's shoulder.

Amsterdam and other cities in the north watched and waited for the Spanish army to arrive, and with each passing day Protestants' terror increased. The Duke of Alva was driving north with a ferocity not seen before, sacking towns and cities even after they had already surrendered.

The Spanish troops crossed the great rivers well east of Amsterdam, and Alva split his army. Some were sent northward to retake Drenthe, Groningen and Friesland provinces. Most stayed with him and his son Don Frederic and marched westward toward Amsterdam, viciously attacking towns and Prince William's garrisons in the provinces of Gelderland and Overijssel.

In the town of Zutphen, they slaughtered the Prince's garrison to the last man. Citizens were stabbed in the streets, hung from trees, and suspended by their feet from gallows to die slow, agonizing deaths. Some were thrown out of the city naked to freeze to death. Five hundred merchants were tied back-to-back and drowned in the river. Every house was burned to the ground. Alva and his troops then moved on to Naarden and destroyed it.

Sea Beggar fleets reached Amsterdam well ahead of the Spanish army and took up positions on the north side of the wide Ij River, opposite the city. While their leaders plotted the next move, the most strident captains organized daily taunting sessions, shaking their swords and yelling toward Amsterdam: "YOU SERVILE PAPISTS! COME OVER AND TAKE US, OR TOMORROW WE'LL COME OVER AND TAKE YOU!"

On November 11, Maarten awoke at 2 o'clock in the morning, eager to get started on the mission he had volunteered for: sending five fire ships across the Ij to destroy enemy warships anchored in Amsterdam's harbor. From the deck of his *Dirck,* he checked the wind. It was coming from the north—perfect. The first mate woke up the men, and nobody complained, even though their muscles ached from hauling weighty barrels of tar and pitch the previous day.

While Maarten and his men rowed out to the fire ship, which he was responsible for lighting, he was giddy with anticipation. Not only was November 11 his name day, Saint Maarten's Day, but it was also the date they would begin liberating Amsterdam.

Once aboard their fire ship, Pieter and the men spread the tar, pitch, and combustibles across the deck and raised the mainsail. Maarten made sure the rudder was tied firmly in place, lit his torch, and watched for the commander's signal.

On the four other fire ships, Sea Beggar captains stood with torches in hand, waiting.

The signal came and Maarten called out "NOW!" Two of his men hauled up the anchor, and Maarten moved around with the torch. Flames were licking up when they all went over the side and into the waiting rowboat.

In unison, the five fire ships started their journey across the Ij River toward Amsterdam.

The Sea Beggars cheered and recited their motto: "Help thyself and God will help thee!" Afterward, the commanders led them in a prayer. By now, the ships were in full blaze and sailing straight at Amsterdam.

BOOM. Amsterdam's cannons commenced firing at the burning ships. Dirck awoke with a start. The Sea Beggars are attacking the city! He leaped out of bed, felt around for his shoes, and raced to the door.

"Dirck!" Betje called out. "Where're you going?"

"I'll be right back." He grabbed his jerkin from the hook.

"Don't you go anywhere!" Betje climbed from her bed.

"*Dirck!*" Hasbrouk said firmly. He was up and putting on his shoes.

Dirck hesitated and then went for the door latch. "I have to go."

Hasbrouk told Catrijn and Nicolaas, who were scrambling to get their shoes on, "Do—not—go—anywhere!" To Betje, he said, "I'll go with Dirck. He'll be fine."

Outside, Hasbrouk called to Dirck, and he reluctantly slowed to let the old man catch up.

BOOM.

Hasbrouk gripped the nine-year-old's hand and walked down dark Kalverstraat toward the blasting cannons. Others came out of their homes, and soon a large crowd was surging toward the harbor.

At quayside, Dirck and Hasbrouk readily discerned what was going on. The city's cannons were shooting at five burning ships coming from the other side of the Ij. At risk were Amsterdam's two warships, which lay at anchor outside the harbor's protective perimeter. The crews of the warships, assembling on shore, were unlikely to get their ships out of harm's way before the infernos arrived.

Dirck grinned up at Hasbrouk, as if to say: We're winning! Hasbrouk frowned back, warning against overt shows of support for the Sea Beggars. Dirck glanced around, worried that someone had seen his indiscretion. But nobody was paying any attention to him, not the concerned-looking men, scared women, kids straining to get a better view, or the horrified Catholic priests. All eyes were on the Ij. Whenever a cannon ball missed its mark, a collective "Oooh neee!" went up.

The fire ships slowed when the wind diminished. By the time the sun came up, they were becalmed. The crowd sighed in relief.

A breeze blew in from the northwest ... moved around to northeast ... back to northwest. The burning vessels changed direction with the wind. Two bumped into each other. When the wind shifted again, four ships turned westward and sailed harmlessly away. The last burning inferno crashed into the Palisade and remained there, until a gust sent it back toward the Sea Beggars on the opposite side of the Ij.

"It's a miracle!" a priest declared. "God is with us!"

Others said, "God's hand was steering those fire ships!"

The Sea Beggar camp grew quiet after the attack, and Dirck feared they might abandon their position, something he could not bear to see. So he quit making daily pilgrimages to the harbor's edge to observe and ponder how to help them, and instead started going to the top of the western city wall to check for signs of the approaching Spanish army.

Mostly Catholics gathered at the wall, hoping the army would arrive soon to put an end to the rebellion. Priests prayed fervently for the army's safety. Families with girls and young women, though, had mixed emotions because Alva might want to billet soldiers in their homes.

Alva's army showed up amid late autumn snow flurries. Advancing from the south, soldiers on foot and on horseback marched in a column, as drummers beat out the pace. Interspersed among them were wagons loaded with boxes and supplies.

That day the whole family went to the top of the wall with Dirck.

Catrijn's first impression was that the soldiers dressed pretty much like Dutchmen. Both wore form-fitting doublets and ballooned-out knee-length breeches, which were slashed to reveal the contrasting color of their shirts beneath. Doublet and pant colors were the same, and stocking and shirt hues matched. But the color combinations were not all the same: some paired red with gold, others blue with yellow, and still others purple with various colors.

"Papa, why do they wear different colored uniforms?" Catrijn asked.

"They're wearing the colors of their regiments. King Philip probably drew regiments from various parts of his vast realm to amass this army."

"Where are their cannons?" Nicolaas asked.

"And harquebuses?" Dirck said. "They don't look very well armed to me."

"Where's Alva?"

"I've been wondering that myself," Hasbrouk said. "The Duke of Alva is known as a supreme tactician, so I suspect he's staging his army's arrival for maximum effect. These advance troops were probably sent to get everyone's attention. War machines will likely come next to instill terror. Then the duke—formidable commander of it all—will make his entrance."

Within a few days, armored men on foot in neat formations appeared, sunshine glinting off their pointy helmets. The sheer number of weapons was frightening—harquebuses, crossbows, pikes, swords, and a new weapon called a musket, which appeared to be a smaller version of a harquebus. Cannons and massive siege machines followed. The intimidating column seemed to be a mile long and took much of the day to reach the camp in front of Amsterdam.

"I've been counting the troops," Hasbrouk said, "and estimate there are about thirty thousand."

"How many zeros is that?" Nicolaas asked.

"Four," Catrijn confirmed. "Three plus zero, zero, z—"

"LOOK!" Dirck shouted. "ALVA!

All eyes went to the impressive retinue of standard bearers with colorful flags fluttering in the breeze, drummers on foot, and buglers on horseback. Behind them were imposing horsemen in head-to-toe gleaming armor.

The Duke of Alva rode alone, haughty and resplendent in shiny black armor embellished with gold filigree. Across his chest was a blood-red sash. Cradled in his arm was his black metal helmet, signaling he had no need of it for he was in full control and feared no one.

Margaretha observed him with contempt, not only because he was a vicious killer, but also on account of his horse treading on her farmland. The land had been purchased many years earlier with part of the inheritance from her father and since been rented to a family who grew crops, providing a reliable income for Margaretha and her Begijnhof work. If Alva's army remained in place through spring, there would be no farming or rent paid, and she and the farmer would suffer.

The city's gate opened, and Amsterdam's government leaders and civil guardsmen went out to welcome the duke. After a brief discussion, they and Alva and a half dozen of his men headed into the city.

"It's time to go," Betje said, and Margaretha clasped Catrijn by the hand. They had previously decided to hide Catrijn away in the Begijnhof as soon as the first soldier set foot in the city.

Hasbrouk led Dirck and Nicolaas to the city gate to get a look at Alva, but could not get close enough. They followed Alva's party at a distance to the City Hall and milled around while the dignitaries were inside. A mayor came out and made an announcement, and afterward Hasbrouk took the boys to the Begijnhof to inform the women.

"Good news," Hasbrouk said, "Catrijn can come home. No troops will be allowed in the city."

"Whew," Betje said, "that's a relief."

Margaretha gave Catrijn a squeeze. "It's nice to have good news for a change."

"Alva will stay in a house on Warmoesstraat," Hasbrouk added, "and his horses and guards will be quartered in monasteries."

"Hmm." Betje's instincts told her that Alva's presence in their midst was bad. "The Inquisitors will be working doubly hard to impress Alva," she said, and her mind raced through the possible consequences. "We're doomed."

Dirck and Nicolaas gaped at their mother. Alarmed, Catrijn turned to her father.

"We're *not* doomed," Hasbrouk reassured them. "We've faced worse before, and we will get through this too."

"How long do you think Alva will stay?" Margaretha asked.

"Probably not long. He intends to lay siege to Haarlem, and the city can't possibly hold out very long with a garrison of only 3,000 to 4,000 men—not against Alva's 30,000 seasoned soldiers. So regardless of whether Haarlem surrenders or resists, it will be over quickly, and Alva will leave."

"Those poor souls," Margaretha said and crossed herself, "they're in for a rough time." She was speaking of Haarlem's 2,000 mostly Protestant residents.

"This will truly be a test of their faith," Hasbrouk added.

On December 10, Hasbrouk and the kids were on the city wall again, after hearing that Haarlem refused to surrender and all the Catholics had fled. The massive Spanish army camp stretching west and south of Amsterdam was alive with activity. Tents were being taken down and bundled onto wagons. Heavy siege machines and artillery were being pushed by soldiers and pulled by horses toward Haarlem.

As they watched, a biting wind kicked up, and Hasbrouk pulled Catrijn and Nicolaas close to shield them. With sadness, he pondered Haarlem, which lay ten miles to the west. Silhouetted against the blue sky, the city seemed as serene as ever.

Bracing into the wind, Dirck pressed the flaps of his beret against his ears and searched for signs of Prince William's army. Rumors said the Prince had recently visited Haarlem to urge its leaders to hold out until he could send reinforcements. Dirck knew his father was out there too, either with Prince William or with the Sea Beggars, and ardently hoped he would somehow be able to help them.

"Can we go to the Ij?" Dirck asked, and Hasbrouk agreed.

At the Ij, Amsterdam's harbor was nearly empty and beginning to ice over. Seeing no movement in the Sea Beggars' encampment, the family went on to the eastern city wall to observe progress on the fleet of shallow-draft gunboats under construction. They were going to be launched in spring under the command of Spanish Count Bossu to clear Sea Beggars from the area. Today, the view was grim. Two more gunboats had been completed, and several others were nearly so.

Haarlem was a poor town protected by an ancient city wall and surrounded by a moat. The Duke of Alva put his son Don Frederic in charge of the siege and predicted Haarlem would fall within a week.

Don Frederick established camps along Haarlem's perimeter, which were widely spaced owing to the long length of the city wall. On December 18, he initiated his assault with a cannon bombardment of the main gate, the Gate of the Cross. His troops cheered as the cannonballs splintered the wooden gate and smashed holes through the surrounding wall.

Haarlem's men, women, and children worked day and night to plug the holes with earth and rocks, and vindictively added statues taken from Catholic churches. They also reinforced a second wall which they had recently built behind the gate.

At dawn, Spanish troops stormed the broken gate, surged through it, and found themselves trapped between the city wall and a second inner one. More soldiers followed, crowding into the already packed space. Rocks came raining down, smashing skulls and breaking limbs. Bodies piled up. Then came the boiling oil ... flaming hoops ... and hot coals. Amid screams and desperate attempts to pull off fiery hoops, terrified soldiers clambered over burning and dead bodies to flee. When it was over, four hundred Spaniards lay dead, including many of their officers.

Don Frederic decided to change tactics. To demolish the city wall, he would dig tunnels underneath and plant bombs. During the weeks of tunneling, Haarlemers watched, noted the locations, and dug their own tunnels to intercept and destroy the bombs. Don Frederic abandoned tunneling.

Meanwhile, Prince William of Orange had amassed his army south of Haarlem and was launching assaults on Don Frederic's troops and also attempting to deliver arms and food to the besieged city. Some were successful but many were not. In an ill-fated one, four thousand of the Prince's men were ambushed by Spanish soldiers in a blinding snowstorm, leaving a thousand dead and hundreds taken prisoner. To demoralize those defending Haarlem, Spanish troops hung their captives on gibbets in full view of the city.

On December 21, the Prince sent seven pieces of artillery with two thousand men to Haarlem. A dense fog rolled in, and the Dutchmen lost their way, despite Haarlemers trying to guide them by ringing bells and making fires on the ramparts. Spanish troops attacked, the Prince's men retreated, and in the melee their captain was captured.

The Spaniards beheaded the captain and heaved his head over Haarlem's wall with a note attached:

> This is the head of Captain de Koning, who is on his way with reinforcements for the good city of Haarlem.

In retaliation, Haarlemers rolled a barrel filled with heads from eleven captured Spaniards into Don Frederic's trenches. The note said:

> *Deliver these heads to the Duke of Alva in payment of his Tenth-Penny Tax, with one additional head for interest.*

Haarlem held out through Christmas ... New Years ... and well into January. In late January, Don Frederic launched a three-day cannon barrage that damaged the gate and wall. At midnight his troops attacked and breached the gate. Inside a new inner wall stopped them, which had been mined. It exploded, killing hundreds. Melted pitch and burning coals wiped out most of the survivors. The rest ran for their lives.

The vicissitudes of the siege were quickly reported in Amsterdam. Catholics were increasingly frustrated, while Protestants secretly rooted for feisty Haarlem. The Duke of Alva was furious. In his forty-five years of fighting battles for Holy Roman Emperor Charles V and King Philip II, he had defeated the greatest armies of Europe. For that, he was known as the Iron Duke.

The Iron Duke summoned his son Frederic to Amsterdam and demanded to know why he had not yet defeated the little city. When Frederic said Haarlem could not be subdued, not without additional troops, the Iron Duke flew into a rage. Full of derision, he threatened to take over the siege, even though he was sickly. If he died, the Duke warned that Frederic's mother would be so embarrassed by her son's failure that she would come from Spain to finish the job herself!

In the end, Alva asked King Philip to send three more regiments from Milan. Until they arrived, Frederic was to stop attacking Haarlem and instead do everything possible to starve the city into submission.

In response, Prince William resolved to keep supplies flowing to the city by turning frozen Lake Haarlem into a thoroughfare. Four hundred of his soldiers and Sea Beggars took to the ice day and night, hauling one hundred and seventy sledges laden with supplies. Even though Prince William controlled much of the lakeshore and could provide cover for the deliverers, it was a risky undertaking. Not only did his men have to brave the elements, but Haarlemers had to sneak out of their city, varying their exit points to keep the Spaniards guessing, and timing it accurately to retrieve the supplies. Fortunately, Don Frederic's soldiers were ill-prepared to counter them, most being from the south and unaccustomed to harsh northern winters, plus few had ice skates.

On a frigid night thick with fog, Maarten and his men loaded the sledges assigned to them. To determine who would pull the heaviest one, Maarten let the men draw from slivers of wood. He and Pieter drew the unlucky short one. The men with lighter loads moved off smartly, and Maarten and Pieter slogged on alone.

That same night, Dirck went to bed with all his clothes on, in order to sneak away as noiselessly as possible before dawn. His goal was to help Haarlem. He slept fitfully until the church bells chimed five and woke him up. He glanced at Nicolaas sleeping beside him ... and at his mother in the other bed. Timing his movements to match her snoring, Dirck edged out of bed and tiptoed to the front room. The room was pitch black. He felt around for the shoes and skates he had left under a chair.

After opening the door with minimal sound, Dirck stepped outside and turned to gently close the door. "Ah!"

Catrijn put her finger to her lips, shut the door soundlessly, and nudged him to get going. She whispered, "I know you intend to help Haarlem, and I'm going with you."

"Nee, you're not." He grabbed her arm. "Girls can't go." Dirck pointed toward the house. "Now do as I say. Go back!"

"If you don't let me go, I'll tell your mother."

Thinking she was bluffing, Dirck puffed up his chest and stepped closer. Catrijn stood firm.

"You can go, but *only* to the city gate—*no* further! Now stay close to me."

Along the way Catrijn put on Nicolaas's beret, and Dirck realized she was not only wearing his brother's beret, but also his leather jerkin. She looks like a boy! Both frustrated and admiring, he muttered to himself, "She's so nervy!"

At Amsterdam's Haarlemspoort gate, they hid behind a wagon and waited. Others arrived and milled around, until gatekeeper Rutger arrived with the key. The gate opened, and the wagon started to roll.

"Stay here, Catrijn," Dirck whispered in his deepest, most authoritative voice, before ducking under the wagon. Hunched over, he walked toward the gate, trying not to be seen.

Catrijn crouched next to the rear wheel and slipped out behind him.

Once outside, she said, "What are we going to do?" her voice full of excitement and tinged with apprehension.

Glaring, Dirck pointed toward the gate.

"What's your plan?" Catrijn asked, ignoring his command.

Seeing her resolve, he said, "If you go with me, you have to do as I say." Catrijn nodded agreement, and Dirck explained the mission, "I'm going to take this to Haarlem," and held out a powder horn he had found at home. "Your father must have forgotten it when he sold his gun."

Catrijn examined the rather ordinary looking horn and barely recalled having seen it. She did remember Papa's gun, though, which he had sold to buy food. Papa had treasured it—not as a weapon but for the beauty of its inlaid handle—and had never fired it.

"Once I get to Haarlem," Dirck said, "I'll do whatever they want. Prince William's troops and the Sea Beggars are out there, somewhere, and need help."

Together they started down the frozen path toward Haarlem. Hearing Spanish voices ahead, Dirck nudged Catrijn toward the dike. The two climbed over, put on their skates, and set off.

After skating through the fog seemingly without direction, Catrijn grew anxious and grabbed Dirck's hand. Her eyes questioned: Are we lost?

Dirck gave her a reassuring look, but had no idea where they were. He gripped her hand and skated on. Impatient to find Prince William's men or at least a landmark to tell him where they were, he let go of her hand and whispered, "We should skate faster."

Muted voices and scraping sounds began emanating from the fog. Dirck threw out an arm to stop Catrijn, hitting her in the chest and knocking her off her feet.

"Who–goes–there?" a man's deep voice said in Dutch.

"W-we're here," Dirck said and immediately chastised himself for his feeble reply. He pulled Catrijn up and stood as tall as possible to face the indistinct outline of a man emerging from the mist.

"What are you boys doing here? Don't you know it's dangerous?" the Dutchman said. Behind him, hazy images of men and sledges appeared.

"I brought this to help Prince William," Dirck said while holding up the powder horn, "and I—"

"I'll see that it's put to good use," the man said and accepted the horn. "Now, you two go home before the fog lifts and the dons start firing." His voice was stern.

"I want ..." Dirck started to plead his case, but stopped, afraid that Catrijn might say something and the men would realize she was a girl. Not knowing what would happen then, he tugged Catrijn back in the direction they had come.

While the men were watching the boys disappear into the murkiness, Maarten and Pieter came up. Maarten rebuked them for standing around, and they defended themselves by showing the powder horn and relating their encounter with the kids.

Maarten held the horn, thought it was vaguely familiar ... turned it over in his hands ... and glanced in the direction the kids had gone. He shrugged and concluded, I've seen a dozen or more like this before, handed it back, and pulled out his compass. After determining they were heading in the right direction, he urged, "We need to get going."

In hushed tones, the men began discussing the courage and stupidity of youth and exchanging tales of their own childhood escapades.

"Pieter," Maarten whispered, "did I ever tell you how I got to Amsterdam?"

"Nee."

"I haven't thought about it in years. I suppose hearing about those boys and being here on the lake made me remember. I was walking from Alkmaar, and a man took me across the lake in his rowboat." Maarten paused, as if sorting out his memories. "I was nine. My father, a herring fisherman, had been lost at sea when I was little. I hardly remember him. Anyway, my mother remarried. He was a big guy ... had three almost grown sons. I guess his previous wife had died. He was so mean, he might of killed her." Maarten let out a sardonic little laugh, as though it was an inside joke. "Nee, nee, I shouldn't have said he killed her. I don't know what happened to her. But him—he was *mean*."

Pieter suspected Maarten was going through some type of soul searching or catharsis because he rarely spoke about his past or feelings. Sensing this could go on for a while, Pieter stopped, unwrapped his scarf, and rewound it around his head and neck to cover more skin.

"Getting cold, eh?" Maarten commented and tugged on his own beret. "As I was saying, I was living in my stepfather's house, and he didn't like me much. I was too small to be of real help. I was really skinny—"

"I never would of guessed it," Pieter interjected, "if Heer Hasbrouk hadn't told me you were a scrawny little kid when he met you."

"It's true. Anyway, back then wild storms came out of the North Sea all the time. The one in '53 broke through the dikes. Water *this* high," his hand went up above his head, "crashed through our village. Carried me away. I landed on a roof ... saw my stepfather go by ... animals ... boats smashing into houses." He swallowed, holding down the bitterest image. "I found my mother ... she was dead. But *he* lived. That's when I decided to leave."

Pieter wanted to offer something consoling and was searching for the right words—

Musket fire sounded in the distance.

"Better move faster," Maarten said.

The sun rose, infusing the fog with a warm glow, and Maarten and Pieter picked up their pace and caught up with his men. He gathered them close.

"We're approaching the rendezvous point," Maarten whispered. "In these conditions of low visibility, Haarlemers will use a signal to guide us to them, so keep your ears open for the password—Safe—or the sound of gentle clanging on a pot."

The men nodded they understood and resumed their march.

Bam. A musket fired not far away. Maarten could not tell where it originated. Bam.

"Arghh!" the man in front of Maarten cried out. "I been hit!"

"Keep moving, keep moving," Maarten quietly ordered, while he and Pieter lifted the wounded man onto their sledge.

Musket fire pierced the air again.

"Detener! Deja de disparar!" Stop! Stop shooting! A Spaniard called out, his voice coming from straight ahead.

"Safe," a Dutchman said softly, also seemingly from directly ahead.

Maarten repeated the password, "Safe," but was baffled. Are there Dutchmen or Spaniards ahead? Should I stop the men—

"Safe ... safe." came a whisper in Dutch, and Haarlemers emerged from the fog.

"I sure am glad to see you," Maarten said. "I thought you might be dons. We heard someone yell in Spanish just before the shooting stopped."

"That was one of the Prince's men," a Haarlemer said and pointed to a grinning Dutchman. "He speaks Spanish and comes in handy at times like this—confuses the dons and buys us time."

After the Haarlemers transferred the supplies, the Sea Beggars departed with the empty sledges. Hearing distant gunfire from behind, Maarten quickened their pace, and he and his men made it all the way back to their base without incident.

Meanwhile, Dirck and Catrijn had returned home just before sunrise. They tiptoed in and silently removed their outer clothes before sitting down next to the front window.

"Catrijn," her father called from his bed enclosed by a heavy drape, "is that you?"

"Ja, Papa."

"You're up early. I thought I heard the door open."

"I'm just sitting with Dirck by the window. We both woke up early." The two grinned at each other. Catrijn touched his hand, and her eyes said thanks. Dirck acknowledged it with a roll of his eyes and wry smile.

The perilous day-and-night procession of sledges succeeded in keeping Haarlem supplied.

Meanwhile, Don Frederic refrained from assaulting the city, but Haarlemers relentlessly tried to provoke him, preferring to die fighting rather than by slow starvation. By day, residents insolently placed altars and statues from Catholic churches on the parapet and paraded around while wearing priests' clothes and shouting taunts. Almost nightly, Haarlem's defenders launched attacks on Don Frederic's camps which were spread along the city's lengthy perimeter, varying the exit gate each time to maintain the element of surprise. In one attack, a thousand men spewed out of Haarlem, killed eight hundred Spaniards, burned three hundred tents, and returned with captured cannons and wagon loads of provisions. Only four of their own were killed.

Haarlem never succeeded in prompting Don Frederic to attack, but the Duke of Alva was so impressed by their gutsy efforts that he wrote to King Philip II: "Never was a place defended with such skill and bravery as Haarlem ... it is a war such as never was seen or heard of in any land on earth."

As winter dragged on, food supplies dwindled and hunger stalked everywhere: in Haarlem, Amsterdam, and in Alva's camps. Supplies from the south were never going to be sufficient to feed Amsterdam's twenty thousand residents plus Alva's entire army, and Prince William's attacks on Alva's Utrecht-to-Amsterdam supply route only exacerbated the problem.

In Haarlem, starving people boiled and ate leather when everything else ran out. In Alva's camps, more soldiers died from exposure, starvation, and disease than in battles.

In the Hasbrouk house, Dirck and Heer Hasbrouk took to the streets to hunt. Today, however, there would be no hunt because Hasbrouk was tending an unwell Margaretha. With nothing to do, Dirck stared at the clay birdhouse hanging outside, hoping for prey to alight, while Nicolaas huddled near the hearth contemplating the shriveled white carrot and precious lone onion, their supper for tonight. Meanwhile, their mother checked the empty mustard and butter pots for any overlooked morsels and was moving on to her containers of ointments.

"Mother," Dirck said, "may I go hunting today?"

"I'll go too!" Nicolaas said, all excited. Heer Hasbrouk never allowed him to go along, saying he talked too much and scared off quarry. Without Hasbrouk, Nicolaas knew Dirck would make it an adventure.

"You can both go," Betje said, "but be careful."

As soon as the two went out the door, Dirck asked, "Think we'll find a bear?"

"Ja—maybe even an elephant!" Nicolaas had heard Heer Hasbrouk's story many times about how an elephant had come to Amsterdam in 1484 in the time of his father.

Nicolaas raced ahead, but screeched to a stop on seeing the body of an emaciated old woman on the edge of the street.

Dirck knelt next to her—there were no signs of life—and looked around for an adult to help him decide what to do. Seeing none, he said a prayer, glanced up and down the street again, and reluctantly walked away.

Where two alleys intersected, Dirck found a promising hunting spot and stationed Nicolaas on one corner. After explaining what to do when an animal came by, he assumed a position on the other corner. With their clubs at their sides and Dirck's sack at his feet, they waited. Dirck pretended to be a bear and pantomimed a growl at his brother. Nicolaas bristled in feigned fright.

Dirck peeked around the corner. A cat! It was prowling for something to eat and heading straight toward them. He raised his club.

Nicolaas lifted his.

As the cat passed between them, Dirck swung his club down as hard as possible. It hit a hind leg. The cat squealed and bolted, and Dirck gave chase.

WHACK. A man further down the alley killed the cat with a strike to the head. "Back off, kid!" he told Dirck and scooped it into his sack.

Grumbling, Dirck searched for another promising location and found one near the Damrak canal. Seeing Nicolaas lag behind, he motioned him to hurry up.

"I'm cold," Nicolaas said.

"You shouldn't have come if you're going to complain." Dirck instructed him, "Here. Stand here," and stood opposite him. Out of the corner of his eye, he glimpsed movement near the edge of the canal. Slowly and deliberately, he brought up his club—"Psst"—and got Nicolaas's attention to raise his.

A rat popped its head up, climbed over the edge of the canal, and boldly rested in broad daylight.

Fuck! Nicolaas said to himself, using his favorite swear word. It's gigantic!

He's awfully big, Dirck thought to himself.

A split second later, the hairy rodent broke into a run and headed right toward the boys.

"Aaah!" Nicolaas jumped back.

Dirck slammed the club with all his might and caught the monster behind the head. One last bash convinced him the behemoth was dead.

Laughing hysterically, simultaneously expelling fear and exhilarating in the conquest, Nicolaas cautiously stepped closer and poked it with his club.

Dirck snatched the rodent by the tail, dropped it into his sack, and slung it over his shoulder. Nicolaas was still giggling nervously, and Dirck showed him his fist. "Stop that *stupid* laughing, *will you?*" When Nicolaas whimpered, he consoled him, "Aw, come on you silly kid. You know I wouldn't hit you," and put his arm around him.

As the two walked along, they spotted grouchy old Heer Jacob leave his house and step into the toilet box over the canal. Normally they would sneak over and throw stones into the canal until water splashed up on his arse and he would start cussing. With the canal frozen over, they had to settle for pelting the outhouse with chunks of ice, and the old curmudgeon did not disappoint. The boys ran all the way home, laughing and repeating his swear words.

With a smirk on his face and the sack held high, Dirck came through the front door and taunted, "Catrijn, are you hungry?" knowing that she found the hunt disgusting, despite understanding its necessity. She waved dismissively without looking up, and Dirck proceeded to the kitchen and plopped the sack on the table.

Betje inspected the contents. It was not the dog or cat she had hoped for, but not the first rodent she had cooked either. "Good work, boys. It'll make a nice roast *and* soup."

Mercifully, spring arrived early, thawing out Dutchmen and Spaniards alike and sprouting tender shoots in gardens. When ice on the Ij and Lake Haarlem melted, Count Bossu eagerly launched his newly constructed fleet of shallow-draft gunboats.

The Sea Beggars also released their own boats into the lake, a hundred in total, with a mission to deliver supplies to Haarlem. They were a mixture of longboats rigged with sails, ships with one to three masts, and galleys with a dozen or more oars on each side, all bearing the orange-white-blue striped flag of the rebellion. Protecting them were a string of Prince William's small forts along the shore.

Today, Maarten was making his third run to deliver supplies, leading a convoy of five gunboats and four supply boats laden with munitions. His first run had gone without incident but the second had been marred by an encounter with a Spanish fleet that left significant casualties on both sides. With skirmishes occurring almost daily, Maarten's convoy had been assigned one extra gunboat. He himself captained the largest one, with two masts, oars, and a cannon. His first mate commanded a sailboat provided by a loyalist from the town of Hoorn and equipped with a cannon.

Prior to boarding, Maarten assembled his captains and reiterated their charge: "The goal is to deliver supplies—not to score victories. We will outrun rather than engage any Bossu boat we encounter. The supplies *must* get to Haarlem." Those were the orders of Commander Dirckszoon under whom Maarten now served, having left his previous commander. Maarten made the change after volunteering for a couple of Dirckszoon's special missions and liking his personality and capabilities. Pieter and the crew were happier too.

While boarding his gunboat, Maarten scanned the lake and

spotted a few dots on the horizon, too distant to worry about. His eyes shifted to Amsterdam and again wished there was a way to reunite with his family. With a sigh, he suppressed the thought, ignored his weariness from hunger and the never-ending war, and went to work.

The convoy set off on a brisk wind, and he put his gunboat in the lead.

They were making satisfactory progress until the wind slowly diminished. When the laden supply boats lagged, their crews brought out oars.

Maarten again surveyed the lake. The distant dots were now unmistakably an enemy squadron, and it was sailing directly at them. He ordered his gunboat captains to begin towing the lumbering supply boats, and let his own drift back to guard the rear.

The defenders of Prince William's closest fort were observing the struggling Dutch convoy and advancing Bossu squadron, and began repositioning their cannons and bringing forth harquebuses and crossbows.

A cannon blasted from one of the Spanish vessels, and the shot splashed into the water behind Maarten. Another sent a cannonball that made a direct hit to the forward gunboat. It started taking on water, and the captain cut the line to the supply boat in tow and signaled to Maarten he was going to shore. With men furiously bailing and rowing, the distressed craft reached land not far from the fort.

Cannons at the fort discharged. One ball flew through the sail of a Spanish gunboat, the second crossed another's deck killing a man, and the squadron veered away to regroup out of range.

Maarten spied two of their gunboats leave the squadron, turn south, and hoist more sails. On their course, they would intercept his convoy at its most vulnerable point: just past the Prince's last fort and when making the final run to Haarlem. He called to his first mate on the closest gunboat:

"*They're going to try to head us off!*" Maarten gestured toward the two Spanish boats picking up speed. "*Follow me!*" To the other captains, he commanded, "*Stay with the supply boats. And keep close to shore for cover!*" With the wind stiffening and more forts ahead, he felt confident they would be safe for now.

Maarten and the first mate set off in pursuit. Their foes kept a steady course and sent desultory fire, but none did damage.

Close now, Maarten called to his first mate to grapple and board the lead enemy boat, while he went after the rear one. To his crew, Maarten signaled to get low and ready their grappling irons, and he took up a position near the bow, crouching with sword drawn. An incoming arrow whizzed over his head and struck the mast. A second one zinged past and knocked off a crew member's hat. Maarten's archers fired back, killing a Spaniard.

"Grapplings!" Maarten ordered, and two men stood and heaved their irons. They clanked on the adjacent gunwale, locking the two boats together.

Maarten and his men leaped across, and he jammed his sword into the closest Spaniard and pushed him overboard. With so many bodies slamming, slashing, and stabbing each other, the boat rocked violently. Maarten steadied himself, until from behind a man crashed into him, knocking the sword from his hand. In a domino effect, Maarten fell against a Spaniard, dislodging his knife, and both toppled over.

The two wrestled while trying to retrieve their weapons, and the Spaniard ended up wedged in the curve of the hull with Maarten straddling him. He found his knife and swung it up, and Maarten pulled back. The blade swiped back, and Maarten raised his knee, knocked the man's arm to the side, and pinned the knife hand to the deck. His fingers went to the Spaniard's throat and squeezed. The frantic man thrashed while his free hand tried to pry them away, but Maarten's thumbs only dug deeper. Almost out of breath, the Spaniard beat his fist against Maarten's head and in a final act of desperation grabbed his hair, yanked down his head, and bit on the closest thing before passing out. Maarten's hand reached for the man's knife and with quick jabs finished him off.

Maarten was getting up and noticed a bloody chuck of something in the man's mouth. His eyes squinted at it, and hand flew to his ear—My ear! He bit off my ear! Then he glimpsed a severed finger floating in a pool of blood next to his knee. His mind snapped. I can't take this anymore—

"*Maarten!*" Pieter called out, "*They're getting away!*" and pointed to the other Spanish gunboat, which had disengaged from the first mate's vessel and was starting to sail away in pursuit of the convoy.

Maarten shouted, "*Back to our boat!*" and stabbed his way past foes to get to a grappling hook. He yanked it up and, before jumping aboard, dragged one of his wounded men to the gunwale, and Pieter pulled him in. The boatswain and another man together cast off the other grappling hook, after slashing the enemy's sail and heaving their oars overboard.

As Maarten sailed past his first mate, he saw several men trying to raise the sail despite the rigging being severely damaged. Blood seemed to be everywhere. He momentarily thought of giving assistance—Nee! I can't, he told himself, must protect the supply boats. He trimmed his sails and set a course on the escaping gunboat. Good, she has only one sail and it's torn. We'll overtake her.

When in range, he commanded, "*Archers! Commence!*"

Several Spaniards were hit, and their archers returned fire.

"*Load shot!*" Maarten yelled. Balls linked by chain blasted from his cannon, tumbling ball-over-ball through the air, and tore through their rival's sail.

"*Load ball!*" Maarten ordered. Getting no response, he swiveled around. The cannoneer was dead, blood still pumping from the arrow in his chest. Maarten quickly took over the cannon and with Pieter loaded the last cannonball. The recoil rocked the boat. The ball smashed into the enemy's mast, splintering the upper part and toppling it over. With its sail dragging in the water, the vessel came to a halt.

Maarten sailed on. Without shot or cannonball, he intended to spend his last arrows before grappling the Spanish gunboat nearest to his supply boats. As he approached, though, the enemy squadron changed direction and started retreating across the lake. Nearby, a cloud of smoke hung over Prince William's fort; its cannons and harquebuses had done their job. Maarten also noticed, with relief, that his convoy was nearing the heavily defended rendezvous point.

"*Prepare to come about!*" Maarten turned back to aid the first mate. Coming alongside, he witnessed a bloody scene. Propped up against the mast was his first mate, his face ashen and eyes barely open. He ordered the injured transferred to his boat and sent several able-bodied men to get the crippled gunboat underway. The two set sail, with Maarten cradling his first mate in his lap. The man's eyes fluttered, and Maarten comforted him with "You'll be all right, mate."

At the rendezvous point, Dutchmen came aboard to help remove bodies to an empty supply boat, including Maarten's first mate who had died en route. They also carried the injured ashore, and Maarten and Pieter set about treating them.

After bandaging gashes, stemming the flow of blood from wounds, and setting broken limbs, Maarten sat down, exhausted. With elbows on knees, he dropped his face into his hands.

Pieter sank down next to him, spent. On seeing the last supply boat being emptied, he turned to inform Maarten and for the first time noticed his half-bitten-off ear. Appalled yet curious, he could not resist touching it. When Maarten's head raised, Pieter withdrew his hand and said, "The supply boats are ready to go back." Seeing Maarten's sad eyes, he added with a wan smile, "At least we were successful," but it came out unconvincing.

Successful? Maarten surveyed the carnage and stared back at Pieter. At a loss for words, all he could do was shake his head at the absurdities of war.

On Good Friday, all was quiet on Lake Haarlem, and Hasbrouk was happy not to have to go to the top of the city wall again to decipher which side was getting the upper hand. So much bloodshed, it sickened him. What he direly needed was a dose of the redemptive qualities of Christianity, as opposed to the divisive ones, and to attend a Calvinist service. No clandestine services were being held with Alva present, so he settled for the next best thing, taking the family on a walk past Catholic places of worship. He set a leisurely pace.

At the Begijnhof's church, a Good Friday mass was in process with soothing and sublime chanting by the Beguines. The Holy Place Church was quiet, and the family went on to the Rokin canal, where Hasbrouk stopped to chat with an old friend docking his rowboat.

Betje and the kids continued on. At the Dam, she perused the merchant stalls that were still open. Meanwhile, Catrijn and the boys knelt down to see sailboats lower their masts and disappear beneath, and then they raced to the other end to watch them emerge, raise their masts, and resume their journeys. The sight was familiar but never failed to entertain them. Though the Dam appeared to the casual observer to be a part of the adjacent Dam Square, it was in fact the top of a dam controlling the flow of water between the city's two main canals: the Rokin, which was fed by the Amstel River, and Damrak that carried the water northward into the sluggish Ij River and ultimately to the Zuider Zee.

Finding no bargains at the stalls, Betje looked for Hasbrouk and spotted him standing in Dam Square, gazing at the Town Hall's tower, from which music was being played. He seemed to be lost in thought. She gathered the kids to join him.

Hasbrouk was staring not at the Town Hall's tower, but at the steeple beyond of the 1400s Gothic Nieuwe Kerk (New Church), and he was reminiscing. The place and the music had brought back memories of marching as a Catholic youth in the annual Miracle Procession, a magical event full of pageantry and passion in celebration of the 1345 miracle.

For a studious boy like Hasbrouk, the Miracle Procession offered a rare opportunity to engage in drama. His first experience had been as a small child parading with friends wearing a devil costume, his soot-smeared face scowling fiendishly. Alongside them were little girls dressed like angels. When older, he and his peers periodically paused their marching to perform a short play about Saint George slaying a dragon. Such drama. Later as a Latin school student, he and schoolmates proudly wore their white robes and sang. The order of the procession was always the same. At the head were guild members carrying candles, banners, and paintings of their patron saints. Then came the children and Latin school adolescents, followed by the archers. The next group consisted of the clergy and barefoot penitents, and bringing up the rear were city government officials.

Hasbrouk could have lingered at Dam Square all afternoon, but Nicolaas was growing restless, so they moved on. Following the Damrak canal northward, Hasbrouk continued to be his congenial self, nodding and tipping his hat to those he knew. A short walk on the bridge over the Damrak took them to the older eastern half of the city and within sight of the imposing 1300s Oude Kerk (Old Church), a medieval masterpiece. Just seeing it lifted Hasbrouk's spirits because Oude Kerk, which was dedicated to Saint Nicolaas, had been his parish church before his conversion to Calvinism. This was where he had received the sacraments—baptism, first Holy Communion, and confirmation—and where family marriages and requiem masses had been held.

In front of the church, Hasbrouk removed his hat, and Dirck followed his lead and also took off Nicolaas's. Bowing their heads, all offered a silent Good Friday prayer.

In Hasbrouk's mind, he could envision the interior of Oude Kerk with its vaulted wooden ceiling and light streaming through those glorious stained-glass windows. And he could hear the chanting of the mass, smell the burning incense, and see its smoke wafting upward. Though un-Calvinistic, the recollections were nonetheless supremely comforting. He was sorely tempted to go inside, but decided not to because it might confuse the children.

Some people were going in and out of the church, while others just milled around and socialized outside. The usual peddlers were selling their wares, and destitute people loitered, hoping for alms.

Seeing the sad-looking alms seekers gave Betje a twinge of nostalgia, for Pieter had always given generously to the needy, though he himself had little. She said a silent prayer for her gentle brother and fervently hoped Maarten was keeping him safe.

Dirck was watching two priests hurrying toward the church with a painting of the Virgin Mary cradled in their arms, an unusual sight. Such objects were rarely seen in public anymore, not since last year when a Protestant mob stormed the church and carried away holy pictures and statues, which they smashed to bits on the pavement. The two priests were almost to the front door, when a shoe came hurtling through the air and smacked into the painting.

A boy ran up to retrieve his shoe, shouting "*Nee graven images!*" A man looped his arm around the boy, sending his arms and legs flailing and him screaming, "*Let me go!*" A crowd started closing in.

Feeling that someone should intervene to protect the boy until the sheriff arrived, Hasbrouk told Betje, "Stay here," and walked alone to where people were swarming. He craned to see the boy, but did not recognize him.

The mob was working itself into a frenzy, taunting the boy and disagreeing. "Get the little heretic!" "Satan's work!" "Leave him alone—he's just a kid!"

Seeing Hasbrouk disappear into the crowd and the sheriff's men enter the square, Betje pulled the children back to safety. Other onlookers were retreating too, and she noticed the Calvinist lay minister scurry past without making eye contact and then break into a run. From a side street, Betje and the kids observed the square.

Hasbrouk raised his hands and tried to calm the crowd. "Gentlemen! Ladies! Be reasonable. He's just a child!"

"Who are you," one man shouted, "his father?" A woman proclaimed, "You're his father!"

"Of course not," Hasbrouk defended himself. "You know me—"

"We should take *you—not* the boy!"

The group shifted its confused wrath to Hasbrouk. Invectives flew.

"*Calm down!*" Hasbrouk demanded. In exasperation, he raised his voice, "CALM DOWN!"

Startled by Hasbrouk's outburst, people standing nearby quit yelling and the noise level dropped.

"*What's going on here?*" a sheriff's man asked as he entered the fracas. "Clear the way." He looked at Hasbrouk. "Are you the ringleader here?"

"Of course not!" Hasbrouk said and started to relate what had happened.

"If you aren't," the other sheriff's assistant said, "why did they quiet down after you yelled? I heard it."

Incredulous, Hasbrouk said, "I was just trying to bring reason to the crowd because he's just a child."

"*He probably put the kid up to it!*" a man in the crowd yelled, setting off another cacophonous round.

"*Enough!*" the sheriff's assistant yelled, "ENOUGH!" and grabbed Hasbrouk by the arm. "You come with me." The other ripped the kicking and screaming boy from the men holding him and dragged him away.

As Hasbrouk was taken away, a man from the crowd punched his shoulder and swore at him. The sheriff's assistant smacked his pike against the perpetrator and shoved at others trying to block their way. Meanwhile, the mob grew angrier, and men started pushing each other.

Hasbrouk frantically searched for Betje and the children. They were nowhere in sight. Good, he thought, Betje must have kept a cool head and gone home.

Betje had to restrain Catrijn and put her hand over the girl's mouth when her father was led off. Hysterical, Catrijn pulled at the hand and tried to break away.

"Stop it!" Betje demanded and shook her. "Get hold of yourself, Catrijn." She glanced around nervously. "You *won't* help him that way. And you'll get us *all* arrested."

Catrijn's plaintive eyes beseeched Betje: We need to help Papa! What are we going to do?

"We'll go to your Aunt Margaretha's. She'll know what to do." Betje straightened herself and firmly grasped Catrijn and Nicolaas's hands.

Dirck watched them leave, looked at the square, and ran back to it.

Betje walked so fast the kids had trouble keeping up. At

Margaretha's house, she paused to catch her breath, and Catrijn ran in and flung herself into her aunt's arms.

"Where's Dirck?" Nicolaas asked.

"What?" Panicked, Betje scanned the street. Dirck was nowhere to be seen.

He had backtracked to the square and veered into the street where the crowd had gone. After jumping up several times trying to see Heer Hasbrouk, he bent down to make himself small and weaved his way through the crowd.

"*Hey*, waddya think you're doing?" a man said and seized Dirck's neck. "Are you one of them troublemakers?"

Dirck shook his head no. "Not me."

A woman glared at him, and another man.

Dirck broke loose, squeezed by a few people, scooted between the legs of two others, and ran all the way to the Begijnhof. He arrived to see his mother and Catrijn sobbing and Margaretha consoling them.

"Dirck! Where have you been?" Betje and Margaretha demanded almost in unison. Betje slapped him hard on the bottom. "Don't you *ever* do that again! When I go, I expect you to follow. Do you understand?"

A bow of his head said yes, and Dirck added, "I saw where they took Heer Hasbrouk. It was the sheriff's office."

"I'll go and see what I can do," Margaretha said. "Betje, you should take the children home. I'll ask one of the sisters to go with you."

Margaretha prayed all the way to the sheriff's office and on arriving found an angry mob blocking the door. Using her cane and relying on people to step aside in deference to a nun-like woman, she pushed her way forward. Inside, luckily a reasonable and sympathetic man, whom she knew, was on duty. She launched into pleading her case.

"Sheriff Johann, you are holding my brother. You know him—he's a good man. He was only trying to help that poor, misguided child. You know I've devoted my *entire* life to bringing such lost souls into Our Savior's love and divine grace. Surely, you don't think my brother would incite violence against anyone."

"I'm sorry, Sister Margaretha. Heer Hasbrouk has been transferred to the Inquisition's jurisdiction ... to the Minor Friar Monastery. The matter is out of our hands." Seeing Margaretha's resolve, the sheriff guided her into an adjacent room to speak in private. "Sister, you saw the mob outside. What else could we do? They call him a heretic. He must answer for himself."

Margaretha knew all too well that her brother's fate ultimately lay with the Inquisitor's most important question: Do you accept Catholicism as the only true, holy, and apostolic faith and renounce all others? To which, he will answer emphatically No! For him, disavowing his Calvinist beliefs was not remotely possible. She stared at the sheriff, not knowing what to say. "I ... we need to ..."

"Sister, please go home," Sheriff Johann advised and gently touched her shoulder to get her moving toward the back door. "Let justice take its course."

Hesitating, Margaretha considered whether to press her case further and decided instead to talk to Father Hein, the head of the Beguines.

Margaretha was able to convince a reluctant Father Hein to intercede, and he went to the Minor Friar Monastery to talk to the Inquisitors. Later in the evening, he returned and found Margaretha in the Begijnhof's church.

"Nothing can save your brother," Father Hein said. "However, I was able to negotiate a merciful death. He will be spared the agony of being burned while still alive." With sincere sympathy, he added, "I'm very sorry, but it was the best I could do," and sat down beside her. Together they prayed through the night.

In the morning, Margaretha found the strength to go to the Minor Friar Monastery, where she was told her brother was with the Inquisitors and unavailable. She proceeded to the Hasbrouk house. Even before her cane hit the front step, Catrijn had the door open and was staring anxiously. The anguish in her aunt's eyes was clear, and Catrijn burst into tears.

Betje ushered them both inside and scanned the street before closing the door. She too could see the news was going to be bad. Near the window, a pensive Dirck stood, with Nicolaas cowering behind him.

Margaretha sat down and clasped Catrijn's hands in hers. "Catrijn, you must be strong. Your father has had a long, happy, and righteous life. The Inquisition has already decided ... there is nothing we can do." She paused and cleared her throat.

Tears were streaming down Catrijn's face. By now, Betje was weeping uncontrollably.

Margaretha continued, "There should be no sadness. No recriminations against those ... who, uh, judge him." The last statement caught in her throat. "Your father does not want that." Margaretha squeezed Catrijn's hands. "Your father will soon take his rightful place with our Heavenly Father. For that, we should rejoice and give thanks."

Betje said an almost inaudible "Amen."

Silently, aunt and niece held hands until the raw emotions receded.

When Margaretha finally saw her brother, they embraced without speaking. Glued together in unbearable grief, neither could move. Hasbrouk eventually relaxed his arms, stepped back, and both sat down. In as calm a voice as he could muster, he recounted the circumstances of his arrest and trial.

He's so composed, Margaretha was thinking, so admirable. But he's scared. I can hear it in his voice. I must be strong for him. Can't cry. Oh I love him so much.

Hasbrouk concluded with, "I've been convicted of heresy and will be punished in the customary way, burning at the stake." For her benefit, he added, "I am not afraid."

"Father Hein has interceded on your behalf," Margaretha said and touched his hand. "A merciful death is promised. You will not feel the flames."

"In these times of few mercies, the heart must be thankful for scraps," Hasbrouk said and sighed.

Margaretha blinked her eyes in agreement and convinced herself that her brother's fear had diminished.

"Margaretha," Hasbrouk said in a changed tone, almost businesslike, "Catrijn will need comforting and moral guidance. I know Betje is a loving godmother and she will do her best. But in the formative years ahead, Catrijn will also require intellectual stimulation and education. I will die in peace if you promise to do those things ... as I would have."

"You have my solemn oath."

Hasbrouk went on to explain his financial situation, what little there was, and his last will and testament, and tried to hide his shame for leaving his only child so ill provided for. He added that, of course, it was too dangerous for Catrijn or the Van der Voorts to visit him. And he certainly did not want his daughter's last memory of him to be in this place or at the stake.

Margaretha stayed as long as the keepers would allow, exchanging memories and praying with her brother.

The Inquisition and the magistrates wasted no time in delivering their brand of justice, and Margaretha went alone to the Dam to witness it. She had already resolved to put her own feelings aside and focus on transmitting love and support to her brother as he departed this life. She had to use her cane to push people aside to get near the two stakes that had been erected, one for her brother and the other for an unknown heretic. There she waited until the prisoners were brought. The buzz of the crowd hardly intruded, until she heard a woman excitedly tell people around her that the little boy heretic had been executed that morning, by drowning in the canal. Margaretha felt tears welling ... one escaped. She dabbed it discreetly.

Heer Hasbrouk stoically walked toward the stake, eyes focused ahead, and climbed the makeshift steps. The other man had already been attached to his stake, and the fire lit beneath him. Smoke wafted up.

Hasbrouk maintained his steely composure while his

executioner finished securing the ropes. Below him, two men ignited the wood.

Margaretha was aghast when the executioner descended the stairs. No! He's supposed to be dead before the fire starts! They promised! She struck her cane against the woman in front of her—"Out of my way!"—and moved forward. By now, the flames were flaring bright yellow.

The executioner climbed the stairs again. He pulled out a knife and skillfully slit Hasbrouk's throat.

Some hissed.

Margaretha let out a weak cry. Her head dropped; she could bear no more. Abruptly, she turned and threaded her way through the boisterous crowd toward home.

For the next several days, Betje lived in terror of what might happen next and was on alert for omens: an odd flicker of a flame, unusual hoot of an owl, or abnormal blemishes on the children's faces.

Meanwhile the boys were growing ever more rambunctious, and Betje agreed to let them go outside. First, though, she poked her head out the front door to make sure it was safe—

Sheriff! Betje shut the door and breathlessly stood behind it, praying: Please Lord, don't let him stop at our house.

The doorknocker banged.

Betje was scared. Oh no, not again. They're going to take this house too.

The knocker clapped repeatedly, and a man's voice commanded, "OPEN UP!"

Reluctantly, Betje released the latch, and the sheriff and his helper forced the door open.

"W-what do you want?" Betje asked.

The sheriff displayed a piece of paper and perfunctorily recited: "For actions by one, Heer Hasbrouk, in defiance of the Council of Trouble," the official name of the Inquisition, "this property is forfeited. You are ordered to vacate it immediately."

"Nee, please, three children live here," Betje implored them. "We have nowhere else to go. *Please*."

The sheriff and his helper stood mute and unmoved. They had their orders.

Betje fell to her knees, ready to beg.

"What's going on here?" Margaretha demanded as she walked up. After knocking one man's calf with her cane—"Step aside."—she scowled at Betje: Stop groveling!

Betje rose to her feet.

"This is *my* house," Margaretha said. "I am a Catholic, a Beguine, and use this house in service to *the* holy church."

Puzzled, the men looked at each other.

"Heer Hasbrouk was my brother—but this is *my* house. And these are *guests* in *my* house." She swung her cane. "Now, be off with you. Go back and correct your records. This is *my* house!" She stepped inside, giving Betje a little shove ahead of her, and closed the door firmly behind.

Margaretha sat down and nervously fanned herself, hoping her stern theatrics would save the house.

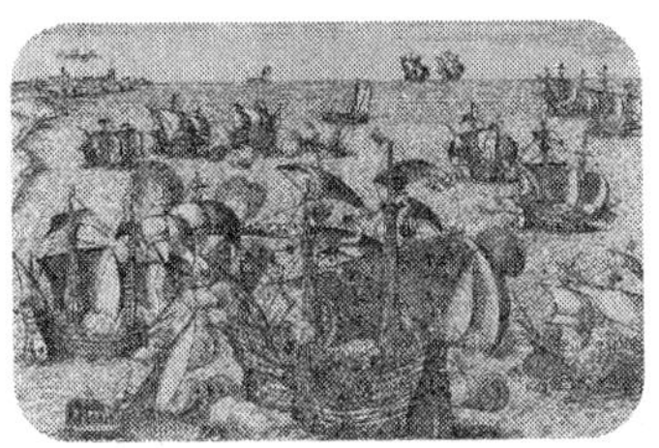

Battle for the Zuider Zee

CHAPTER 3

Expel Spain – 1573-1575

On May 28, 1573, the Sea Beggars' successes on Lake Haarlem came to an end. Count Bossu launched a massive attack, using all his gunships plus others that had been cruising the Zuider Zee, and overwhelmed the Beggar fleet. Twenty-two boats were captured. Thousands died. Bossu went on to seize every one of Prince William's forts. With supply lines to Haarlem cut and Lake Haarlem under his control, the Duke of Alva knew that victory was within his grasp.

Haarlem continued to hold out, though their situation was dire. In June, their desperate leader sent a carrier pigeon to Prince William with a message written in his own blood, saying they could not survive much longer. The Prince replied with a promise to raise money and provide help soon.

The city's fate was sealed when Prince William sent a pigeon to inform Haarlemers that 4,000 reinforcements would arrive on July 8. One of Don Frederic's soldiers shot down the bird, intending to have a meal, and found the message. On July 8, Don Frederic's troops lay in wait, and the Prince's inexperienced volunteers were easily routed.

After enduring the siege for seven months, Haarlem surrendered on July 12 on Don Frederic's offer of mercy. In the week that followed, Don Frederic mercilessly hanged, beheaded or drowned the entire garrison and all of Haarlem's 1,000 town officials and residents. Claiming their spoils of war, his soldiers rampaged through the city and plundered everything.

The Duke of Alva selected 16,000 men from his army and set his sights on the next target, the rebel town of Alkmaar with 1,000 adult residents and Prince William's all-volunteer garrison of 800.

When the sheriff did not return during the three months following Margaretha's rebuke, Betje decided it was time to resume normal life. That is, as much as was possible with ruthless Alva still in their midst and Amsterdam being called Murderdam for the Inquisition's deadly toll. As part of her routine, Betje took daily walks to the city wall, which Heer Hasbrouk had done and the kids liked so much. On some days, Margaretha or Hasbrouk's old friend Heer Nostrand accompanied them.

Today as Alva's troops prepared to leave for Alkmaar, all of them were at the western wall jostling for a view. Rumor had spread that the soldiers refused to march on Alkmaar until paid, and Amsterdammers wanted to see for themselves whether violence was going to erupt. Though Alva had lost 10,000 men in the Haarlem siege, his troops still numbered 20,000. If they mutinied, even Amsterdam might not be safe.

After observing that the army camp was calm, Betje and the youngsters went on to the harbor. There, the kids exchanged giddy glances while watching the Sea Beggars set up a blockade by sinking old vessels in the Ij to create a navigational nightmare for ships trying to leave Amsterdam, and positioning their own ships to attack any that made it through.

Betje was staring in vain at the distant figures, hoping to spot Maarten. In the last five years she had heard nothing from him, but knew in her heart that he was alive. She made a silent plea—Oh

Maarten, if you're out there, please let me know!—and dispatched it with a kiss on the wind.

The top of the eastern wall was their final vantage point, and the view was alarming. Count Bossu was building a new fleet, and for the first time they comprehended just how threatening it was. Large three-masted ships were in varying stages of completion, and neat rows of ominous cannons lay nearby. Sea Beggar ships were no match for these.

October 1573 was shaping up to be a month of reckoning for both the Sea Beggars and Alkmaar.

Alkmaar was bracing for yet another assault by Don Frederic's troops. During the last two and a half months, the beleaguered town had repulsed three major attacks by pouring boiling water, hot oil, pitch, molten lead, and lime on the attackers and by relentlessly pushing their siege ladders off city walls. Though many more Spaniards had lost their lives than Alkmaar's defenders, the residents' situation was nonetheless dire, totally isolated and growing ever more hungry.

In Amsterdam, Count Bossu was preparing to launch his thirty new ships. His order from the Duke of Alva was to hunt down and destroy the Sea Beggars, once and for all.

The Sea Beggars were cruising the Zuider Zee, and Maarten made an emergency stop in Hoorn, a seafaring town loyal to Prince William of Orange's cause. While he arranged for needed repairs to his *Dirck*, Pieter recruited sailors to replace those who had perished in the Lake Haarlem battle. Several other ships of their fleet were anchored nearby, doing the same thing. Work on the *Dirck* had barely begun when a fellow Sea Beggar ship, the *Resolute*, sailed into port with its men yelling: *"Alkmaar won!" "The siege is over!"*

Cheers erupted on land and ships.

After the *Resolute* set its anchor, townspeople and Sea Beggars went aboard to hear more. The *Resolute's* captain reported that Alkmaar had cut its dikes at the perfect time when the wind was strong and coming from the sea. Surging sea water raced through the openings and straight into Alva's camp. His troops panicked, broke ranks and ran for their lives.

Everyone declared it a great victory and cheered wildly.

The *Resolute's* captain also carried orders from Commander Dirckszoon. All Sea Beggar ships were to rendezvous on the other side of the Zuider Zee as soon as possible. Count Bossu was launching a threatening new fleet, and every Sea Beggar ship was needed, regardless of its condition.

Maarten returned to his *Dirck* unsettled. The coming lopsided contest with Bossu was giving him a bad feeling. Unless most of his fleet foundered on the old hulks sunk by the Sea Beggars, Bossu was going to defeat them, and even worse than on Lake Haarlem. Also weighing heavily on his mind was the fate of his hometown, Alkmaar, for in cutting their dikes they had inundated their farmlands. He knew that long after the euphoria of victory had faded, Alkmaar residents would be toiling to rebuild those dikes, drain the seawater, and replenish the soil to grow crops again. In the meantime, famine would stalk.

After darkness fell, Maarten and Pieter took the sea chest and slipped over the side of the *Dirck* to bury it, ensuring its safety in case the ship sank in battle. The chest contained all that remained of their prize money and loot taken during the last five years.

Pieter had been able to recruit only two additional crewmembers while in Hoorn, and one of them, experienced seaman and skilled crossbowman Rykaard Beekman, seemed a likely replacement for Maarten's long-time first mate, who had fallen at Lake Haarlem.

The *Dirck* sailed off undermanned and in fragile condition to join the Sea Beggar fleet riding at anchor on the far side of the Zuider Zee. When all ships were present, Commander Dirckszoon summoned their captains for a briefing.

"I am sorry to report that Count Bossu's entire fleet somehow managed to navigate through the obstacles we placed in the Ij." Seeing the dejected looks on their faces, he added, "Bossu has had a string of good luck, but it can't last."

The captains said, "He's right!" though few were convinced, for they already knew the enemy ships outnumbered theirs and were larger and better armed. The most formidable was Bossu's *Inquisition*, which reportedly carried 300 men and 34 hefty cannons, and possibly had metal armor on its hull.

"Count Bossu is somewhere in the Zuider Zee with his fleet," Dirckszoon said, "trying to find us. When he does, he'll line up his ships and pummel us with cannon fire. Well, I don't need to tell you ... they will destroy us. We can't match them cannon for cannon. But we *do* have advantages: our speed and agility. So we must sail straight at them to give the smallest and fastest-moving target possible. Closer in, we distract them with cannon and small arms fire to break up their line. If they won't break ranks, we have to force them. Wear them down. Sail around them. Sail through them—harass—until they do. And when they try to change positions and drift apart, we divide up and surround their ships and grapple. *Then*, we board and fight hand-to-hand. That's how we'll win. Hand to hand."

The captains exchanged confident looks, knowing that Sea Beggars excelled in fierce man-to-man clashes. They were fighting for their homeland, while Count Bossu's Spaniards and mercenaries were just paid combatants.

"Of course, we can expect to take many of Bossu's ships as prizes," Dirckszoon said as an added motivation. "Any questions?" Hearing none, he finished with "We sail tomorrow, if the wind is right."

Maarten went away in a miserable mood, knowing this encounter was likely to mean the end of the Sea Beggars, despite the commander's upbeat message about advantages. Their mishmash fleet of 24 ships, some new and others in various states of disrepair and with only 700 men, was no match for Bossu's 30 brand new, well-armed warships carrying 1,300.

As he rowed himself back to his ship, Maarten wondered how he was going to pump himself up for this battle, let alone inspire the men. The usual rallying cries—For Prince William! To Victory!—felt gratuitous. While searching for ideas, his thoughts wandered back in time, recalling books Papa had read to him. A quote came to mind, "Men in exile feed on dreams," and another, "Tame the savageness of man and make gentle the life of this world."

Maarten went to bed with those sage words swirling in his head. At dawn, he awoke and checked the wind. It was favorable. Today, October 8, was going to be their day of reckoning.

After the crew had stowed away their bedding and eaten, Maarten gathered them on deck. In stark terms, he laid out the odds and related Dirckszoon's strategy for engagement, emphasizing the Sea Beggar's agility and hand-to-hand advantages.

The men asked no questions, accepting their fate.

Maarten turned philosophical. "We are exiles. For years, we've been forced to face every day as though it might be our last. Danger is everywhere ... from the wild seas to the savageness of other men. How do we go on, day after day? What keeps us from giving up?" He looked from face to face. "It's our dreams. Dreams of reuniting with our families. Of our children growing up in a less brutal world where there is no war. Where we can be friends with our neighbors again, without worrying whether they have the same beliefs as us. Where ducats are spent on food, learning, caring for each other—and not on armaments." Maarten paused and gazed across the Zuider Zee. "Today, let us exiles feed our dreams. Let us make gentle this world we live in. Let us resoundingly defeat Bossu and his savageness." He raised his fist, emphatic but not militant. "To dreams! To Prince William and tolerance!" His expression was both determined and hopeful. "We can win this."

Energized, the men pumped their fists. "To dreams!" "To our children!" "To no more war!"

The fleet set sail on a light eastern wind, and the *Dirck* assumed its position on the southern flank, near the *Resolute*. With Dirckszoon's ship at the center, the fleet moved into the Zuider Zee.

After the sails were trimmed and the *Dirck* on a steady course, Maarten sent a man to the crow's nest.

"*Bossu!*" the lookout yelled, "*straight ahead. They're between Hoorn and Enkhuizen!*" Soon the same call came from other ships.

"*How many?*"

"LOTS, and the Inquisition is REALLY big!"

Maarten ordered the men to prepare for battle. Cannoneers stacked their balls, while Pieter and others went below to retrieve their weapons. From the helm, Maarten kept an eye on the line of Dutch ships. All were keeping a reasonable distance from each other to avoid giving Bossu's cannons concentrated targets. Faster ones were moving ahead.

BOOM. One of Bossu's cannons fired. The cannonball fell short of the Dutch ships. More cannons erupted. The Spanish ships maintained their positions. Dirckszoon's fleet continued on course.

BOOM. A cannonball splashed in the water on the *Dirck's* starboard side. The next whizzed over the deck, tearing through a section of rigging. Two men raced to haul in the trailing lines. Maarten kept his course.

Other Dutch ships were taking fire. The swiftest ones were nearing the opposing fleet and soon would be in range of their archers and harquebuses.

As the *Dirck* edged closer to the Spanish line, Maarten gulped hard, realizing just how big those ships were. "*Ready cannons!*" he commanded and nervously checked to see how nearby Sea Beggar ships were doing ... none seemed to have sustained serious damage. His eyes returned to the closest enemy ship and saw crossbowmen in chain-mail coats amassing at her bow. "*Aim high!*" he ordered. The enemy came into range. "*Fire!*" Maarten watched with satisfaction as one cannonball took out a chunk of the prow and another blasted into its gunwale, driving the crossbowmen back. "*Good aim, men!*"

BOOM. Flying through the air at the *Dirck* came shot: balls linked by a chain. One tore through the edge of the mainsail.

"RETREAT!" came Dirckszoon's order, which was relayed from ship to ship. "RETREAT!"

Maarten announced, "*Ready to come about!*" and considered himself lucky to be escaping with so little damage to his *Dirck.*

At a safe distance from the enemy, Dirckszoon's fleet came together, and word was passed along that many Dutch ships had been damaged, but all remained seaworthy. Tomorrow, they would try again.

Two more days of skirmishing left nearly every Dutch ship impaired, several sunk, and Bossu's disciplined line beginning to break down. All the while, vessels were coming from nearby towns to resupply the Sea Beggars with ammunition, food, and reinforcements, and to ferry injured seamen to shore. Maarten prayed for better wind, because the *Dirck* was sailing sluggishly from a hit to her already weakened hull.

On October 10 the wind blew strong, and the Dutch fleet charged the enemy. The speedy ships proved to be difficult targets for Bossu's cannon volleys, and most of them reached the Spanish line unscathed.

Maarten steered between two hostile ships, and his harquebus and crossbow men commenced shooting at their opponents. Shots were returned and enemy cannons blasted, but the *Dirck* reached the end of the gantlet unharmed. Maarten guided his ship around the stern of one—"*Whoa!*" Ahead, was the *Resolute* heading straight toward them, having sailed between two other ships and just changed course. Maarten veered the *Dirck* away, barely avoiding a collision. As the two passed, Maarten yelled "CLOSE CALL!" and the *Resolute's* captain saluted and let out an adrenaline-filled laugh. Maarten circled his *Dirck* around to make another run. Archers and crossbowmen resumed firing.

The nimble Dutch ships continued their harassments, and soon small supply boats from nearby towns arrived. With so many vessels swarming the waters, their hulls sometimes scraped against each other, Dutch and Spanish alike. Under the relentless badgering, the Spanish ships attempted to block their passage, but moved too slowly to be effective. Their formation breaking down, Bossu's ships drifted apart, with Sea Beggars in pursuit. By three o'clock, individual battles of two and three ships were raging on the Zuider Zee from Hoorn to Enkhuizen.

The *Dirck* and the *Resolute* converged on the same ship, each trying to avoid her cannons, which were discharging at an alarming rate. Maarten sought refuge near the stern, and his men heaved a grappling hook toward the gunwale, requiring several attempts before locking it in place. The *Resolute* sailed to the prow and set its hook. Neither captain had any idea how they were going to board such an immense ship, so for now they contented themselves with serving as a drag and pummeling its hull with their cannons.

Each time a Spaniard appeared at the gunwale and attempted to cast off the grapple, he was targeted by one of Maarten's archers. When dozens of them amassed and sent down a rain of arrows, Sea Beggars took cover. The Spaniards loosened the grappling hook, tossed it overboard, and cheered "Hurrah!" Maarten's men recommenced shooting.

With arrows and harquebus bullets flying in both directions, Maarten's men tried desperately to reset the grapple but were unsuccessful. The enemy ship began sailing away, leaving the *Dirck* in its wind shadow and Maarten struggling to get her underway. As the Spanish ship gained speed, a becalmed *Dirck* came in direct line of its cannons. The cannons opened fire.

"*Down!*" Maarten yelled. A cannonball crossed the deck and smashed into the mast, and a round of shot tore through her mainsail. Meanwhile, archers on the Spanish deck stepped up their barrage, killing a man next to Maarten and grazing Pieter's arm. Another ball dealt a final blow to the mast, and it came crashing down along with the sail. Maarten's cannoneers pushed the fallen sail from their cannons, and men one by one emerged from under the sail with their harquebuses, bows, and crossbows. Maarten ordered them to fire at will.

"*We're out!*" one of the cannoneers shouted. "*Us too!*" men with harquebuses proclaimed.

CREEAAK. The Spanish ship shuddered. Her guns went silent. Archers quit shooting.

"*She's hit a sandbar!*" Maarten exclaimed.

The *Dirck* drifted toward the grounded ship and soon came to rest on the same sandbar, with the two hulls almost touching.

The Spanish ship groaned loudly and listed, putting her cannon ports nearly level with the *Dirck's* deck.

From the ports, Spaniards stared. Rykaard shot his crossbow

with deadly accuracy, and they retreated. Archers appeared in one of the ports and were met with a spray of Sea Beggar arrows.

With sword raised, Maarten put one foot on the gunwale. "*Prepare to board!*"

A Spaniard sprang from his port. Maarten jumped out of his way, turned and slashed the man's back, and he collapsed. Another leaped onto the *Dirck* and ran into Pieter's outstretched pike. After yanking out his weapon, Pieter followed Maarten's vault to one of the ports. Met by a line of knife-wielding foes, Pieter jabbed his pike and Maarten swung his sword to push them back.

Seeing more ferocious Dutchmen come in through the ports, several defenders retreated up a ladder. More followed.

The Sea Beggars pressed forward and fought their way to the ladder. Maarten led the charge up. Emerging on the main deck, he glanced toward the bow. The *Resolute's* men were meeting fierce resistance. His eyes shifted to the stern, just in time to see a man running at him with a sword. Maarten lurched sideways, but it was too late, and the blade sliced through his thigh. As he staggered backward and fell, one of his men tackled the attacker. While trying to staunch the flow of blood from the wound with his beret, he surveyed the deck and spotted the commander of the ship near the mast. With effort, he climbed to his feet.

The captain caught sight of Maarten advancing and pivoted to face him, a dagger in one hand and sword in the other.

Maarten lunged at him with sword outstretched. His leg gave way, and he tumbled to the deck. Seeing the Spaniard's sword swing up, he rolled aside—the blade slammed down next to him—and he rolled up and onto one knee and shoved his sword into the captain's belly. It came out as fast as it went in, and the captain collapsed, dead.

Seeing their captain fall, men nearby dropped their weapons and retreated to the opposite side of the deck with their hands raised in surrender. Some jumped overboard.

Noticing Pieter and Rykaard hemmed in at the capstan, Maarten charged their assailants from behind. With a two-handed rake of his sword, he cut down two of them. Another spun around and wildly jabbed his dagger, driving him back. When Maarten slipped on the bloody deck and landed on his back, Rykaard arrived and slayed the Spaniard with a well-placed stroke of his knife and then pulled Maarten to his feet.

After giving him a nod of thanks, Maarten paused to scan the melee. Sea Beggars from the *Resolute* had advanced to mid-deck and were fighting side by side with his own men. Some Spaniards continued to oppose them, but most were laying down their weapons and withdrawing to where their compatriots were surrendering. Several were teetering on the gunwale, ready to jump, while below small Dutch vessels were corralling those already in the water. The Sea Beggars had won.

The *Resolute's* captain and Maarten ordered their men to disarm their rivals and lock them up below. The battle over and the adrenaline surge fading, Maarten felt the pain in his leg. Grimacing, he sat down to inspect it, and Pieter, whose mouth was bleeding from having lost two teeth, came to help. After Pieter tore a piece of cloth from his shirt and tied it around Maarten's leg, the two went on to help others. Meanwhile, a flotilla of supply boats arrived and delivered food and water to the exhausted Dutch fighters.

As twilight descended, the *Resolute* sailed off with fresh reinforcements to join an ongoing assault on another ship, while Maarten and the wounded remained behind to guard the captives. By nightfall, several Spanish ships had been captured, some were retreating to Amsterdam with Dutch ships in pursuit, and others continued to fight on in scattered locations on the Zuider Zee.

Bossu's *Inquisition*, which had been drifting with three Sea Beggar ships grappled to her prow and sides, struck a rocky shoal. Throughout the night, Bossu's men repelled those who attempted to board. In early morning, one man succeeded in reaching the deck but was killed while attempting to take down the *Inquisition's* flag. Bossu finally surrendered at 11 o'clock after realizing he could not win. His ship was unable to get away, his fleet was nowhere to be seen, and he was battling an enemy with a seemingly endless supply of reinforcements and ammunition.

Maarten and the boatswain boarded the *Dirck* and after

inspecting the damage agreed that she was beyond repair. Afterward, they and the men removed everything of worth and gathered their dead. Reverently they committed their bodies to the sea.

Five captured ships were brought to Hoorn amid cheers, and prisoner Count Bossu stepped ashore to jeers. The ships were destined to be sold as prizes, and Bossu was going to be held in Hoorn until Prince William of Orange traded him for Dutch patriot Philips van Marnix, who had recently been taken prisoner.

Admiral Dirckszoon and many Sea Beggar ships left Hoorn before the snow flew and the Zuider Zee iced over. Others remained behind to recover from the toll on their ships and crew.

Maarten's most pressing need was to find a replacement for his *Dirck*. After retrieving the strongbox, tallying the coins in it, and ascertaining his likely share from the sale of the prizes, he set off with crossbowman Rykaard, a native of Hoorn, to search out available ships. They found a half-finished one at a shipyard on the edge of town whose builder had run out of money. It was a boeier design, the same as his *Dirck*, but was an upgrade with slightly larger hull and two masts, rather than one, yet the price was affordable. Maarten specified a few modifications and struck a deal. While the shipbuilder did his work, Maarten and his crew settled into housing in Hoorn, intending to stay there for winter and in spring rejoin the Sea Beggar fleet.

In November news came that King Philip II had recalled the Duke of Alva to Spain and his army would retreat to the south. That got Maarten thinking about trying to sneak into Amsterdam to visit his family, reasoning that there would be no Spanish troops to contend with, the Inquisition might be less active with Alva gone, and he may not be this close to home again for a while because the Sea Beggars undoubtedly would go south in spring to join ongoing battles there. He also wanted to deliver what little money he had to Betje.

Maarten arranged for a fishing boat to take him to a dike

outside Amsterdam, from which he would walk to Haarlemspoort city gate. He planned to wear beggars clothes to blend in with the multitudes displaced by war and also carry a few apples and pretend to want to sell them, in case beggars were denied entry to the city.

When the time came to leave, Maarten put on beggar rags and wrapped a well-worn cloth around his neck and pulled it up to cover his chin and cheeks. The addition of a hat, yanked low over his eyes, completed the outfit, and he inspected the results in a mirror. No, *that* doesn't work! Too obvious I'm trying to hide my face. He glanced down at the beggar purse stashed in his pocket that contained gold coins to be given to Betje—that's *not* safe either. Staring into the mirror, he thought for a moment. The hat and scarf came off. The rag went under his chin and up and over his ears and was tied at the top of his head. After stuffing coins into his mouth and creating a bulge in his cheek, he grimaced and peered into the mirror again. Good, looks like I have a tooth ache. Now all I need to do is moan.

Everything went as planned, and Maarten entered Amsterdam through Haarlemspoort gate, moaning and surrounded by somber people in various stages of malnutrition and weariness. He wanted to cry out—I'm home!—but instead concealed his joy and with head down walked briskly toward his house. En route, he paused at the spot where he had first encountered Aunt Margaretha at the tender age of nine. Even today he could recall in vivid detail how it happened:

That lousy scoundrel Rijp Dekker was instructing me on what to do after he snatched a rich lady's purse, and I was hating every minute of it. At first, I believed him when he said he was my friend and wanted to help me—but came to realize he really didn't care about me. He just wanted to make me a crook like him. I despised having to learn his gang's tricks for stealing and then covering up the evidence. But what could I do? I had no money, nowhere to go, and I was starving. So I stood there, behind him, while he peeked around the corner looking for a rich-lady victim.

Someone grabbed my hair and started pulling me backward. It hurt like heck, and I twisted to see who it was. A nun! At least she resembled one. Rijp grabbed my feet, and I thought they were going to pull me apart, until she smacked him with her cane, and he let go. She warned me "I'll hit you too, if you run!" I was too scared to move. When Aunt Margaretha led me away, Rijp yelled "You're too cowardly for my gang anyway!" And he never stopped making fun of me for letting a crippled old lady capture me, or quit trying to convince me to rejoin his gang. Rijp never could understand that I was glad to be rid of him and that I was the lucky one. Meeting Aunt Margaretha and being adopted by Papa were the best things that ever happened to me.

With a warm feeling inside, Maarten quickened his pace in anticipation of a happy reunion with his family, something he had envisioned innumerable times.

Betje will cry and bury herself in my arms, and I'll feel those voluptuous breasts against my chest. The boys might be unsure at first, but they'll come around. They'll be strong, maybe showing signs of virility. Papa, he'll be overjoyed, and both of us will probably cry. Aunt Margaretha ... well, she'll be Aunt Margaretha, loving yet firm and with lots of questions.

Around the corner and down the street, Maarten's modest home came into view. It was a welcome sight, despite the nagging memory of money still owed on it. The door opened, and Maarten expected to see his loving wife or one of the boys emerge. A man came out instead and casually sauntered away. Who is *he*? Why is a stranger visiting *my* house? Maarten stormed across the street, intending to barge in and demand an explanation from Betje but halted when the door opened again.

A woman stepped out with a broom and began sweeping the steps. Betje had done the same thing every day before Maarten went away, but this woman was not Betje. The woman noticed the beggar staring at her and swung her broom to shoo him away.

Maarten had no idea who the woman was, and rather than make a scene he retreated, bewildered. Where's Betje? He went on to Papa's home, hoping to get some answers, but it was quiet. Should I knock on the door? He opted instead to wait across the street until someone came out or went in. Thirty minutes passed, and no one did. Concerned that his presence was arousing suspicion, he walked around the block and took up a less conspicuous position in a dark doorway opposite the house. There he squatted and shivered until darkness fell. When no candles were lit, he concluded, they must not be home.

On to Aunt Margaretha's house he went, slapping his arms around his body to warm up. The gold coins were cutting into his cheek, and he was starting to think it was not such a clever hiding place after all. Using his tongue, he maneuvered them to the other cheek.

At Aunt Margaretha's house, faint light emanated through the cracks of the shutters. He slunk cautiously toward the front door, vowing to play dumb and beg for food, if someone other than his aunt answered. Before he could knock, the door creaked open, and the light of a lantern sent out a warm glow.

He withdrew and plastered himself in the recess of the next doorway.

"Are you certain you'll be all right?" an unfamiliar woman's voice asked from within Margaretha's house.

"I'll be perfectly fine," Margaretha's familiar voice answered, and she stepped out with a lantern and strode in Maarten's direction.

"Aunt Margaretha ... it's me," Maarten said softly as he stepped forward, trying not to startle her. "Maarten van der Voort."

Margaretha stopped and raised her lantern and cane. "Maarten?" Skeptical, she demanded, "Show yourself!"

Maarten pulled the rag from his face, spat the coins into his hand, and gave her a warm smile.

"Maarten! It *is* you! I feared you were dead."

He dropped to his knee to be at eye level with her.

Margaretha embraced him, and then anxiously gestured for him to stand up. "We need to move along." She glanced at an upper window. "Prying eyes."

"Where's Betje?" Maarten whispered. "I went to my house—a strange man and woman came out—is she all right? And the boys?"

"Betje is fine, and the boys too," Margaretha reassured him, "but much has changed." While they walked, Margaretha explained as succinctly as possible that she was now staying at Papa's house to protect the family, the house was probably dark because Betje was conserving candles, and that many problems had befallen all of them. Impatient, Maarten kept interjecting questions. When informed of Papa's fate, he had to stop to compose himself.

By the time they reached Papa's house, Maarten's mind was a jumble and fomenting irrational thoughts. I'm so thin ... what will Betje think of me?

On seeing a beggar walk into the front room behind Margaretha, Betje jumped to her feet and recoiled. The boys and Catrijn were too shocked to move. Maarten removed the hat and rag from his head, and Margaretha lit a candle. Betje's eyes widened and hands flew to her mouth.

Maarten said, "I missed you terribly, Betje," and enveloped her in his arms, while thinking how pale and drawn she had become. Gone were the easy smile and plump, curvaceous figure.

"It's been five looong years." Betje sank into his embrace and realized his body was thin, but hers thinner. I'm so skinny, he must think I'm ugly. She began to cry.

Maarten mistook the tears for a sign of happiness and caressed her head lovingly. Over her shoulder, he caught sight of the kids staring at him.

"Dirck," Maarten said, "such a big guy now. Ten, eh?"

Dirck nodded yes, and thought: Father has blue eyes—just like me. And freckles, same as Nicolaas. I'd forgotten.

Nicolaas blurted out, "Sea Beggars *really* are beggars!"

"Nicolaas," Maarten said with a chuckle and reached out to embrace the boy, but his son stepped back, confused. Maarten tried to coax him forward. "Nee, it's just a disguise. I don't usually dress like this—"

"Where's Pieter?" Betje asked, her eyes full of fright.

"In Hoorn ... overwintering. All of us are. Don't worry, he's fine."

"Hoorn—that's where you defeated Bossu," Dirck said.

"Sure is."

All the while, Catrijn was staring at Maarten, trying to reconcile his haggard appearance with her fuzzy memory of the big, jovial man who had left Amsterdam when she was six years old and used to carve wooden toys for her and the boys.

Maarten noticed his goddaughter. "Catrijn—you've grown."

Her eyes blinked yes.

"Maarten," Margaretha said, "you look tired. Why don't you go to bed and get some rest." She turned to Catrijn. "You can go home with me, and the boys can use your bed, so their parents can have the kitchen bed to themselves and get a good night's sleep."

In bed, Maarten put his arms around Betje and snuggled her close.

"While you were gone," Betje said, "much happened. My mother died ... four years ago next week. Then Heer Hasbrouk. There hasn't been much to eat ... as you can see."

"I'm sorry," Maarten said and stroked her head. "I know it's been difficult. I'm sorry."

Betje's head nodded in appreciation, and she sank into his embrace, taking comfort in the beating of his heart. She reached up to tenderly touch his cheek and pressed her lips to his.

The next kiss was full of passion, and Maarten's hand slid down her body. "I missed you terribly."

"Me too." She had almost forgotten the feeling of being loved and making love. He rolled on top of her.

The next morning, the two slept until well after the sun had risen. Maarten was the first to awake and get out of bed. While he splashed water from a basin onto his face and upper body, Betje rolled over.

Maarten beamed at her. "Morning." After giving his chest a final wipe with his shirt, he sat down next to her. "How're you feeling?"

"Terrific."

While she lounged in bed, he put on his clothes and went into the front room where he found Margaretha at Papa's desk, listening to the children take turns reading Latin. He tousled the boys' hair and touched Catrijn's head.

"What's to eat?" he said, "I'm starved."

"A few root vegetables," Betje called from her bed, "and they have to last all day."

"Where did I leave the money?" Maarten glanced around the room.

"Here!" Nicolaas pointed to the pile of coins and beggar purse on Heer Hasbrouk's desk, which he, Dirck and Catrijn had hardly taken their eyes off all morning.

"Aunt Margaretha," Maarten said, "can you take the kids and buy us a feast?"

The children scrambled to their feet and raced to put on their coats. After they left, Betje dressed and joined Maarten at the table.

"So, Betje," Maarten said, "who lives in our house?"

"Uh ... er ... Rijp, Rijp Dekker." Betje said the name cautiously, cognizant that the two never got along, even when they were kids.

"*Bastard!* How did *he* get it?"

"I don't know. I guess the Inquisition or whoever took our house rented it or sold it. They never told me, and I was too afraid to ask."

Maarten's eyes conveyed that he understood and was saddened by what Betje had to endure. Nonetheless, he still wanted to know more about the house. "If Rijp lives there—who was the man I saw coming out? He wasn't Rijp."

"Probably his wife's *visitor.* People say she's a slut—sells her body to anyone. If you ask me, I'd say he got what he deserves."

Disdainful of gossip, Maarten made no response, though he was fuming inside, not only about the loss of the house, but about Rijp, who he knew had a perverse, nasty streak. I wouldn't put it past him to get hold of my house on purpose. He'd love the irony of me the good Calvinist losing my home, and him the clever crook winning out.

There was great fanfare when Margaretha returned with fresh bread, cheese, pickled herrings, salt, and a live chicken, and reported that the line to buy bread had been very, very long.

The children jostled to be the one to help Betje unwrap each parcel, until Margaretha dispatched Dirck to the kitchen with the chicken to tether its leg to the table and warned Catrijn, "Act like a young lady."

While Betje and the youngsters prepared the meal, Maarten went into the front room with Margaretha for a private conversation. He wanted to learn about Papa's situation over the last five years as well as the circumstances of his arrest and execution. As Margaretha stoically recounted the events, Maarten sensed still raw emotions and a smidgen of vulnerability in her, neither of which he had ever seen before. For the first time, he was seeing Margaretha as a real person, not just a figure of authority.

When Margaretha finished the last painful detail, the two sat in silence.

"Aunt Margaretha," Maarten said, "I never asked you. What happened to your leg? You always used a cane. I never asked why."

"*That*, Maarten, is because youth are too self-absorbed to think of others." A faint smile crossed her lips. "I'm pleased you asked because it's a sign you've matured." She went on to explain her disability in matter-of-fact terms. "I was born with two good legs, but, when I was twelve, I jumped from my father's boat to tie off the line and slipped. The boat kept moving and crushed my leg against the dock. It's all still there, but quite misshapen."

Maarten nodded knowingly and patted his own leg. "I was cut from here to here." He drew a finger down his thigh. "A don's sword."

"Hmm, I noticed the limp," Margaretha said, "and the missing piece from your ear too." She laughed. "Looks as though someone took a bite out of it."

On hearing that, Nicolaas scampered in and touched his father's ear. "Did a Spaniard bite you?"

"That's *exactly* what happened."

The comment drew Catrijn and Dirck in, followed by Betje.

Maarten related the battle, his body moving instinctively with the action, and finished with, "I had the Spaniard by the throat; wouldn't let him break my hold. He was desperate. Grabbed my hair—yanked my head down. I felt a tug on my ear. Didn't know what happened 'til I felt blood dripping and saw a chunk of my ear in his mouth."

"Eew," Catrijn said, "that's disgusting."

"Did you kill him?" Nicolaas wanted to know.

"Had to. It was him, or me."

For Dirck, the story was more exciting than he could have ever imagined, and his father went up another notch in his esteem and now occupied a rarified realm.

Nicolaas started asking more questions.

"Let's eat first," Maarten said, "talk later."

Betje served the meal, and while Maarten devoured his food, Nicolaas started in with questions. "What do you wear in battle?"

"Regular clothes ... sometimes a metal helmet and chain mail I captured from a don."

"How did you capture Brill?"

Maarten wiped his mouth with the back of his hand and launched into an account of how easily the town had been taken.

"Do you still have the *Dirck*?" was Dirck's next question.

"Nee, lost her taking a Spanish ship in the Zuider Zee.

"Will you get a new one?" asked Betje. "A new *Dirck*?"

"A new one's being built in Hoorn right now. I'm thinking of naming her *Nicolaas.* The first one was for my first son—this one's for the second. What do you think?"

"I like it!" Nicolaas was ecstatic. "*I love it!*"

"I do too," Betje said. "Saint Nicolaas is the patron saint of Amsterdam and sailors, so he will keep both you and Pieter safe." Though Calvinists eschewed saints as popish idolatrous inventions, Betje did not. To her, they had a rightful place in her mélange of Calvinist and superstitious beliefs.

The next day Maarten found an appropriate time to speak privately with Catrijn about their father. By now, he had discerned she was blessed with a rational mind and a fair bit of maturity for her age, which would make the conversation easier.

"Catrijn," Maarten began, "you suffered a great loss—so did I. I was lucky your Papa adopted me ... treated me as his own flesh and blood. Did you know that my own parents died before I was nine?"

Catrijn shook her head no and felt empathy with her stepbrother, for there was genuine shared sadness in his voice.

"I know you're my step-sister, of course, er, by adoption," Maarten continued clumsily. "I want you to know I'm grateful for our Papa ... what he did for me, and my family. And I, uh, feel more like a father to you. I *am* your godfather." He touched her hand. "I want to assure you I'll try, I mean, I *will* act in your father's place. I will look after you, as if you were my *own* flesh and blood."

Catrijn smiled, for Maarten's compassionate eyes reminded her of Papa. Though she was aware that he and Papa were not related by blood, the similarities between the two told her she could trust Maarten.

Maarten patted her hand again. "I realize it's been difficult for you. I'm sorry." He leaned forward and kissed her on the forehead before getting up.

Relieved that the conversation was over, Maarten braced himself for the next difficult discussion he knew was coming. It occurred the following evening when Margaretha cornered him after supper.

"Maarten," Margaretha said in a stern voice, "were you involved in those Sea Beggar attacks on monasteries and murdering of priests and monks?"

"We did plunder monasteries and churches. I'm not proud of what I did, but we had no other way to support ourselves ... keep our ships afloat, feed our crews. If we could've made an honest living, believe me, we would've. Mostly we captured Spanish ships and sold them as prizes, and *always* gave a share to Prince William of Orange to support the rebellion."

"And the killing of priests and monks?"

"Nee." Maarten shook his head. "Never. Some Sea Beggars did ... some for revenge, others just cruel. I once tried to stop our commander from killing priests, but wasn't successful. I eventually transferred to another fleet, whose commander didn't do those things. Prince William of Orange is doing everything he can to stop such murders, but even *he* can only do so much." Saying the Prince's name made Maarten realize again how important the man was to the rebellion. "We're lucky to have Prince William. He spent his fortune on our cause, risks his life every day ... demands religious tolerance. He's a *great* man." Maarten looked down at his hands. "But men like me? We're just trying to survive ... and make mistakes."

Margaretha rested her hand on his and squeezed it approvingly.

At the end of his stay, Maarten said he did not know when he would return, because in spring he had to rejoin the Sea Beggar fleet in southern Holland. As soon as he had more money and was back in the north again, he would try to visit. There were tears, kisses and long embraces. He started to put on his beggar disguise again.

"Ahem." Dirck got his attention. "Father, do you think I could go ... I mean, go with you? I could help ... do all sorts of things."

"I'm sure you could," Maarten said with a look of sincere appreciation, while trying to ignore the scowl on his wife's face, which he took to mean: You better *not* take the boy with you! "But you're the man of the house now, Dirck. Your mother relies on you, as do I. You're needed here." He stuck out his hand to shake.

The following year in autumn 1574, Maarten returned to Amsterdam and encountered a crowd outside the gate, clamoring to get in. Gatekeeper Rutger recognized him and warned that a food riot was underway and everyone was being scrutinized to keep out troublemakers. And such scrutiny was only likely to intensify as cold weather set in. Maarten could not risk being identified, so he went back to Hoorn and asked first mate Rykaard to deliver his letter and money pouch to Betje.

Wearing his best clothes, Rykaard arrived in late-November and found the house Maarten had described. He removed his hat and knocked on the door.

Margaretha opened the door a fraction and suspiciously eyed the tall, rugged-looking man.

"Does Betje van der Voort live here?"

"Why do you want to know?"

"My name's Rykaard Beekman," he whispered, "I'm Maarten's first mate, and I have something for her." He presented the letter.

Margaretha recognized Maarten's handwriting and stepped aside. "Please come in."

Rykaard handed Betje the letter along with a sack of coins and explained, "Maarten tried to get into Amsterdam, but it was too dangerous with the riots going on. It's safer for me to come, because I'm from Hoorn and Amsterdam's Inquisitors don't know me. And my cousin is Rutger—"

"Rutger!" Nicolaas said. "We know him—he's the gatekeeper!"

"Ja he is," Rykaard said and chuckled inwardly at the boy's exuberance. "Maarten is in Hoorn overseeing repairs to the *Nicolaas,*" he said and went on to relate how the ship had been damaged last year in a battle near Antwerp, which the Sea Beggars had won. He also confirmed that Calvinists still controlled Antwerp, even though the Spanish army had plundered the city after mutinying for not being paid for three years.

Betje set down a bowl of soup in front of Rykaard and began reading the letter.

Between big appreciative gulps, Rykaard told how the Sea Beggars had also helped Prince William's army break the five-month siege of Leiden. Again, the decisive factor had been cutting dikes, which sent the Spanish troops running for their lives.

"Maarten says," Betje interjected, while holding up the letter, "he's able to trade in salted fish sometimes. He buys them in the north and sells them to starving people in the south."

"But it's risky," Rykaard noted.

"He says he hopes to come back north to patrol the Zuider Zee soon." Betje blinked back a tear and wiped her nose with her finger. "Says he's sick of war—wants to come home."

"Prince William wants us to keep helping Antwerp and free the south," Rykaard said, "but Maarten and me think Antwerp and the south will be lost, eventually, and don't want to spend any more time fighting there. I'm lucky, I can go home. Maarten can't, so he reckons the next best thing is to come to the Zuider Zee whenever he can get away from the Antwerp blockade for a while. The blockade is now our main job: keeping supplies flowing to the city and preventing Spanish ships from attacking."

"Your father has a job for you, Dirck," Betje said. "He wants you to go to Alkmaar next summer to help rebuild dikes. He says it's *very* important work."

Seeing Dirck's eyes light up, Rykaard could not resist patting his shoulder and saying, "Lots of other *men* are volunteering, so you'll be in good company. My son Rykaard Jr. will be there too."

In spring 1575, Rykaard arrived in Amsterdam to deliver more money to Betje and take Dirck to Alkmaar. He explained to Betje that he and Dirck were going to cross Lake Haarlem by boat and walk the rest of the way to Alkmaar, where his son will be waiting. After finding a work detail and lodging for all three of them, he will help rebuilt dikes until Maarten picks him up to sail south and rejoin the fleet. Dirck and Rykaard Jr. will return home at the start of the new school year.

Betje gave Rykaard explicit guidelines to ensure the boy's safety, and Margaretha instructed Dirck about good behavior. The only thing that would stick with and fascinate the thirteen-year-old, though, was the warning to avoid those who would drag him into sins of the flesh.

When Dirck was ready to leave, he teased his brother, "Goodbye, Saint Nicolaas."

Nicolaas hugged him and hung on, dreading the first separation of their lives.

"Take good care of yourself," Catrijn said. "Remember, you won't have me to help you."

Dirck rolled his eyes and walked out the door.

"*We'll miss you!*" Catrijn called from the doorway, as a sense of emptiness swept over her.

On a warm autumn afternoon, Dirck returned to Amsterdam nearly five months after leaving. Gatekeeper Rutger vouched for him at the gate, and he went straight home.

Margaretha was the first to see him come through the door. "Mary, Mother of God, look at you! You've grown!"

Betje embraced him tearfully, and Nicolaas flung himself at his brother and smothered him in a bear hug.

Catrijn hung back, viewing Dirck with fresh eyes. He seems so much older.

"Hi, Catrijn," Dirck said, while twisting Nicolaas's arms to extricate himself. She's even prettier, *and* her body has curves.

Their eyes met, not just as best friends, but something more.

"Hi, Dirck."

The newfound feelings of the thirteen- and fourteen-year-olds for each other did not go unnoticed by Betje, and she vowed to prevent them from evolving. In Betje's mind, her good reputation would be ruined if children in her care, who were often mistaken for brother and sister, acted on their emerging desires.

"Tell me *all* about it," Nicolaas said and dragged his brother to a chair and sat down next to him. "Did you see the *Nicolaas*? Any Spaniards? Was it—"

"Nee Spaniards, but I did see the *Nicolaas*—she's a beauty!" Dirck went on to relate a summer of toiling, punctuated only by eating, worshiping, and sleeping. The best part was making friends with Rykaard Jr., with whom he shared a bed in the home of a Calvinist minister and his wife, who were very poor and extremely strict. There were many more dikes to repair, and he was eager to return next summer.

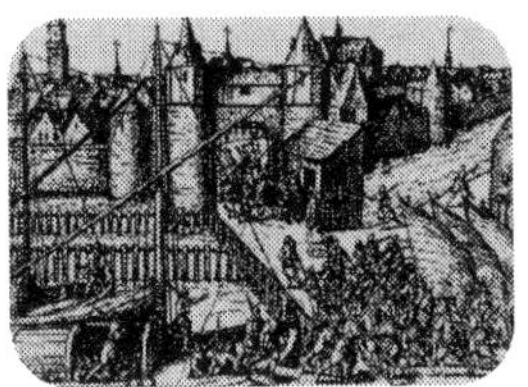

Sea Beggars at Amsterdam's Haarlemspoort Gate

CHAPTER 4

Amsterdam a New Jerusalem? – 1578

For two more summers Dirck went to Alkmaar to rebuild dikes, but by early 1578 a return seemed unlikely, because rampaging Calvinist extremists were making travel hazardous. They had swooped through southern Holland, taking one Catholic town after another, sacking churches, and banning the Catholic religion. Prince William of Orange tried to rein them in, but could do little to curb the violence. Now those zealots were showing up outside Catholic-controlled Amsterdam, Haarlem, and Utrecht, prompting their city fathers to send urgent messages to King Philip II asking for troops to protect them.

Maarten had heard of the extremists' exploits from reports and gossip trickling into Hoorn, where he and his men were overwintering again, and he was wondering how much of a threat they posed to Amsterdam's Catholic leadership. If there was a chance that Amsterdam might fall, he wanted to know, and, if possible, help bring it about. So he decided to go and see for himself.

Soon, Maarten was shivering outside Amsterdam's Haarlespoort gate, wearing his toothache disguise and doubting that he would get in. Civil Guardsmen were interrogating every male and rejecting most in an effort to keep Calvinist militants out. After observing for a while, however, he noticed that those leaving the city, mostly Catholics fleeing with belongings strapped to their backs and piled high on carts, were pretty much ignored. If he waited for a sizable group to exit, he might be able to weave his way through the horde and sneak into the city unnoticed amid the hubbub.

Soon such a crowd came forth, announcing itself with a cacophony of hooves pounding the pavement, creaking wheels, a baby crying, low grumbles, and exclamations: "That's my hen!" and "Stop pushing!"

Maarten leaned forward and fought his way through the human tide. A man elbowed him and growled, "Watch it!" He shouldered past another. A cart came rumbling by, forcing him against the wall and on tiptoes. Maarten received a jab to his side … a cough in the face … a foot stepped on … and he was inside the gate.

"*You there!*" a guardsman called.

Maarten kept walking with his head down.

"*Hey, you!*" The guardsman grabbed Maarten by the collar and swung him around.

His eyes downcast, Maarten moaned and put his hand to his cheek. A momentary glance upward brought his eyes in contact with Gatekeeper Rutger's.

"He has a toothache," Rutger said. "Why don't we let him pass. He's in pain … probably wants to get a tooth pulled."

Maarten nodded yes and exaggerated the pained expression on his face.

"We don't need no more beggars in Amsterdam," the guardsman said.

Maarten held out his apples.

"Are you trying to *bribe* me?"

"Nee," Rutger said, "I think he's just showing us he has apples to sell. He's not a beggar."

"All right." The guardsman nudged Maarten's shoulder. "You

can go—but leave as soon as you're done. And don't come back again! You hear me?"

Maarten's head went up and down, and his eyes met Rutger's and said thanks. Rutger blinked an acknowledgement.

Near Papa's house, Maarten observed Catrijn ushering out three youngsters. Catrijn noticed him and flashed a warm smile. After the kids were out of sight, she let him in, kissed his cheek affectionately, and sank into his fatherly embrace, before explaining:

"Those boys you saw are my students, Protestants whose parents don't want them going to a Catholic school. I've been tutoring for several years to earn money."

"Father!" Nicolaas scampered in, and Betje followed.

After the usual tearful reunion with them, everyone sat down at the table, and Betje brought out a pot of soup and bowls.

"When will you attack the city?" Catrijn asked.

"Everyone thinks you're going to take over," Nicolaas said.

Maarten raised a brow and shrugged. "There's no organized effort I'm aware of, just mobs of Calvinist extremists rampaging from city to city. I'm not involved with mobs and don't condone them. Neither do the Sea Beggars. So where does that leave us? We're not like Alva. We don't lay siege and we certainly don't want to bombard our hometown. I'm not sure what'll happen next. That's why I'm here, to reconnoiter and figure it out."

Nicolaas was disappointed, but Catrijn understood his dilemma.

Between gulps of soup, Maarten glanced around. "Where's Dirck?"

"He's staying with Margaretha at the Begijnhof," Betje said, "to protect her."

"Funny, isn't it?" Nicolaas commented. "Aunt Margaretha used to live here to protect us. Now we have to defend her."

"All the monasteries and convents have guards now," Betje said. "They're afraid the rebels will overrun the city before the king sends troops."

After he finished eating, Maarten donned his toothache disguise and went to Margaretha's.

She answered the door and teased, "Oh, no, not *that* disguise again." Maarten hugged her and shook Dirck's hand.

"When will you attack the city, Father?"

Maarten gave the same answer as earlier.

"When the rebels come back," Margaretha asked, "will churches be sacked and Catholics killed? Catholics are terrified of that. Father Hein—he's the one who helped your father, remember?—he barely sleeps. I spend many nights praying with him."

"I will do everything I can to prevent attacks on Catholics. Prince William has ordered everyone to show tolerance, and I'm certain most will."

"You remember, don't you, Maarten, when you left with the Sea Beggars in '68? The Catholics showed you respect and gave you a nice sendoff."

"Ja, they were glad to get rid of us," Maarten said, his voice full of resentment. "But things were different then. No one had any grudges. This time, we'll come back knowing how much was done against us ... unforgivable things."

"Maarten, it troubles me to hear you talk that way. You must find within yourself the capacity to forgive. Otherwise, you will be eaten up by hatred and thoughts of revenge."

"Don't worry, Aunt Margaretha. I'm not eaten up by anything. I just want to come home and live in peace."

The two sat in silence, and after a few minutes Maarten rose. "I have something to do. I'll see you later." He kissed his aunt on the cheek and returned to Papa's house, where he found Betje alone and eager for his embrace. They spent a loving afternoon together.

Dirck came home for supper and brought with him a request from Heer Nostrand for Maarten to meet him at Aunt Margaretha's house at noon tomorrow.

Maarten had little appetite for supper, knowing that tomorrow was going to be his day of reckoning. He owed Nostrand a considerable sum for his house and the *Dirck*, both of which he had lost. He's going to be an awfully unhappy man when he learns that I can't pay him, he lamented.

That evening, Maarten spent the final hours sitting at his old desk, tabulating the amount of principal plus interest owed and writing out a pledge to repay the money in two installments. The first was to be paid when he retrieved the remaining gold coins from his strongbox, and the second in the future after resuming trade. That was the best he could do, and he wasn't proud of it.

With great trepidation and his toothache rag tied around his head, Maarten trudged through the freshly fallen snow to meet his creditor. Margaretha was not at home, but had left a note saying she and Dirck had gone to the Holy Place Church. He sat down at the table near the hearth and placed the pledge on it. After rereading it and confirming there were no errors, he leaned back and waited. He repositioned the piece of paper to square its edges with the sides of the table. A knock came at the door.

"Uncle," Maarten said, using the term of endearment Nostrand always insisted on, though they were not related. "I'm so happy to see you." He was also pleased to see that the twinkle in the kindly gentleman's eyes was undiminished, even though his thin body bore the signs of hardship and his hair was now snow white.

"Maarten, I'm so relieved to see you're alive." Nostrand shook Maarten's hand, before leaning into him for a big hug. "We've all been worried sick about you."

"Come, Uncle, please sit by the hearth. Warm yourself."

While Nostrand settled into a chair, Maarten remained standing and said, "Uncle, I'm sorry I've been remiss in making payments to you. I'm mortified to come to you today—"

"What?" Nostrand looked up at him, not comprehending.

Maarten pushed the paper toward him. "I plan to make it right."

"Oh ... that. *That* can wait."

"But ..."

"Please sit down, Maarten. We have much more important things to discuss."

Maarten took the seat opposite him.

"I didn't come here to collect money," Nostrand said and patted Maarten's hand. "I came to talk about your future—*our* future." He pushed the paper away and smiled warmly. Maarten relaxed.

"It is inevitable that you and other exiles will be allowed to return to Amsterdam," Nostrand said. "The City Council has learned that King Philip is deploying his army to the Mediterranean to fight the sultan and cannot send troops to help keep you out. And more importantly, the council in essence already agreed to let Protestants come back when it ratified the agreement between Holland States-General and Prince William, which restores the prince as our governor and *requires* freedom of religion."

"Then why haven't they let us in?"

"Fear. Fear that extremists will flood into Amsterdam along with returning exiles and start attacking churches and monasteries and killing Catholics, and maybe try to unseat the City Council. I've been meeting with my Protestant and Catholic friends to determine how to allay the council's fears and have concluded that practical Protestant men need to be empowered to help control the fanatics. They, like Catholics, don't want to see extremists rampaging through their city. So we're trying to convince the City Council to appoint responsible Protestant exiles to the council, and we're preparing a list of names for them to consider. I want to put your name on the list."

"Me?" Maarten shook his head no. "I don't know anything about the City Council, and I just want to return home and go back to being a merchant." With a final shake of his head, he added, "I'm not qualified either."

"Maarten, you're the perfect candidate. You meet *all* the qualifications: honorable, notable, wise, and never been bankrupt. Being rich is normally required, but what Protestant is wealthy after having had his property and livelihood taken away by the Inquisition? Without question, you're honorable—everyone knows Heer Hasbrouk's good reputation. You're notable—a hero of the revolt. You're wise—Margaretha says you've matured and show wisdom. And your convictions are right for the position: you embrace Prince William's belief that religion is a matter of conscience and has nothing to do with government, and you're *not* a religious fanatic."

"Perhaps I do qualify, if that's all it takes," Maarten said. "But I don't know anything about running a city."

"You won't have to; you'll be just one of twenty-four city councilors. The council itself doesn't operate anything and merely meets once a year, on February 1, to select the people who do."

Once a year? That's not bad, Maarten told himself, warming to the idea.

"The four mayors are the ones who run the city. They're selected from the ranks of the council and are responsible for overseeing the government's operations and recommending candidates for treasurer, aldermen who make the laws, and the sheriff who upholds them and carries out the magistrate's orders to seize debtor's property. They also nominate people for jobs, such as the gatekeeper and the Palisade manager, who closes the floating beams at night."

"Would I be expected to hold one of those positions? They'd take a lot of time."

"Nee, we older men will fill them so younger men like you can carry on with business and generate tax revenues to support the city and the rebellion."

"Is your name going on the list?"

"Ja."

"Hmm. Well, I don't see how I can say nee. The sooner the list is submitted, the sooner I'll be coming home."

"Good. I knew I could count on you." Nostrand slapped his hands on his knees and stood. "I'll send you word in Hoorn to let you know when you can return." He put out his hand to shake and ended up giving Maarten a hug.

While Maarten waited in Hoorn, news spread of the negotiations underway in Amsterdam, and exiles who were sheltering in nearby towns came to Hoorn to learn more. Discussions ensued, and all vowed to do everything possible not to jeopardize this long-awaited opportunity. They readily agreed to bar zealots from returning with them and upon arrival to conduct themselves peaceably and with goodwill, but whether to bear arms generated discord. Sea Beggars insisted on carrying weapons in case of duplicity by the

Catholics. Others argued that most cities require men to surrender large knives and weapons upon entry, for the safety of their citizens, and carrying pikes and harquebuses would surely be seen as a sign of aggression. After a testy exchange, an accord was reached. Only concealed weapons would be allowed, and Maarten in his prerogative as captain could wear his sword, though it was discouraged.

When Nostrand's letter arrived, it instructed Maarten and fellow exiles to return to Amsterdam on March 16 and enter through Haarlemspoort gate.

On the appointed day, Sea Beggar ships docked near the gate, and captains ordered, "Tie her off!" "Lay down the plank!" Men came streaming down gangplanks.

The sheriff's men and civil guardsmen observed them from within the open city gate and the guardhouse.

The exiles assembled and formed an orderly column while keeping their boisterousness in check. Some carried Sea Beggar flags bearing ten coins, and a few displayed banners with hastily painted renditions of Amsterdam's coat of arms. The column advanced, paused at the gate, and met no resistance. "HURRAH!" Inside, a contingent of civil guardsmen awaited, and Maarten and the other Sea Beggar captains ordered their men to quiet down and stand at attention.

The captain of the guard stepped forward, made eye contact with each Sea Beggar captain, and scanned their men. Returning to Maarten, he glared at his sword. Maarten hoped he would not be asked to surrender it, something he would never do, and was relieved when the captain instead commanded:

"FOLLOW ME."

The exiles were led through Nieuwendijk Straat, and wary residents scurried out of their way. Women dropped brooms and disappeared into houses. Doors and shutters slammed shut.

At Dam Square, the captain halted and motioned for the exiles to join Heer Nostrand and his colleagues, who acknowledged the rebels with confident nods. In front of them was the two-story Town Hall, its warm yellow color casting a mellow glow. In the portico stood the sheriff and more guardsmen.

When nothing happened, the exiles began shifting nervously from foot to foot. Some shot quizzical looks at each other, and a few whispered to Heer Nostrand and his colleagues, "What are we waiting for?"

In the portico a man appeared, who was wearing a government medallion and official robe and holding up a scroll. He announced it was a proclamation of the Amsterdam City Council and read it aloud.

"First, Protestant Amsterdammers are free to return, and there will be no persecutions. Second, they are free to practice their religion, but will not have a dedicated church for worship. Third, they are urged to resume their businesses."

Cheers went up. Maarten flung his hat into the air, waved his arms wildly and howled like a dog, "*Ahr-ooooo!*" It was so unlike him, but he could not stop himself. After ten long years, he was finally home! Free at last to walk the streets of his city. Free to practice his religion. He bounded over to a tearful Pieter and threw his arms around him. All around, men embraced and many wept openly. Hats fluttered to the ground.

Maarten wanted nothing more than to race home and sweep Betje into his arms, plop her on the bed, and smother her in kisses—but reality set in. He was a Sea Beggar captain and Prince William loyalist. He had responsibilities. So he gathered his men, shook every hand, wished them well, and reminded: "There will be *no* icon bashing—*no* attacks on Catholics—and *no* looting. Prince William of Orange commands it."

After the men dispersed, Maarten pivoted and ran home, with Pieter close behind. He burst through the door, grabbed Betje and gave her a huge hug, rocking back and forth. She was delirious with joy. When she saw Pieter, she did not even notice his battle scars: cheek disfigured by the slash of a dagger, teeth missing, and lopped off finger. Maarten dropped to his knees and squeezed the kids. Tears of happiness flowed.

Now that Maarten was home for good, his first responsibility was to settle up his debt, and he made a visit to Uncle Nostrand.

"Ah, Maarten, please come in." He clasped Maarten's hands in his and said, "Congratulations on being home."

"Thank you, it's great to be back. And I owe it to you and your colleagues who convinced the City Council to let us in."

"I was pleased to help," Uncle said with a nod, "but I'm truly sorry the council chose not to give Protestants a role in government."

"Oh, *that*. I'm not concerned about that, Uncle, because those things have a way of working themselves out eventually." Maarten added with a wry upturn of the lips, "I came to talk about something more important, for you and me."

Nostrand winked, appreciating the reuse of his phrase.

"I'm here about my debt, Uncle." Maarten retrieved the sack of coins concealed within his doublet and handed it over along with his pledge. "I'm sorry I don't have enough to pay off the loan, but promise to give you the rest after I sail north to trade."

Heer Nostrand went to his desk, counted the coins, and marked the pledge PAID for that amount. He paused ... put the coins back into the sack and gave them to Maarten. "You'll need this money to buy goods to trade. Consider it an investment in your future. Your Papa would have done the same, God rest his soul. Anyway, I've lived so long without money that I can't think of anything to spend it on."

"Thank you, Uncle. I promise to pay back everything soon ... with interest. Promise."

"Good. Now sit down. We need to talk." Both pulled chairs up to his desk.

"I've given considerable thought to the City Council's action," Uncle said, "and concluded my colleagues and I naively overestimated the councilors. We thought they'd realize that sharing power with returning exiles was in the best interest of the city. It would help heal old wounds and give Protestants a stake in stemming the violence. Instead, they did what was expedient—allow former residents to return without threat of persecution, which was required anyway—and let the Civil Guard and the sheriff deal with the extremists."

"It makes sense, from *their* perspective," Maarten said. "The councilors retain power, and the rebels can come back as long as they act like nothing happened during the past ten years. We're supposed to restart our businesses, be good citizens, pay taxes, and hold our religious services in the fields again. Easy."

"Right, and I don't know what would persuade them to do otherwise," Uncle said, resigned. "Some of us had hoped the Civil Guard might be able to help, but they can't. They're just a militia of civic-minded volunteers, who have never been involved in politics. The City Council does in fact consult them once a year, as they do the guilds, but have no obligation to take their advice."

"So nothing can be done," Maarten said, neither disappointed nor resentful. For him, serving on the city council would have been an unwelcome distraction from the vital work of restarting his business.

After sharing a few beers with Uncle, Maarten headed home to Papa's house. The word *home* stuck in his mind, and he lamented: How I wish I could get my old home back. While walking along, nostalgia filled him as he envisioned himself working at his desk, sleeping in his bed, and eating food cooked at his hearth during happier times. The vision altered, and Rijp began replacing him at his desk, in his bed—anger exploded. I'm going to throw that louse and his whore wife out! With jaw set and fists clenched, he veered toward his home. Almost there, he stopped. What am I doing? I've just been let back into the city, and the first thing I'm going to do is assault a citizen? That's the stupidest thing I could possibly do. Shaking his head, he swung around and trudged back toward Papa's house.

Along the way, he passed Town Hall and decided a better option was to go inside and learn about Rijp's tenancy. With beret in hand, he requested to see the records of property transactions under the Inquisition. He was told none were available.

Grumbling to himself, he returned to Papa's house and decided to put his old home and Rijp out of his mind. He had more pressing things to do, in particular getting together with other returning exiles to organize a trading trip north. Captains usually sailed their ships in convoys to allow for their goods to be spread among numerous ones, thus avoiding a complete loss if one ship went down. Convoys also offered safety in numbers against enemy ships and pirates.

To plan their convoys, merchants typically met in a pub and usually included Catholics and Protestants alike, but Maarten decided to exclude Catholics for the time being and not to meet in a pub or other public place. Over the next several days, he and Pieter set about identifying returning exiles who might be ready to join a flotilla, and Papa's house ended up being the best place to meet. A date was set for the following week.

In the meantime on Sunday, over one hundred Calvinist families joyously gathered for their first service in the glaring light of day. It was in an open field west of the city, and there was no sunny glare, only darkening clouds that promised rain. With spirits high, the celebrants broke into hymns. Just when the minister was about to begin his sermon, the clouds let loose a deluge. Unfazed, he continued with his heartfelt message of David triumphing over Goliath and Calvinist exiles returning to a new Jerusalem. The flock prayed and sang fervently and loudly. Betje lifted her face to the rain, which for her symbolized a cleansing in preparation for a bright new future. Maarten tried to ignore getting drenched and sang enthusiastically. When the service ended, the congregants marched back into Amsterdam feeling renewed, and Maarten could not help but notice that while they were soaking wet, the Catholics were filing out of Nieuwe Kerk nice and dry.

On the day of the merchants meeting, one Lutheran and ten Calvinist sea captains showed up at Papa's house. Most owned ships in various states of repair, but a few had lost theirs and needed to buy or build a new one. The problems they faced in resuming trade consumed much of the conversation, from the lack of capital to the need to clear hulks from the Ij the Sea Beggars had sunk. That segued into a discussion of obstacles in general to rebuild their lives after ten years in exile.

"I tried to get back my old house," the Lutheran said, "but the Catholic who occupies it refuses." He added sarcastically, "He complained that he too suffered greatly over the years because he couldn't trade after the Sea Beggars blockaded the harbor ... poor man."

"Can you force him out?" Maarten asked.

"I don't know. He says I can't."

"There must be a way," another man said. "What about Town Hall? Can the sheriff or someone else help us?"

"They say they have no Inquisition records," Maarten told him.

"Of course, why would they keep records? Those rich councilors and monks got all the money," said a merchant whose homeless family was now living aboard his ship.

"Bastards!" another man chimed in.

"Did you see the new ship in the harbor?" the homeless man said. "Belongs to one of those mayors."

"Ja, another bastard."

Others added to the rancor. "Someone ought to pay for what they did to us." "Why isn't anyone being punished?"

"What about the Minor Friar monastery?" one man said. "That's where they took my father."

"My brother too," a Calvinist added, his face red with anger. "How come those monks are still there, fat and happy?"

"It's getting late, gentlemen," Maarten said to bring the discussion back around to business. "When should we sail north? When will you be ready?"

"In three weeks. What about you, Maarten?"

"Two weeks is good for me."

"We shouldn't have any trouble getting crew with more and more exiles returning," one man said, trying to introduce a little optimism.

"I can't go anywhere 'til I get a new ship," the Lutheran said. "Anyone know where I can borrow some money?"

Heads shook no.

"Should we try to include Catholics in the convoy?" Maarten asked.

"I'd rather burn in hell," the homeless man said, and was joined by others, saying, "Me too." and "Over my dead body."

Another round of griping started, which moved on to the joys and misery of their first Calvinist service in the rain, and questioning "Why can't we have our own church?" Maarten tried to avoid joining in, but, with each successive round, sank deeper into their morass of bitterness and confusion. In despair, he finally called the meeting to an end.

In anticipation of the voyage north, Maarten had the boys clean out the second floor and basement in case they were needed to store grain until it was sold. Though he was unlikely to need additional storage space, Maarten went for a walk around the city to scout available properties.

At the Dam, he breathed in the fresh air of freedom and savored the sight of lighters busily ferrying people and supplies to and from ships in the harbor. From there, he headed south onto Kalverstraat (Calf Street). To his right, the edge of the Saint Lucien Convent came into view, which was situated just north of the Begijnhof. At the Holy Place Church, he skirted a clutch of Catholics praying at the corner fireplace, which marked the exact spot where the 1345 miracle host had been tossed into the fire and would not burn. He was relieved that Aunt Margaretha was not among the worshipers, because this spot, which Catholics considered the holiest of holy places, was undoubtedly a prime target for Calvinist extremists.

After mounting the bridge over the Rokin canal, he rested his elbows on the railing, took in familiar sights of the nearby large Convent of Poor Clares and southern city gate, and then lazily watched the waters of the Amstel River pass under the bridge

Strolling on, he went by Gebed Zonder End Straat (Prayer Without End Street) and crossed two more bridges over canals before turning northward. To his right were Sisters of the Lilies Convent and Bethany Cloister, whose nuns he recalled sold their renowned oxen at the Kalverstraat market. On the other side of the canal was Saint Agnes Monastery. While gawking at all the walled edifices, he realized for the first time just how much land was occupied by Catholic institutions and their orchards, gardens and paddocks. More importantly, those compounds seemed more like places of business than where God dwelled. Annoyed, he moved on.

Finding himself near the stairs leading to the top of the city wall, Maarten decided to go up, something he had not done since childhood. The view was expansive. The churches and their steeples soared above everything else. Each house and tree was visible. He found Papa's house ... his ... and the Begijnhof. Everything seemed to be as it was before he left. The Damrak and Rokin canals were the dominant features: wide, busy with traffic, and bisecting the city from north to south. Other smaller canals formed an interesting pattern, one he had not discerned at street level. The two canals coursing through the older east side were symmetrical with the two on the newer west side. He studied them with interest, not knowing that each canal was a former moat, which had been incorporated into the city through successive expansions. He did, however, remember Papa telling him that the current moat, which he now realized mirrored the curve of the canals, had been dug a century earlier to allow more land to be added to Amsterdam and that the present wall had been built to enclose the newly enlarged city.

When Maarten descended from the city wall, he was confronted with the imposing Minor Friar Monastery, home of the odious Inquisition. There was an eerie stillness about the place. A knot formed in his stomach. He tried to walk away, but his legs felt leaden, as though some malevolent force were keeping him there. Faint noises filtered out. He strained to hear them ... muffled cries ... innocents under torture ... Papa's voice ... an ear-piercing scream. They grew louder. From beneath the massive front door came a trickle of blood. It headed straight toward him and turned into a torrent. He jumped back. The blood kept coming, and the voices seemed to be within it. Unable to bear any more, he slammed his eyes shut and covered his ears. When he opened them, the blood was gone. The sounds were no more. He shook his head. Got to get hold of yourself.

Clink. The latch moved, and the monastery door creaked open. A well-fed friar stepped out. He noticed Maarten and slipped back inside.

"Coward!" Maarten shouted, his fists clenching.

From there, he went on to Saint Nicolaas Church and saw a rowdy crowd forming in its square. He glimpsed a familiar face, a moderate Protestant he wouldn't have expected to get mixed up with extremists. Next to him was a Calvinist zealot Maarten knew from Hoorn, who espoused hateful theories about Catholic clergy not being human and needing to be eradicated. He was a dangerous man. Maarten strode into the crowd, intending to confront the zealot. He slowed ... maybe it would be more productive to talk to the moderate. He stopped. No, you can't risk getting involved. He exited the square.

Maarten returned home, and Betje thought he seemed agitated and offered consolation in the form of soup. Food was her remedy for everything. She also reminded him that they were all going to the Begijnhof to have their evening meal with Margaretha and Dirck.

Maarten was still out of sorts when he arrived at Margaretha's house, but she did not notice, for she was equally so. He placed the pot of soup on the table, Catrijn filled the bowls, and they ate in silence.

"Have you noticed all the ruffians coming into the city?" Margaretha asked.

Maarten nodded yes and thought to himself: Who couldn't notice them?

"Yesterday, a man grabbed Sister Geertruyd and snatched her cross and yelled obscenities. He thought she was a nun. Father Hein is too afraid to go out anymore. All night long we hear 'Death to papists!' This *can't* go on. Something has to be done."

"Hmm." Maarten kept on eating.

"Maarten, you're a Sea Beggar leader. You *must* do something."

"*Me*? Why do *I* have to do something? I have no power. What about the City Council? What about the Minor Friar monks? The Inquisitors? What're they doing? And why aren't *they* being held accountable for anything? Someone needs to be held accountable! Someone needs to be punished!"

Margaretha was aghast, not only at the tone of Maarten's voice but also the disturbing look on his face.

Maarten desperately wanted to scream! Cry! Pummel someone! Do anything to get the anger out! Seeing the shock on Margaretha's face, he instead buried his head in his hands.

Minutes passed while Maarten's fingers kneaded his hair, and Margaretha stared at the little red flowers painted on the wall. The family sat mutely, including Nicolaas, perhaps for the first time in his life.

"Maarten," Margaretha said, "I'm sorry ... I—"

"*Nee* ... I'm sorry. I shouldn't have spoken to you that way." Maarten rolled his head back, working out the kink that had formed in his neck. "It's just that we're—us exiles—are having a difficult time putting our lives back together. And all we hear is how rough it is for the Catholics. Honestly, it makes me sick."

Margaretha blinked away a tear. "You're right, Maarten. And I haven't been ... I'm sorry."

Maarten grunted an acknowledgment and returned to his soup.

More silence.

"Maarten, would you go with me to the chapel tonight? We pray and chant ... it calms us. I'd appreciate your joining me."

Maarten suspected what that was about. Margaretha was a mystic, and, as far as he could tell, so were the other Beguines. Mystics tried to commune with or become one with God through chanting or ecstatic singing. He never really understood it, nor did Papa, and evidently the Catholic Church didn't either, because Margaretha often complained that the church hierarchy didn't appreciate her brand of Catholicism. Maarten exhaled slowly, not wanting to go, yet feeling guilty for having been harsh with her. "All right, I'll go."

During the time needed to put the soup away and walk across the courtyard to the chapel, Margaretha instructed him.

"When you're listening to the chanting, Maarten, you must focus on the sound alone. Clear everything else from your mind.

And eventually you will no longer hear it and will be in a silent, tranquil place where all the cares of the world are irrelevant. To arrive there, you must find your own path. Some people hum; others make a soothing sound. Catrijn, who I brought after your father's death, used a rosary. She didn't say the prayers, just fingered the beads, and soon the fingering matched the rhythm of the chant, and I believe it brought her a degree of peace."

A final word of advice came when Maarten reached for the latch of the chapel door.

"Remember, Maarten, revenge is never satisfying. It's like spitting into the wind—you only foul yourself. If you must have it, then the best revenge is to be *unlike* the person who injured you. That's what Marcus Aurelius said."

While in the chapel, Maarten tried but never achieved the peace his aunt spoke of. However, all the sitting and relaxing did work out the stiffness in his neck. For that, he could honestly tell her he had found some relief.

After Maarten returned home, Aunt Margaretha's ideas began to sink in. It started the next morning when he went to Betje's linen cabinet and retrieved his beggar purse, which reminded him of the Sea Beggar motto: Help thyself and God will help you. He realized he needed to somehow use "help thyself" to achieve justice, if he was to overcome his overwhelming desire for vengeance. But he had no idea how to do that.

Maarten might not know how to solve the problem of his and other Protestants' bitterness and need for justice, but he could stop fantasizing about taking revenge on Rijp Dekker and instead do something about it. So he went to his old home, straightened his jerkin, spit on his hands and tamped down his hair, and knocked on the door.

"Maarten! Great to see you, you old bastard!" Rijp held out his hand to shake, ushered his guest inside, and slapped him on the back. "*This* calls for a drink! Sit down, Maarten. Sit."

While Rijp poured two drinks, Maarten surveyed the statues and paintings scattered around the room.

"To your return!" Rijp said and gulped down his drink.

Maarten took a sip and put down the glass.

"You noticed my collection," Rijp said with pride. "I trade in antiquities now ... see great opportunity in *the* trade." He struck a pose, which in his mind was gentlemanlike. "I'm what you'd call a 'gentleman of opportunity.' "

To Maarten, Rijp had always been an opportunist, but only as a small-time thief. He doubted that Rijp could carry off honest dealings with people who could afford such fineries.

Rijp read Maarten's skepticism and defended himself, "Nee, I'm legitimate. This business is above board and smart too. Refugees'll be coming from the south—lots of rich sons of bitches—and I'll help 'em get settled ... sell 'em stuff they're accustomed to."

"I'm sure moneyed gentlemen from the south will be charmed by your colorful language. But I didn't come here to talk about you. I came to get my house back. The Inquisition stole it—and I want it back."

"I bought it fair and square, *and* I can prove it."

"Regardless of what you prove, it was still stolen from me." Maarten's voice was stern, but he was worried. If a bill of sale did exist, the city magistrate would want him to honor it and for the two of them to work out a satisfactory settlement.

"Don't worry, Maarten," Rijp said, his tone softer. "I'm ready to move on anyway ... my wife's tired of this place." He looked Maarten in the eye. "I'll do you a favor. I'll sell it back to you. Just name your price."

This is *way* too easy, Maarten told himself. His eyes narrowing, he said, "Show me your bill of sale, and I'll think about it."

"I'll have it for you tomorrow."

"Good."

"Hey, I'm sorry about ole Hasbrouk," Rijp said as Maarten went out the door.

Maarten returned the next day and was given the bill of sale. With an impatient Rijp looking on, he sat down and scrutinized the discolored document. The sale price was disappointingly high, more than Maarten had originally paid for the house. Rijp's signature was legible, but a well-placed water stain obscured the seller's name. "How do I know this is authentic?"

"Maarten, Maarten," Rijp said, shaking his head, "you *never* trust me." He placed his hand over his heart. "May God strike me dead, if I haven't been fair with you." His attitude turned conciliatory. "I don't want to argue with you, Maarten. Just name your price, and the house is yours."

Maarten had no inkling of Rijp's motives in making that statement and really did not care. All he knew was that he could not afford to buy back the house for the price Rijp had paid for it, and Rijp would accept nothing less. "I can't afford to buy it. Thanks anyway." He rose.

"Don't go, Maarten. Just name a price. You're a hero of the revolt—you deserve a break. Just name your price."

With a sigh, Maarten reread the price and halved it.

"It's yours!" Rijp said, as though conducting an auction. "Cash?"

Again, Maarten thought to himself, this is too easy. Something's wrong. But he put the concern aside because he really wanted the house. "I can give you a deposit of one-third now and a promissory note for the rest. I should be able to pay off the note when I return from trading in the north."

"Good. You can pay me in ducats, or even grain—I can always sell it." Rijp put out his hand to seal the deal. "My wife and I can leave as soon as you want. Tomorrow? Next day?"

As they shook hands, Maarten asked himself: How does a man move out of a house in just one or two days, especially with all this stuff? He glanced around the room again. I'll be glad when I'm done with Rijp. He makes my head hurt.

Maarten decided not to share the news with his wife until after money had changed hands and a move-in date agreed upon. When Rijp vacated the house promptly after receiving the one-third deposit, Maarten informed Betje. She squealed with joy.

The Van der Voorts moved back into their old house with great excitement. Betje was the first one in and broke down in tears.

There in the front room was her old linen cabinet. Rijp had left it behind. There was nothing special or fancy about the cabinet, but it was hers.

"Did this cabinet always sit so oddly?" Maarten wondered aloud, while maneuvering Papa's desk past the linen cabinet with the help of Nicolaas and Dirck. The boys looked askance at it, as they followed their father outside to get Catrijn's linen cabinet. Catrijn carried in her clothes and other personal belongings, having left nothing behind in her own home. It had been put up for rent to provide needed income for both her and Maarten, who were co-owners under Papa's will.

Neighbors came out to renew old acquaintances, and a few arrived to help, including Catrijn's student Matthys and his older brother. Catrijn said "Hi" to her student and tried to ignore his obsequious sibling.

"Lucky us," Matthys's older brother commented to Catrijn. "Now I, er—Matthys won't have far to go for his lessons."

Through the open window, Betje heard the young man flirting with her goddaughter and anxiously listened for her response. When Catrijn cut the conversation short and exchanged smirks with Dirck as the two went back into the house, Betje fretted that the seventeen-year-old was never going to get married if she didn't stop being so picky about suitors. Dirck's attitude was not helping either.

With the family happily ensconced in their old home, Maarten turned his attention to the upcoming trading voyage to Gdansk, which was only days away. While he searched for goods that could be sold in the north, Pieter procured provisions, chiefly dried fish, cheese, and bread. Dirck and Nicolaas were put to work filling water barrels and helping the crew transport them and the provisions to the ship and stowing them away. Finding no goods to sell, Maarten ordered sand loaded into the hold as substitute ballast. The preparations done, everyone went home for a good night's sleep before setting sail in the morning.

That evening, Maarten noticed Betje was edgy. Assuming it had to do with the boys going to sea for the first time, he tried to assuage her fears by again recounting the convoy's route of travel.

"We're going to sail straight up the Zuider Zee, stay inside the North Sea barrier islands, and make our first stop in Emden." For his sons, he confirmed, "That's our old Sea Beggar refuge. We'll replenish water and food there, and I'll speak with Commander Dirkszoon to let him know that I won't be joining the fleet in the south this year. He won't mind, I'm sure, because fewer ships are needed to protect Antwerp now that King Philip has withdrawn most of his army to fight elsewhere."

"From Emden," he continued, "we'll go up the Jutland coast, down the Oresund strait, and make a stop in Sweden so some of the captains can purchase timber. Then it's on to the Baltic Sea and Gdansk to buy grain." He winked at Betje. "The route is so familiar, I could sail it blindfolded."

In the morning, the wind was blowing directly from the north, making it impossible for their ships to leave the harbor. So rather than go aboard, Maarten and the boys stayed home. The following day, he and the other captains spent the day quayside near the Schreierstoren tower, watching and waiting for a change in the wind. It did not come. The following day brought even stronger wind out of the north, and more of the same the next. A week went by, and Maarten ordered the perishables, the bread and some cheese, to be removed from the *Nicolaas*. Other captains did likewise.

The ensuing week and a half brought more adverse conditions, and with each passing day the captains' frustrations grew. A storm during their Sunday worship service in the soggy field west of the city further added to the misery. Maarten's euphoria about getting his house back faded away, and soon he was commiserating with others about the unfairness of not having a church of their own and questioning why Inquisitors were not being punished.

After returning from the quay one day and in a foul mood, Maarten found Uncle Nostrand sitting with Betje in the kitchen.

Uncle's smiling face and twinkling eyes lifted his spirits immediately, and Maarten could not resist giving him a hug after shaking his hand. He joined them at the table, and Betje poured a round of beers.

"Betje gave me a tour of the house," Uncle said, "and it's just as I remember, comfortable and homey. And her stew smells delicious, as usual."

"It's nice to be back in our home again," Maarten said and exchanged satisfied looks with his wife.

Uncle raised his beer. "Here's to better wind, and soon."

"Here, here!" Maarten clinked glasses with Nostrand and Betje and then leaned back and crossed his legs. "What brings you here today, Uncle. Anything special?"

"Well, ja, something significant did happen, and I came to discuss it with you. The captain of the Civil Guard paid me a visit last week and asked me to arrange a meeting with some of my Protestant friends. He said the guard was having trouble controlling Calvinist zealots and the City Council was offering no guidance and taking no action."

Lately, Maarten had given little thought to the council or the extremist problem, being so engrossed in getting the ship and convoy ready and all the frustrations since.

"At our meeting, the captain wanted to know what could be done to placate former exiles. If he knew, he would ask the City Council to make some concessions that hopefully would lower the level of Protestant anger. My colleagues and I agreed to talk with men like you and report back."

Maarten answered eagerly, "First, we want our own church."

"We all agree with you."

"And there needs to be justice. The Minor Friar monks—everyone who helped the Inquisition—need to be punished."

"Oow, *punished* is a harsh word, Maarten. Do you mean kill them?"

"Well ... nee. If we did, we'd be just like *them*, judging people and creating our own justice." Maarten shook his head. "Nee, I don't want that." He thought for a moment. "Yet, I wouldn't mind if they were roughed up a little ... and thrown out of town."

"The Catholics could possibly agree to that, I suppose, at least the ones who aren't fanatical. But you must remember, Maarten, how precious Amsterdam's religious buildings are to Catholics, including the monasteries."

"Well, either something is done about the Inquisitors and their supporters, or things will get worse. Eventually extremists, and maybe even moderates, will do something rash. Start killing nuns in the streets. Storming cloisters. We exiles can't—won't put up with those fat and happy Inquisition monks enjoying their easy lives. Not while we cope with the loss of loved ones and struggle to put our lives back together."

Heer Nostrand's head was moving up and down almost continuously, agreeing with everything, though the level of Maarten's resentment startled him.

On May 25, the wind finally cooperated and Maarten's eight-ship convoy rushed to depart. Fresh bread was carried aboard, goodbyes were said, and Maarten told Betje he'd be back before August, weather permitting.

As the captains and crews made ready to raise sails and pull up anchors, cheers went up. "*Hurray!*"

From a lighter approaching the ships, Pieter called out, "*Maarten, captains, don't go! There's going to be a protest at Town Hall tomorrow to demand a church of our own. Heer Nostrand wants all of you to come.*"

"*Pieter, we can't,*" Maarten said. "*We have to leave.*" As much as he wanted a church, he needed money even more.

"*Heer Nostrand said it's important! You have to come,*" Pieter pleaded.

One captain called to Maarten, "*I'm willing to stay, if it means getting our own church.*"

"*I am too,*" another added his voice. "*This could be our only chance. And with luck, we'll merely be delayed by a day or two.*"

Frowning, Maarten reluctantly agreed. "*We'll stay too.*"

The next day, the eight captains and their men converged on

Town Hall and joined other Protestants already gathered there. Heer Nostrand and his colleagues were standing in the portico, and civil guardsmen were positioned all around Dam Square. The crowd started out orderly. When it grew in size, men began chanting, "*We want a church!*"

Heer Nostrand stepped forward with raised arms and urged everyone to quiet down. They did, but low grumbles continued.

The captain of the Civil Guard came out of Town Hall, and he and his men escorted Nostrand and colleagues inside.

In the City Council chamber, stern-faced councilors waited.

Coaxed by the captain, Heer Nostrand stepped forward, removed his hat, and said:

"I am a Calvinist, and there is a crowd of peace-loving Protestants outside. I am here to respectfully request that you designate a church for our worship within the city walls."

The council's response, "Nee," came quickly.

Heer Nostrand returned to the captain, expecting to be led away, but instead was told to wait. The captain strode to the council table and in a resolute voice declared, "The Amsterdam City Council is dissolved." Councilors protested and refused to leave, but were forced to stand, shoved toward the door, and led down the stairs.

Maarten watched in disbelief as the councilors stumbled out of Town Hall and were marched toward a waiting barge in the Damrak canal. As they passed by, Protestants jeered, a few spit at them, and Maarten shouted, "*Good riddance!*"

From the steps of Town Hall, the captain of the Civil Guard asked for everyone's attention and held up a proclamation. He read it aloud:

"The Amsterdam City Council has been dissolved and a new one will be formed with 30 Protestants and 10 Catholics." After naming each new councilor, including Maarten and Heer Nostrand, he finished with, "Nieuwe Kerk will become a Protestant church."

Hats flew into the air. Cheers went up. A column of guardsmen marched off to Nieuwe Kerk, followed by a group of boisterous Protestants.

Maarten walked through the jubilant crowd, shaking hands and receiving congratulations for his council appointment, until it dawned on him that Protestant zealots might be emboldened to attack Catholic cloisters and mistake the Begijnhof for one of them. He took several of his men to check on it. Though they found nothing threatening, he nonetheless positioned guards at every entrance and warned the Beguines to stay inside their homes

When Maarten returned to Dam Square, he saw two roughed-up priests being loaded onto the same barge as the deposed city councilors. Added to them were half-naked and bloodied monks, who had come from the direction of the Minor Friar Monastery and were being pushed along by a rancorous mob. With perverse pleasure, Maarten stepped forward and flashed obscene gestures at all of them. There he remained and silently bore witness to justice being served, as the barge full of bigots and wanton murderers made its way down the Damrak. And slowly his pent-up anger, frustrations, and vengeful urges drained away. With renewed vigor, he walked briskly across the square to Town Hall and jogged up the stairs to the council chamber, where new councilmembers were gathering. He joined his contemporaries and from across the room observed Heer Nostrand, who was deep in conversation with his Catholic and Protestant counterparts.

Heer Nostrand's coterie was discussing the Civil Guard's action. All agreed that the guard had no choice but to act decisively in response to the council's dithering, and, if guardsmen had not done so, religious violence would undoubtedly have engulfed Amsterdam. Nevertheless, they feared that an ominous precedent had been set. Never before had Amsterdam's Civil Guard acted against its own government, and measures needed to be taken to ensure it never did again. Jointly, they devised two laws to be enacted: one to bar the city council from ever consulting the guard again on any matter, and another requiring guardsmen to surrender their weapons each night, to be kept under lock and key, until needed again for designated patrols.

The Civil Guard captain arrived and reported that the barge was on its way to drop off the councilors, priests, and monks at a dike east of the city. From there they could walk the twenty-six miles southward to Montfoort, where other Catholics were taking refuge. Though the Minor Friar Monastery had been plundered, no one had been killed. There were no other disturbances or attacks on Catholic facilities anywhere in the city. Upon completion of the captain's report, a magistrate swore in the new City Council.

The date, May 26, 1578, became known as the Alteration, the day Amsterdam inextricably shifted from a Catholic city to a more Protestant one. Calvinists believed it marked the beginning of their new Jerusalem, and Catholics hoped the change would bring peace.

The next day, the council met again. Mayors were chosen, several councilors volunteered to work with the sheriff to identify extremists, and instructions were given to the Civil Guard to establish specific patrol routes in support of the sheriff's work.

That night the wind became favorable, and Maarten and his convoy set sail on the early morning tide.

While Maarten and the boys were away, Aunt Margaretha's birthday rolled around. This year was her sixty-third, a crucial one in most people's opinion, because, if you were lucky enough to live to that ripe age, you were assured a long life. Betje invited her to the house to celebrate, promising that Catrijn had a surprise in store.

On arriving, Margaretha knocked and no one answered, so she let herself in.

"Hello ... is anyone home?"

Betje awoke with a start. "Oh, Margaretha—I ... I must of dozed off."

"Of course, we're home." Catrijn came in from the kitchen and kissed her aunt's cheek. "I'm so sorry no one was here to greet you, especially on your birthday."

Margaretha pshawed, as if to say, that doesn't matter.

"It *is* important, especially on *this* birthday, your sixty-third. I want to have you around for many more years."

Catrijn returned to the kitchen, and Margaretha observed

Betje listlessly walk to her linen cabinet. Betje tugged on the cabinet door, braced her hand against the edge, and gave a good yank.

"Having trouble?" Margaretha said and went to help.

"This darned cabinet," Betje complained, "I don't know what's wrong with it." Finally, with the two pulling, the door swung open. "Catrijn's cabinet door sticks too. I think it's due to the way we filled them ... maybe too much on one side."

Skeptical that linens could cause such a problem and wondering whether Betje was thinking straight, Margaretha asked, "Are you all right? You seem tired."

"I'm not sleeping well. Some nights I'm fine, but others ..."

"Maybe it's because you miss Maarten." The two sat down. "He should be home soon, shouldn't he?"

"Hopefully next month." Betje rested her head on her hand. "It's this old house ... it seems to have a mind of its own. Creaky one night, quiet the next. I guess it's just something to get used to again ... it's probably always been like this."

Catrijn joined them again, proudly displaying plump herring she had bought with her own money—

Creeeeaak ... CRACK.

"Dear Lord, help us!"

Upon returning to Amsterdam, Maarten was pleased that his first trading voyage to Gdansk had gone so well. Supplies of Polish wheat had been plentiful, his hold was full, and there had been no damaging storms, just the usual choppy seas. Dirck was elated, knowing he had found his calling at sea. Nicolaas was queasy.

While helping to take down the mainsail, Dirck again marveled at his father's deftness at directing the men and Rykaard's skill as first mate. Their knowledge of the sea was immense, from knowing that a change in the water's color might warn of a sandbar, to watching surface ripples for clues of changing winds. They maintained accurate charts and a rutter (a book containing navigational details), were decisive in crisis, and firm, yet fair, with the crew. And he was only just beginning to learn.

Nicolaas eagerly assumed his position to assist with the anchor, for the sooner it was set, the sooner he would be on dry land. There was nothing he liked about being at sea, not the mountainous swells, or the eerie creaking and cracking of timber, or shaking masts when gusts hit. And the seasickness! The only enjoyable times in the entire trip happened on land, where there were things to do and plenty to talk about, especially with seamen about pleasures of the flesh that Aunt Margaretha had warned against. Despite the allure of Gdansk's pleasures, Nicolaas made a vow to himself never to go to sea again.

As soon as the *Nicolaas* was securely anchored outside the Palisade, Maarten left Rykaard in charge and took the boys home, assuming Betje would be anxious to see them.

At their house, Dirck reached to open the front door. "It's locked."

Maarten rapped on the door. Again, more loudly.

Dirck noticed young Matthys, Catrijn's pupil, watching them and called to him. Matthys bounded over.

"No one seems to be home, Matthys," Dirck said. "Did you see them go out?"

"They moved."

"They *moved*?"

"It's the house." Matthys put one forearm on top of the other to form a platform. His eyes crossed, and slowly the platform tilted. "Creeeaaa—K!" After getting the reaction he wanted, Matthys said, "My father says it shifted. Bad foundations."

"Where did our family go?"

"All of them went to live in the Begijnhof. I go there for my lessons now."

Maarten and Dirck stepped back and inspected the house. Sure enough, there was a decided tilt to portside.

At the Begijnhof, Margaretha and Catrijn were relieved to see them.

Betje broke into tears. "God has punished me."

Maarten put his arms around her. "Why would—"

She pulled back. "Why? So you *do* think I'm being punished."

"*You* said—I just—" Perplexed, Maarten appealed to Margaretha, his expression saying: What's going on here?

"Everyone's nerves are frayed, Maarten," Margaretha said with her eyes directed at Betje, "with the loss of the house—*again*. The house is tilting. The foundations are the problem, I'm told. They're rotten, or sinking. I had Betje and Catrijn move in with me, in case it moved further—or collapsed."

Maarten had heard of such things happening because the city sat mostly on reclaimed land. "I'd better take a look and see what I can do." Betje handed him the house key, and he departed, saying, "I'll be back before dark."

By the time he and Dirck arrived at the house, Maarten was agitated. Why me? I still have *two* mortgages to pay off. He unlocked the door, and, when it wouldn't open, the two threw their bodies against it and forced the door ajar. The evidence inside—light streaming through a wide crack in the wall, a dislocated wooden beam, and debris littering the floor—confirmed the shift had been substantial. "This house isn't safe to live in."

Maarten found a warehouse to rent, borrowed a cart, and he and Dirck began moving their belongings. Meanwhile, Maarten grew angrier and angrier. Rijp knew about this. That's why he accepted a low price and moved out in such a hurry. I'm going to strangle the bastard!

That night an infuriated Maarten banged on Rijp's door.

Rijp opened it and took a step back. "Hello Ma—"

Maarten barged in and grabbed Rijp's lapel. "You knew it, you crook! You knew the house was sinking." He shoved the bill of sale in Rijp's face. "I want my deposit back!"

"Maarten, a deal's a deal. Cross my heart, I didn't know."

"You're a liar!" Maarten could barely contain himself, until a pungent scent wafted into his nostrils. It was familiar ... something rare and expensive ... ah, ja, I remember. A faint smile formed. "Is that cinnamon and lemon I smell?"

"Nee, I don't smell anything."

"I do," Maarten said with a sly grin, "and wouldn't the sheriff be interested to know." Maarten had learned during his brief time with Rijp's gang that cinnamon and lemon were good for cleansing jewelry, if you suspected it had been robbed from a grave. The combination supposedly removed bad odors and deadly grime.

"You wouldn't."

"Ja, I would." Maarten's head went up and down. "I would love to let the sheriff know what you're up to."

Rijp snatched the bill of sale from Maarten's hand and, at his desk, scrawled CANCELED across it. After retrieving a pouch of gold coins, he counted out Maarten's deposit without saying a word.

In the coming days, Maarten profitably sold his Polish wheat and hunted for a new house. He found a suitable one on busy Nieuwendijk Straat, which offered good exposure for his business. It was a bit of a stretch for his budget, but the success of the first trading voyage had left him feeling confident. The front room of the house had the customary high ceiling, tall windows, and a door that could be left open at the top to be welcoming to customers. Maarten thought the room would easily accommodate all their furniture—three desks, two linen cabinets, chairs and a table, and built-in bed—without looking crowded. Maarten told the owner he would buy the house, if his wife liked it too. Later that day, he brought the entire family to inspect it.

"The house is very nice," Betje said. "The kitchen is good, and so are those little cubicles upstairs; you don't see them very often in a house. They'll be perfect for the kids to sleep in."

Catrijn smiled. "It would be nice to have my very own room. And I'm pleased that this front room is so spacious; it'll easily accommodate all my new students."

"Uncle Pieter and I," Dirck said, "are impressed with all the storage space in the partial basement, on the second floor, and there's even more in the attic." Pieter nodded agreement.

"Good," Maarten said. "I'll tell the owner right away that we'll buy it. While we're here, I thought I'd mention that I've been thinking about setting up a schedule for this room, especially with our business growing and Catrijn getting new students. In the mornings, we four men will work here, while Betje and Catrijn go to the market. In the afternoons, Catrijn can have the room for tutoring, while Dirck and Nicolaas are at Latin School and Pieter and I go out to do business. Evenings will be the same as always; we'll all use it."

"Good plan," Betje said, and everyone concurred.

When they were leaving the house, Betje noticed a shadow cross her path and looked up. A large bird was circling above.

"L-look!" Betje said, her hand gesturing wildly. "It's a stork. *It's a stork!*"

Maarten's eyes lifted and followed the bird until it landed on the roof. "Yup, it's a stork."

"Don't you *see*? The stork is building a nest on *our* new house—it's an omen. It'll bring us good luck."

Oh boy, Maarten thought, more stupid superstitions, or as he liked to call them, *stupidstitions*. Somehow over the years, he'd forgotten how much Betje believed in them.

The stork's nest, however, became something of an attraction for Amsterdammers in the coming weeks. Some regarded it as a novelty, and others just wanted a little dose of good fortune to shine down on them. Storks were sacred birds, whose nests were protected by law and morality. All the attention shown to the house was fine with Maarten, because it meant more people saw his new sign: VAN DER VOORT & SONS.

On returning from his second voyage to Gdansk, Maarten was steering the *Nicolaas* into Amsterdam's harbor, when he heard rumbling sounds coming from within the city. After the sails were taken down and the anchor set, he hailed a lighter and asked its skipper:

"What's going on?"

"Calvinists. They're attacking the monasteries. Mobs everywhere."

Maarten's first thought was of Aunt Margaretha. "Dirck, come with me," he said and selected his strongest men to accompany them.

As the lighter made its way down Damrak canal, the din of mobs tramping through the streets filled the air. Maarten had the skipper drop them off at the lower part of Rokin canal, and, from there, he and the men jogged the few blocks to the Begijnhof. The courtyard was empty, except for a man loitering near the chapel. Maarten knocked on Margaretha's front door, while keeping an eye on the man. No answer.

"*Aunt Margaretha! It's me, Maarten!*" He knocked again.

A woman's voice came from the window of the adjacent house, "Sister Margaretha is at the Holy Place Church."

By now, the suspicious character near the chapel had disappeared; nevertheless, Maarten left four men to guard the Begijnhof and went with the rest to the Holy Place Church, where an irate crowd blocked the entrance. He pushed his way to the front door and turned to address them.

"*Go home! Let the City Council and Civil Guard deal with the Catholics.*"

"*Says who?*"

"*Says me—Maarten van der Voort—City Councilor!*"

"*Don't listen to him!*" a man shouted, and others started egging each other on. "*He's nobody!*" "*How do we know who you are?*"

Maarten had no proof he was a city official, so he pointed to the Sea Beggar pin he had recently bought and regularly wore for times such as this. "*I'm a Sea Beggar! I command you to go home!*"

"*They can't make us go!*" a woman said and encouraged the others. "*Don't listen to him!*"

"*Those lousy papists must pay!*" a man with only one arm shouted.

One man shook his fist in the air. "REVENGE! WE WANT REVENGE!"

"LISTEN TO ME!" Maarten said. "*Revenge never solved anything! Go home! If you want revenge, then the best revenge is NOT to act like the Catholics. Don't do to them what they did to us!*"

The crowd quieted, digesting what he had said.

"*That's stupid!*" an old man declared, and more joined in the hectoring. "*Ja!*" "*That's not revenge!*" "*What's he talking about?*"

Maarten gave up and took his men to the rear door, dispersed the small crowd there, and knocked loudly. "*Aunt Margaretha!*"

"What?" came her voice from within.

"*Open the door.*"

Margaretha stuck her head out.

"What are you doing here?" Maarten said in exasperation. "It's not safe. You should be in the Begijnhof—or at my house."

"Nicolaas is here to guard me."

Nicolaas, who had remained in Amsterdam rather than go to sea with his father again, came to the door and shook his head and shrugged as if to say, she doesn't listen to me.

"I have to stay with Father Hein," Margaretha said. "You remember him, don't you? He helped your Papa. He was here alone and scared. I had to come. I couldn't let the mob get its hands on him *or* the holy relics."

Not having time to argue with her, Maarten posted Dirck and his men outside and went to Town Hall. His arrival created a quorum, and a meeting was called to order.

The mayors reported that several monasteries had already been sacked and the Civil Guard was confronting mobs at others. Catholic councilors were outraged and demanded the marauders be brought to justice. Others argued that mobs were unruly by nature and difficult to control. All agreed the attacks would continue inasmuch as the buildings were easy targets. They held expensive items and were poorly defended with so many friars and monks having already fled the city.

The mayors interrupted and reminded the councilors that decisions needed to be made without delay because the Civil Guard and sheriff were awaiting orders on how to handle the mobs, and what to do with cloisters under siege and those that had fallen. The councilors debated various ideas, asked the mayors for recommendations, and debated again. A decision was finally reached and voted on, with Protestants outvoting the Catholic minority.

Maarten returned to the Holy Place Church with Sheriff Johann and a contingent of civil guardsmen, who immediately went to work disbursing the crowd. Maarten and the sheriff went inside.

To Father Hein and Margaretha, the sheriff said, "By order of the City Council, the Holy Place Church must be surrendered to the city government because it cannot be defended against the mobs. To preserve the sacristy's holy items, they will be transported under guard to the Begijnhof, and the Beguines will become their custodians." The sheriff seemed uncomfortable with the order and left promptly.

Father Hein's hands shook as he gathered the vestments and chalices, all the while mumbling to himself and looking dazed.

"I'm sorry, Aunt Margaretha," Maarten said. "The council voted, and it was the majority opinion." He was surprised when she accepted the news with such equanimity.

"It was inevitable," she said. "This is the holiest of holy places for us Catholics, and I know Protestants hate it—call the miracle a papal contrivance. In these times of small mercies, the heart must be thankful for scraps."

"Uh, the council also voted on a few other matters," Maarten said.

Both Margaretha and Father Hein ceased what they were doing and stared at him.

"Some monasteries have been plundered and others are likely to fall." He cleared his throat. "We decided ... the council voted to take over all of them and later convert the buildings to non-religious uses, maybe orphanages. Not the Begijnhof, of course, because it's private, not church property."

"W-what about the friars?" Father Hein asked. "What's going to happen to *them*?"

"They will be given pensions and allowed to remain in the city."

"But where? Where will we live? We can't survive outside the protection of cloisters. If we go into the streets—they'll attack us."

Before Maarten could answer, Margaretha said, "Father Hein, everything will be fine. Let me help you pack this." She faced Maarten and put her finger to her lips: Don't say anything more.

After the Holy Place Church contents were safely stored in the Beguine's chapel, Margaretha asked Maarten to stay with her while Father Hein napped.

"Father Hein *really* needs help. I fear he's losing his mind. Before he came here, he was persecuted in Alkmaar, barely escaping with his life. He's convinced he won't survive this time. If you can arrange passage to Montfoort, he will go because other Catholics are already there."

Maarten disliked the whiny priest, but knew he had no choice, so he thought about how best to do it. "Montfoort's twenty-six miles away—too far to walk for someone in Father Hein's condition. He'd do better riding in a wagon." He thought further. "If you know other priests or monks, even nuns, who want to leave, I can arrange for a wagon to take them to Montfoort. Dirck and a few of my men can go at least partway ... make sure no one bothers them. I think they all should wear regular clothes to not attract attention. Can you help find some? Clothes, I mean."

"Ja," Margaretha said and put her hand on his arm. "Maarten, you're a good man. I knew I could count on you."

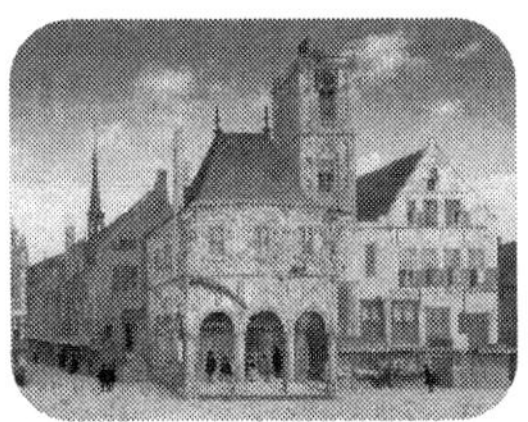

Amsterdam Town Hall

CHAPTER 5

The Immigrants – 1581-1583

Catrijn had just rounded the corner onto Nieuwendijk Straat when she saw a tall man standing next to a cart in front of the house across the street from hers. He appeared to be an ordinary Dutchman wearing a hat and dark cape, and her thoughts returned to the new students she had agreed to tutor. Being a warm day, she paused to push up her sleeves, and the man caught her attention.

He had just removed his cape and was artfully draping it over one shoulder, revealing a sumptuous brocade doublet, over which was a royal blue sleeveless jerkin with a deep-v-front and made of silk, rather than the customary leather. The royal blue knee-length, puffed-out pants had the usual slashes, but instead of merely revealing the shirt below had tufts of silken cloth poking out. At his neck was a large white ruffled collar.

Catrijn was awestruck. No man I've ever seen dresses with such flair! And that collar! So lavish.

Closer now, she glimpsed his face. He has such fine features ... must be from the south. At her front door, she was straining so hard to steal another look that she tripped on the front step and dropped her basket.

The man turned and took a step toward her. His fingers landed on the handle at the same time as hers. Their eyes met.

"Thank you, heer," Catrijn said. They lifted the basket together.

"Miss," he replied, with a respectful touch to the brim of his hat and faint smile.

Once inside, Catrijn hurried upstairs and positioned herself discreetly next to the window. He's so elegant and calm, and sophisticated. Yet there's a seriousness about him. Oh, there's another man coming out of the house ... handsome too, and much younger. His son?

While Catrijn watched, a second cart arrived, was unloaded, and driven away, and a third.

Why would he come with chests but almost no furniture? she wondered and conjured up an explanation: I'll bet he's a refugee and left a magnificent, well-furnished home behind.

The new neighbor, Konrad Teller, glanced at the house across the street before entering his new home. In the upper window he saw the young woman peeking out and thought: These provincial women are so bold.

Konrad and his nephew Jacques freshened up and went outside again, this time to reconnoiter their new city. Neither had been there previously, but had gleaned vital facts about it. With 30,000 residents, Amsterdam was by far the largest city in Holland province. It was much younger—less than 400 years old—than other European cities, and was best known for a miracle that supposedly had taken place in 1345. No king had ever held court here, serfdom never existed, and the number of people with titles was miniscule. For the past 250 years, Amsterdam governed itself through a city council drawn from the merchant class.

They also knew that in 1579 the United Provinces of Netherlands, commonly called the Dutch Republic, had been formed by seven northern provinces—Holland, Zeeland, Utrecht, Gelderland, Overijssel, and most of Friesland and Groningen—plus Antwerp and several other southern cities. The Republic at that time still acknowledged King Philip II as its ruler, but this year had officially renounced allegiance to the king, euphemistically referring to him as the prince: " ... the prince is made for the people, not the people for the prince ... the prince, who treats his subjects as slaves, is a tyrant, whom his subjects have a right to dethrone, when they have no other means of preserving their liberties ... ."

Konrad and Jacques had read the document creating the Dutch Republic and knew it gave the provinces and their cities control over their own internal affairs. To Prince William of Orange went the powers to tax and make war and peace, provided he had the approval of the States-General, which was the representative body of all the provinces. The document also provided for religious freedom: " ... each person shall remain free, especially in his religion, and no one shall be persecuted or investigated because of their religion ..." But *that* freedom was left to the discretion of the provinces and their cities. Amsterdam, in its discretion, had recently chosen to make Calvinism, known as the Reformed Church, its official religion and barred Catholics from serving on the City Council and worshiping in public.

Armed with their knowledge, Konrad and Jacques started their tour of Amsterdam. After reading the sign on the house across Nieuwendijk Straat—Van der Voort & Sons—they headed northward. The air was fresh from the previous night's rain, puddles of water were everywhere, and the street buzzed with activity. Kids were playing, housewives were sweeping their stoops, and businesses had their doors open for customers. The building with a sign depicting an oven was particularly busy, and Konrad took in the rich aroma of bread baking and realized another scent was in the air. It was the distinctive odor of peat burning in hearths, as opposed to the ever-present smoky scent of burning wood in other cities.

Ahead were two establishments, which Konrad made note of, in case needed in the future. One was a doctor's office with the customary urinal pot hanging above the door, and the other a surgeon's with the familiar white-red-blue striped pole. White indicated he pulled teeth and set broken bones, red that he let blood, and blue gave shaves.

Down the street a commotion started, and a squealing pig came charging at Konrad and Jacques, ran between them, skidded sideways, and slammed into a front stoop. Confused, the pig scurried into the open door of the house—squeals and a "*Shriek!*"—and dashed out again, with a woman smacking it with her broom. When the pig's owner ran up, she whacked him too out of frustration. The owner resumed his chase, and Konrad and Jacques, amused, continued toward the harbor. Though the harbor was busy, the scene held little interest, and the two walked eastward.

At the Anthonispoort city gate, the gallows was not in use, but there was an acrid smell of burning flesh in the air and a raucous crowd. The crowd parted, and a burly man emerged yanking a filthy boy by the arm. The boy was holding a hand over his branded cheek and cursing at everyone while being dragged to the gate. The burly man pushed him outside and warned him never to return. Though Konrad and Jacques had witnessed such mutilations before, imposed by magistrates for even modest crimes, they nonetheless found it disquieting that a juvenile was marked for life and would forever be barred from entering Amsterdam or any other city or town.

The crowd dispersed, and Konrad and Jacques noticed people standing atop the city wall and decided to go up. To reach the stairs, they had to pass by makeshift lean-tos and numerous homeless people huddled against recesses in the wall.

The view from the top was expansive and confirmed to Konrad and Jacques that Amsterdam indeed occupied a watery world. To the north lay the Ij, which looked more like a bay than a river. Beyond was the Zuider Zee, and even further was the North Sea, which at 50 miles away could not be seen. To the east, the land was flat, low-lying and wet looking, quite different from the drier farmland they had seen on the western side. From the southeast came the Amstel River. It journeyed northward through the city's moat and flowed through Amsterdam's five canals, all of which emptied into the Ij River.

The sun was casting long shadows when the men finished their touring. By now, it was clear to them that Amsterdam was a city without pretense or trappings of wealth. Buildings were mostly one-, two-, or three-stories and unembellished. Half were wooden, in contrast to other cities where wood had largely been replaced by brick to lessen the fire hazard. Hovels sat next to nice homes. Absent were the grand mansions and dazzling architecture of other European cities. The only prominent structures, other than churches, were former convents and monasteries.

Nonetheless, Konrad and Jacques liked what they saw. The buildings were cheery with doors and shutters painted shiny red, green, brown or white. The streetscape too had a certain charm with its mixture of straight-fronted wooden structures and gabled brick ones jauntily leaning forward to allow goods to be hoisted to upstairs windows without damaging the facade. Most importantly, the town exuded industriousness and friendliness. Everywhere, businesses bustled with activity and people sat on benches in front of houses chatting and doing chores.

Back on Nieuwendijk Straat, the men sought out an inviting tavern. After sitting down at a table next to the wall and ordering wine, the two leisurely took in the scene. On the opposite wall was a freshly painted image of a jovial sea captain holding a diminutive Spanish ship in his hand. In the back of the room, one table was occupied by two men huddled in conversation and another by a man sitting alone, humming to himself. At the closest table, eight men who appeared to be sea captains were having a serious discussion. Konrad and Jacques sipped their wine and eavesdropped.

"So it's decided," Maarten said, "we'll have ten ships on the next voyage. Mine'll have a cannon, and the others will carry the usual: bows, crossbows and harquebuses. We ought to be fine. No reports of Spaniards, or pirates. We'll do the same as last time. Buy grain, maybe timber and, if grains aren't plentiful, then fish." He looked at the other men, who were nodding in agreement.

The men rose, shook hands, and most left. Three stayed behind and ordered another round of drinks.

"Maarten," Hendrik said and leaned forward with shoulders hunched, "you know I'm pleased to be joining your convoy. Like old times, it doesn't matter whether we're Catholics, Calvinists, Lutherans ... or whatever."

"But we want to talk to you about the City Council's decisions concerning us Catholics," Willem said.

"Frankly, Maarten," Hendrik said, "we're disappointed that you, er, the City Council voted to take over *all* our churches, or let mobs do it. Couldn't you leave us just *one*?"

"And you banned us Catholics from city offices," Willem added. "*That's* not right either."

"What did *we* ever do to you, Maarten?"

"Me? Uh, nothing. I mean, you didn't do anything in particular to me." The question caught Maarten unawares. He paused to gather his thoughts, and they were angry ones. "Maybe nothing directly—but you didn't stop the Inquisition either. Not when they took my house. Kicked out my family. Killed my father." Maarten was starting to fume. How dare they complain? Calm down, calm down, he told himself and inhaled deeply and exhaled slowly.

Hendrik and Willem looked down, chagrined.

"I just want you to know," Maarten said in a calm voice, "I did *not* vote to take over your churches, or to ban you from the city council. Or to make Calvinism, uh, the Reformed Church, the official religion. Neither did many other city councilors, including Heer Nostrand. We didn't want to do to you Catholics what you did to us. But we were outvoted." He looked into Willem's eyes and then to Hendrik's. "You have to understand how outraged Calvinists are ... by the loss of property and loved ones, and *ten* long years in exile. And sometimes people who are angry overreact." He didn't want to complicate the matter by also noting the desire by many to make Amsterdam into a New Jerusalem, in which government, Calvinists and business leaders forge a moral society, similar to what was tried in Geneva.

"Ja, I understand that," Hendrik said with a frown, "but I don't like it any better."

"Me neither," Willem said.

Maarten shrugged. "At least you Catholics are a lot better off than we were. Some of those Catholic city councilors—those guys who the Civil Guard kicked out of town—they're already back in

Amsterdam. And their ships might just join our next convoy. And *they* helped the Inquisition. Is that right? So you see, none of—"

Crash. A carafe of wine shattered on the floor.

Maarten turned to look, as did Hendrik and Willem.

A flustered waitress was apologizing, "I'm sorry, heer, so sorry," while trying to mop up the wine she had spilled on her customer.

"*Non—s'il vous plaît—non.*" Konrad rose and used his hand to brush off the remaining wine. "It's nothing, please." He attempted to sit down again, but the seat was wet.

Maarten stood up and said, "Heer, come sit with us." He pulled out two chairs. "And the young man too." Maarten was eager to end the discussion of religion anyway, and these two well-dressed strangers offered a convenient diversion.

Konrad Teller introduced himself and his nephew, and the sea captains did the same. All shook hands.

"I heard your accent and you speaking French, Heer Teller," Maarten said. "You must be from the south."

"Antwerp. We just arrived today."

"From Antwerp, today?"

"Nee, from Italy. I left Antwerp when the Inquisition arrived."

Maarten nodded knowingly. "Well, as you may have heard, we Protestants can worship in peace here."

"So I've heard, and I also understand Prince William of Orange wants everyone to have the right to his own beliefs."

"Here! Here!" Hendrik strongly agreed.

"Heer Teller," Willem said, "you're a well-traveled man. Perhaps you can help us with a discussion we were having earlier. You may be aware that we, the Dutch Republic, severed our relationship with King Philip." Konrad Teller nodded yes. "Well, Prince William and our States-General seem to think we need a royal to replace him, and asked the king of France to send his brother and an army."

"The Republic doesn't need a royal," Hendrik added, "because we already have the Prince to lead our army."

"And the provinces make all the decisions for themselves anyway, and so do the cities."

"What we want to know is, do all provinces and places similar to our Dutch Republic have a king?"

"That's an interesting question," Konrad Teller said and thought for a moment. "There are examples of city-states without kings, such as Florence, Venice ... and Geneva. They're republics and have magistrates or ruling families ... or some could be considered to be an oligarchy, like Amsterdam."

This word, oligarchy, was unfamiliar to the Dutchmen, and each made a mental note to learn its meaning.

"And Savoy," Jacques noted, "it's led by a noble similar to Prince William of Orange, but not a king. Right?"

"I believe so ... hmm ... but Savoy is only one province. I'm not aware of any example of several sizable provinces voluntarily banding together without a king to represent them in the royal courts of Europe."

On Sunday, Maarten took the family to Nieuwe Kerk, and Betje guided them to stand next to Heer Nostrand, hoping to spark a romance between his eye-catching grandniece Kaatje and eighteen-year-old Dirck. Pieter was nearby, standing with his fiancé and her family.

After the service, Kaatje and Dirck went outside together. Betje beamed at them as she gravitated toward the group surrounding the minister, whose words of wisdom for the day she was eager to hear. Ministers, for her, were messengers to this world from the next. When the minister launched into a diatribe about young people coming to church to socialize rather than to hear the word of God, Betje looked for a way to make a gracious exit.

Catrijn's attention was riveted to the crowd. I wonder who the girl is that Nicolaas is trying so hard to entertain. She chuckled to herself. I'll have to remind him that it's not polite to stare at a girl's breasts, even if they *are* huge! Oh no, there's Kaatje with her perpetual grin of delight batting her eyes at Dirck. Someone ought to tell her to be more subtle. Ugh, he's taking it all in. Hmm, there's the new neighbor, and he's talking to Maarten.

Maarten finished his conversation with the neighbor and extracted Betje from the crowd around the minister, explaining that the family had guests coming to lunch and Betje must leave.

When out of earshot of the minister, Betje demanded, "Who's coming to lunch?"

"I invited our new neighbors, Konrad Teller and his nephew Jacques Poortvliet." Maarten saw Betje's face contort. "Don't worry. I said it will be a typical after-church family meal, nothing special."

At home, Catrijn changed her clothes twice and fretted about her pitiful wardrobe: two well-worn, drab outfits. The neighbor wears bright blue! All the while, a frantic Betje was calling her to come down and help clean the house.

Konrad Teller and Jacques arrived punctually.

Catrijn was captivated by Teller's stylish large white collar with intricate lace, but was relieved to see that his beautiful purple doublet bore signs of long use, like everyone else's clothes.

Introductions were made, with Konrad noting that his nephew was from his wife's side of the family, and Maarten mentioning that Betje was a native of Amsterdam, but he himself was not. He commented that both his sons worked in his business, that Dirck had just joined a night-watch militia group, and two family members were absent: Betje's brother Pieter and aunt-by-adoption Margaretha. Regarding Catrijn, he said, "I'd like to present my sister by adoption and goddaughter, Catrijn. Her mother came from Antwerp; perhaps you know her family, the Wynkoops."

Jacques shook his head no, and Konrad said, "Nee, I'm sorry we do not. Do you still have family there?"

"Nee, I'm told my mother was the last of her line. She left in the late '50s to marry my father and move to Amsterdam, and died just after I was born."

As Catrijn spoke, Konrad recognized in her appearance both Hollandish robustness and the refined features and brown hair of someone from the south.

Looking nervous, Betje brought out beer, and Maarten served it.

"I'm lucky," Maarten said, "Betje is an excellent cook, as you'll soon see," and was pleased to see his comment had put his wife at ease, for she was supremely confident in her culinary skills.

"I must hire a cook," Konrad said and turned to Betje. "Do you have any recommendations?"

Betje's eyes darted nervously, for she had never had a cook, or servant of any type. "I must think about it ... make inquiries."

Maarten poured his guests another beer. When they were comfortable and at ease he asked Konrad, "How long ago did you leave Antwerp?"

"Briefly in '66 when my wife died, and permanently in '74 with Jacques after most of our immediate families perished. You may recall, that year the Spanish army mutinied—they hadn't been paid in three years—and sacked Antwerp. I thought of visiting in autumn of '76, but the soldiers again returned, burned half the city and killed more than eight thousand." He paused. "Yet in spite of everything, I'm astonished that Protestants still control Antwerp."

Understanding looks went around, for everyone knew that Antwerp and other southern holdout cities were isolated within Catholic-dominated provinces that had recently made peace with King Philip II. Now, only Prince William of Orange's army and admiralties, funded by the Dutch Republic, stood between those Protestant cities and annihilation.

"Where've you been living since you left?"

"For a while in German towns along the Rhine when Prince William fled there. Later in Geneva, and briefly in southern France ... then Venice, until the plague struck. Finally in Naples, where my cousin Lodewyk had a business."

"Naples?" Betje said. "Isn't that a dangerous place for Calvinists?"

"We conceal our faith, of course, and avoid drawing attention to ourselves."

"After living in so many *fascinating* places," Catrijn said, "why did you choose to come to Amsterdam, Heer Teller?"

"Ja, why?" sixteen-year-old Nicolaas chimed in.

Konrad smiled inwardly—only young people think new places are automatically better than home. "I chose to settle here because I believe Amsterdam is ascendant. The great Hanseatic League cities—Lubeck, Bruges—passed their peaks more than a century ago. Rich trading centers like Venice and Genoa have had their run. Their dominance in the Eastern Mediterranean is over, now that the Ottomans control it. My own Antwerp? Sadly, it will never be the preeminent trading port it once was."

Konrad's eyes shifted to Maarten. "But Amsterdam, it has access to the sea, relative safety from Spain, and is hospitable to most religions and importantly to Calvinists. Wealthy Protestants ... perhaps some Jews and disaffected Catholics ... will flock to it, as the south sinks into an economic morass. That is why, in my humble opinion, Amsterdam is ascendant. It will be the next great city of Europe."

"You put that so well, Konrad," Maarten said with a bit of awe in his voice. Befriending this exceptional man with all his European connections is going to serve me well, he told himself.

Catrijn was speechless, mesmerized by the worldly concepts and words—ascendant, preeminent, morass—that so effortlessly rolled off Heer Teller's lips. His language was pregnant with ideas and images, like her father's had been.

"You must have had a fairly large fleet of ships in Antwerp, Heer Teller," Dirck commented.

"Nee. We owned *no* ships. We Antwerpers were manufacturers and traders with vast warehouses ... middlemen, so to speak. There were plenty of foreign ships to carry our goods to and from the city."

"Hmm." Dirck had never imagined being without a ship. In his world, trade and ships went hand in hand. He was going to learn much from this gentleman and his nephew.

"So," Maarten said, "what do you plan to do in Amsterdam?"

"I was in the business of dying and finishing cloth and intend to establish a factory here. One reason I chose Amsterdam was because it has no restrictions on starting a new enterprise, unlike other cities that require a newcomer to first become a citizen or join a chartered company. Amsterdam's openness is very appealing to new arrivals like us."

Betje came back into the room from the kitchen. "Enough talk of trade. A man needs nourishment. Please, gentlemen, come have a seat at our humble table."

After returning home, Konrad and Jacques shared their impressions of the day, something they had done since departing Antwerp together. Though Jacques was only twelve years old at the time, Konrad knew that the youngster would need to serve as his confidant, business partner and intellectual soulmate if they were to survive. So he cultivated Jacques's intellect, encouraged candor, and taught him everything he knew about people and business.

"I like Maarten," Konrad said. "He's a nice family man. Seems honest and thoughtful."

Jacques nodded, agreeing. "I like Dirck too. He's a forthright guy. I asked him whether the van in Van der Voort meant they were aristocrats, assuming it might be similar to the German von, French de, and Italian di. Dirck just laughed and said, 'Not likely,' and figured van," meaning from, "probably just indicated his ancestors had come from an area where there was a voort," ford in a river.

"Now *there's* an honest fellow. It's refreshing."

"Did you know his father was a Sea Beggar? That's what Dirck told me."

Konrad's brow arched. "Hmm, a Sea Beggar. They had quite a reputation and not all good. Perhaps there's more than meets the eye with Maarten van der Voort." He rose from his chair. "Nonetheless, I think a celebratory drink is in order."

While his uncle rummaged around for a bottle of sherry and glasses, Jacques continued to think about the Van der Voorts, and an image of Catrijn's pretty face and pleasing figure formed in his mind. She was joined by other girls he had seen in church; Kaatje stood out among them. More entered the lineup, all enticing, but the ones he favored most were the striking beauties with sun-kissed skin from Naples, the place where he had come of age.

Konrad handed Jacques a glass of sherry and raised his own. "To new friends!"

"New friends!"

Konrad sat down again. "Perhaps you'll have a friend in Dirck. Someone to show you around and introduce you to young people." Konrad sensed that Dirck, like Jacques, was mature beyond his eighteen or nineteen years due to experiences in life, but at heart both were still just young guys who wanted to meet girls and have fun.

"Perhaps," Jacques said, withholding judgment to avoid getting his hopes up. In the past, it always seemed that just when he was beginning to make friends, he and his uncle had to move to another city. This time, he hoped they were settled for good.

On market day, Catrijn left the house with a basket jauntily dangling from her arm and glanced across the street. I wonder how the neighbor is doing. Haven't seen much of him in the last few months, except in church and when those two desks and chairs were delivered.

The door opened and Konrad Teller stepped out. He touched his brim. "Miss Catrijn."

"Good morning, Heer Teller." They met in the middle of the street. "Are you enjoying your new home?"

He nodded affirmatively. "I hope you've been well."

"Very well, thank you."

"I couldn't help but notice girls and young ladies coming and going from your house. Are you a tutor or teacher?" He assumed the subject must be needlework and womanly arts.

"Ja. I teach Latin, some Greek, and classical works. French also."

"*Impressionnant, mademoiselle.*"

"*Merci, monsieur.*"

He glanced at her basket. "I'm going in the direction of the market. May I walk with you?"

"*Certainement.*" As they strolled away, Catrijn explained, "During the revolt, my students were all Protestants and mostly boys. Now they're all girls, both Catholic and Protestant, who want classical educations. If girls were admitted to Latin school, they'd be going there instead." She surprised herself by speaking so comfortably and freely to this older gentleman, who was little more than a stranger to her.

Konrad Teller marveled again at the incongruity of an intelligent and attractive young woman speaking in the coarse Amsterdam dialect. He had to admit, though, her mellifluous voice made the dialect sound quaint, even charming.

When the two disappeared around the corner engrossed in conversation, Betje stepped back from the window, perplexed. Is Catrijn interested in Heer Teller? I'd have thought she'd go for handsome Jacques. After all, she did say Jacques was debonair. Though Betje did not know the meaning of the word, she assumed it was a compliment. Shaking her head, she confirmed again, Catrijn is a mystery to me.

After saying goodbye to Heer Teller near the vegetable vendor, Catrijn's eyes followed him as he walked away. Hmm, everything about him is so interesting.

When finished shopping, Catrijn left the market humming to herself.

"Catrijn! ... *Hi, Catrijn!*" Heer Nostrand's grandniece Kaatje called out. "I saw you at the market, but you left before I could say hello."

"Hello."

"Remember your student Matthys? You'll never guess what his older brother did." Kaatje giggled and scrunched her nose. "He tied a flower to the knocker of our door." Her eyes widened with excitement.

"That's *so* romantic," Catrijn said dreamily, for she knew it was a request to begin courtship. "What're you going to do?"

"He's cute ... but I don't know." A circumspect look came over

Kaatje's face. "I kind of like Dirck. Do you think your brother likes me?"

"My *brother*? Dirck's *not* my brother—he's my nephew—but not *really* a blood relative. He's the son of my stepbrother, uh, by adoption—"

"But does he *like* me?"

"How would I know?"

"You know Dirck better than anyone."

"Well, I don't know." But if he asks my opinion, she thought to herself, I'll tell him he'd be crazy to get involved with a mindless flirt like you. Catrijn tried to suppress her irritation, but was losing the battle. "I'd better be going. It's getting late, and I need to stop by my aunt's house before I go home."

Inside the Begijnhof, Catrijn paused in front of the Beguine's sturdy chapel with the sad sign, NO ENTRY, tacked to the door. I don't understand why it had to be closed, she grumbled. Protestants aren't going to use it anyway, not here inside the Begijnhof.

At Aunt Margaretha's door, Catrijn thought she heard voices inside ... perhaps chanting. She knocked gently. The sound ceased.

Margaretha opened the door a crack. "Catrijn, it's you." She glanced around the courtyard.

"I've come to ask you to supper tonight," Catrijn said, while staring into the dimly lit room. She realized: The Beguines are holding a clandestine Catholic service! Just like we Calvinists used to do.

"Ja, I will come tonight ... but you must leave, Catrijn."

Catrijn's eyes told her aunt that she understood.

Upon arriving home, Catrijn heard Maarten's exasperated voice filter through the front door. At the mention of Nicolaas's name, she realized the harangue could go on for a while because Maarten was fed up with Nicolaas's poor grades and truancies at school. She sat down on the bench and began shelling peas.

"Nicolaas," Maarten was saying, "you *will* finish Latin school this year, and you *will* find productive work. God requires it of you, and all of us. I understand that you don't like going to sea. That's fine; it's not for everyone. And you don't seem to care for bookkeeping either, even though your Uncle Pieter tells me you're good at it."

"It's boring," Nicolaas said, his face contorting to indicate it made him gag. Actually, he did like the challenge of checking coins to find fake ones, but did not want to let on that there was anything positive about bookkeeping.

"Well, what *would* you rather do?"

"I don't know. I like people ... and they like me. Maybe you can find me a job along those lines."

"I can't pay you to like people."

Nicolaas thought for a moment. "Well, remember when I was in a tavern and a sailor told me a fleet from Hoorn was coming to Amsterdam with their holds full of timber?" Maarten blinked a yes. "That was useful information, wasn't it?" Maarten blinked yes again. "Our ship had just returned with grain and timber, and you sold the timber as fast as you could at the highest price—before the Hoorn fleet arrived. If I hadn't talked to the sailor, you wouldn't have made as much profit."

"Let me get this straight. I should pay you to hang around taverns, drink with sailors, and listen to gossip. Right?"

"Something like that. But there must be a better name for it."

"As I said, I want you to figure out how to use those talents God gave you, *and* also finish Latin school."

From his perch atop sacks of grain, Dirck was instructing the lighter captain where to dock along the busy Damrak quay, when he noticed Jacques walking nearby. "Jacques!" he called out.

Jacques waved and met the lighter where it came ashore. The two shook hands. "Successful voyage?" he asked, though the answer was obvious from Dirck's high spirits.

"Ja," Dirck said as he bent down to tie off the lighter's line. "So what are you up to?"

"Just observing and learning how business is done in

Amsterdam—duties, costs, and shipping—while Uncle Konrad searches for machines for our cloth business."

"Maybe you want to see our ship ... learn how we do things. I'm going back to her as soon as someone gets here to unload this lighter."

"I'd like to."

Pieter arrived and asked, "How was the voyage?" While Dirck gave him a report, Nicolaas bounded up, looking excited.

"Hey! Did you hear?" Nicolaas said. "King Philip took over Portugal and now he's king of both Spain *and* Portugal! Father just heard it at a special council meeting. Says it doubles his navy *and* empire."

The news was unsettling, but not surprising. King Philip II was known to have been scheming for Portugal's throne for the last three years, ever since its King Sebastian had died heirless.

"Father says," Nicolaas added, "the king's so big-headed now he might just send those extra troops Parma's been asking for." The Duke of Parma was King Philip's current military commander in the Netherlands, and he had requested 60,000 additional Spanish troops to help fight Prince William's forces in the south.

Nicolaas's comments drew a crowd, and Dirck and Pieter stepped away.

"I'll take care of these, Dirck," Pieter said, pointing to Dirck's lighter and the other one being tied off nearby. "Nicolaas," he called, "time to get to work!" Their job was to oversee unloading and transport of the goods to the Waag, the weigh house near Town Hall, to be weighed and taxed.

Dirck hailed a rowboat. When it arrived, he grabbed hold of the line and said, "Ready, Jacques?" Jacques gingerly stepped into the boat, trying not to use the dock to steady himself, but ended up spreading his arms anyway for balance. Landlubber, Dirck thought to himself and exchanged a knowing smirk with the oarsman.

"Jacques," Dirck said, "you haven't been on many boats before, huh?"

"Actually, almost never, except for an occasional river crossing."

"Almost never?"

"Europe isn't the watery world Amsterdam is. Elsewhere, travel is mostly overland, especially when river traffic is under Spanish control."

"Hmm." Dirck scolded himself, next time don't be quick to judge. You sound as though you know *nothing* about the world.

As the oarsman made his way through the Damrak, Dirck commented, "Catrijn's father, Heer Hasbrouk, told me that the Rokin and Damrak canals were the original harbors, until ships became too big to fit. Now seagoing ships anchor in the harbor."

Ahead was a high wooden bridge and after that the harbor, where numerous ships were tied up to the Palisade or bobbing at anchor.

"There she is," Dirck said and proudly pointed to their two-masted, single-deck ship.

"When I was a child in Antwerp," Jacques said, "I remember seeing ships with bright patterns painted on their sides similar to yours. My father told me they were from the northern provinces and brought wheat, fish and timber. He said they purchased goods we manufactured in Antwerp, as well as products delivered by ships from elsewhere: Lisbon, Genoa, and towns along the Maas and Rhine rivers. Mostly cloth, salt, fruit ... and wine and spices too."

"It seems that Antwerp was a pretty important link between north and south trade."

"That's how it was described to me, but I didn't experience it directly because the rebellion had already stifled trade when I lived there."

"I didn't either, not until my father came home."

Once aboard the *Nicolaas*, Dirck introduced Jacques to Rykaard, noting he had vast knowledge of the sea and was the captain, while he himself was Rykaard's first mate. He proceeded to show his guest around, which did not take long. There was a peek into the tiny cabin he and Rykaard shared, a quick descent into the cargo hold which was still being emptied, and a glance at the area above the cargo where the crew slept. Back on deck, Jacques took in the view.

"I never realized how much diversity there is in boats, Dirck.

Look at those ungainly ones with really stubby fronts and the variety of sails: triangles, squares ... and some so puffed out, they barely seem attached."

"That's right, and it's because ships and sails are related to the work they do. Those with unusually stubby fronts are *busses*, fishing vessels. The shape helps them avoid damaging each other while fishing in close quarters. All *busses* look pretty much alike, but have slightly different features according to the shipbuilder's design and construction methods and a captain's preferences. For example, some captains prefer masts that can be lowered, essentially folded back, to prevent the ship drifting toward another when their nets are out. Features created by builders are harder to detect because they tend to keep them secret to prevent copying.

"Sails also reflect their purpose. *Busses* have big powerful squares because they need to get from place to place quickly." Dirck scanned the harbor. "See the ship with two big triangular sails? Those are called lateens and are good for going upwind."

"I see." Jacques studied Dirck's ship for a moment. "What type of ship is yours?"

"Basically a boeier. Designed to maneuver pretty well in all wind directions. All our sails are down, so you can't see the variety we have." He searched the harbor. "That ship coming from the Zuider Zee is similar to ours. Both have loose-footed gaff mains—"

"Dirck, Dirck. I have *no* idea what those words mean. Can you say it in simple Dutch?"

"Ja, sorry. The main sail has a gaff, a diagonal piece of wood on the upper edge, which gives the sail form. Above it is a square topsail that gives extra power. In front of the mainmast are two triangular sails; they balance the mainsail and allow it to be bigger."

"That's all quite complicated, and must be the reason you have so many crew. I counted twenty-three. Never expected that many on a boat this size."

"You're right, but, actually, our full complement is closer to thirty, including Rykaard and me."

"Crew must be a major part of your costs."

"For sure."

"If you had a larger cargo hold," Jacques speculated, "you could carry more goods, and the cost of sailors wouldn't be so high ... relative to the larger amount of goods."

"Ja, but the ship would sink!" Dirck said with a laugh. "She's made of oak, which is heavy. So if you increase her size and add more cargo, she'd have trouble staying afloat and certainly would run aground in the Zuider Zee—it's shallow."

"Ah, there you have me," Jacques conceded. "That's why you're a captain—er, first mate—and I stumble around boats, uh, ships."

After the two returned to shore, Dirck invited Jacques to join him for a drink at a nearby tavern, where, in the presence of a curvaceous waitress, the two started vying for her attention. At first, she enjoyed toying with the frisky young men, but eventually lost interest. The contest over, the men relaxed and focused on their beers and plate of herring.

"Jacques," Dirck said, "I've been wondering how you and your uncle managed to survive while you were moving around. I mean, how did you make money? We had a tough time, but at least always had a roof over our heads."

"It *was* difficult. At first, we had Uncle Konrad's money from his business, and some that my father gave to me in '74 before he died. When it dwindled, Uncle Konrad worked as an agent, matching buyers and sellers of imported goods in cities where we lived. Of course, it took quite a while for him to learn the suppliers and prices of goods and the buyers and their preferences. He'd master it, and we'd do well for a while. Then a threat would arise, a plague or something else, and we'd have to move, and he'd have to start all over again. Uncle Konrad always manages to get by because he gets along well with people, understands their motives, and knows how to strike the best deal for all parties. And he's a sponge for information ... always comprehends which goods are in demand, which aren't, when there's going to be a glut, and whether prices will rise or fall. I learn from him, but I don't have his knack. Mine is numbers, so I became our record-keeper. Uncle Konrad isn't good with numbers—he's the one with the ideas. We make a good team."

"I know about agents. We use them in Gdansk to help us buy

wheat. Without them, we'd have to spend months there learning about the grain producers and the quality and amount of their supply. My father goes to Gdansk at the beginning of each season to establish a relationship with an agent and explain what we want."

"I believe," Jacques said, "you're always better off having someone from your own business serve as your exclusive agent. It's a luxury, but ensures someone is looking out *only* for your best interests."

"We can't afford it now, and no one in our family would be willing to spend the entire trading season in Gdansk. But having our own agent would be worth considering when we have more ships."

The waitress came back, and each tried to win her attention, but to no avail. The two returned to their beers.

"I noticed you and your friend Kaatje in church," Jacques said. His brows arched, indicating he thought she was quite something. "Is she your girlfriend?"

Dirck would normally have denied it, but instead said, "Sort of," to discourage the competition. He gulped down the last of his beer. "Ready to go?"

In the lead up to the 1582 trading season, the owners of Van der Voort & Sons assembled in the front room to discuss what they might do differently this year. It was a bitter cold February day, and Betje passed around steaming cups of broth to ward off chills.

"I've been thinking," Pieter said, "I can handle the record-keeping by myself… Nicolaas doesn't like it anyway. So maybe he should work with you, Maarten, learn the buying and selling side of the business. He likes people, seems suited to the work."

Nicolaas's lips turned up at the corners, for he had planted the thought.

"Good idea," Maarten said, thinking it was a way to reward his son for completing Latin School.

"I've been thinking also," Maarten said. "We've had three very profitable seasons." Betje knocked on the table for good luck. "So,

I think we should consider buying another ship." He turned to Dirck. "You've proven your capabilities at sea. This should be yours to command."

Dirck nodded and said in a calm, businesslike manner, "Good," but his eyes danced with delight.

"Rykaard Jr. can be your first mate. He has enough experience now. Rykaard and I will start training his next son—"

"And the next, and the next ..." Nicolaas said, his index finger rolling over and over, "the next, and—" He burst out laughing, because Rykaard had seven sons who were all destined to become seaman. And another child was on the way.

Nicolaas's laughter was so infectious that even Betje chuckled, though she was worried about Rykaard's wife. Eight children!

When everyone quieted down, Maarten returned to business. "Money," he said and turned to Pieter. "I've already talked to Uncle Nostrand, and he's agreed to reinvest part of the loan I paid off. If we combine that with our cash, I think we can afford to buy a used ship. Maybe even have a new one built. What do you think?"

"A used one," Pieter said, "but probably not a new one. Not now." While scratching his forehead with the tip of his quill pen, he examined the ledger. "But if profits are good from the first two voyages this year, we should be able to afford a new ship by mid-summer."

"Good," Maarten said, "Dirck and I'll start looking for a used ship. If we don't find one, we'll have a new one built, which will take until late summer to complete anyway."

A suitable used ship was not found, and Maarten dispatched Dirck and Pieter to Hoorn to order a new one from the builder of the *Nicolaas,* and to include Rykaard in the discussions.

Dirck explained to the shipbuilder that his father wanted the same type of ship as his two previous ones, a boeier. He and Rykaard had already discussed that the *Nicolaas* did not maneuver particularly well in high winds and asked whether something could be done to remedy the problem in the new ship. The shipbuilder proposed various design changes, Rykaard and Dirck weighed in on each, and they all agreed that the best solution was to add a third mast with a lateen triangular sail. Pieter negotiated the price, and the deal was sealed with hand shakes and a deposit.

Meanwhile in Amsterdam, Nicolaas started his new position as Maarten's assistant, and a few days later his work ended in frustration.

When Dirck came back from Hoorn and noticed Nicolaas's despondency, he put his arm around his brother. "Why so glum? I thought you were excited about the new job."

"I was," Nicolaas said, "but after following Father around looking for salt, wine, pepper, and cloth—things he used to sell in Gdansk, but aren't available—we ended up buying almost nothing. And he's not even concerned and just said it's because Spanish troops at our southern border continue to prevent goods from reaching us. Now he's getting ready to sail for Gdansk with almost nothing in the hold." He shook his head. "That might be fine for him, but where does that leave me? I've got nothing to do now and guess I'll have to start working with Uncle Pieter again ... boring."

"What did you expect? Don't you understand that buying grains in Gdansk is where we make our money—not selling goods to the Poles? And if commercial quantities of items Father normally sells to the Poles aren't available, what else can he do?"

"Try some other stuff. Maybe we could start making money, if we found something the Poles like."

"Well, instead of staying here, you could always go to Gdansk to find out what the Poles want *and* learn the grain trade. This time of year, Father interviews agents to represent us for the season, and you'd learn a lot. Of course, you'd have to go to sea again, which you said you will never do."

"Nee, I will *never* go to sea again."

"Too bad, because someday, when we have more ships, we'll need to have our *own* agent stationed in Gdansk, someone who looks out *only* for our interests. I thought you might become our agent, if you learned about the grains, suppliers, and prices. And if you were willing to go to sea twice a year: once at the beginning of the season, and again at the end."

Nicolaas feigned disinterest but mulled it over while nibbling on a piece of cheese. In Gdansk, I'd be on my own, do what I want, under no one's thumb. "I guess I could tolerate going to sea twice a year, if it would help our business."

"Good, I'll suggest it to Father. I'm sure he'll approve."

Maarten embraced the idea and complimented Dirck for his forward thinking.

While the ship was being readied for the voyage, Nicolaas scoured Amsterdam one last time, hoping to find something, anything, to sell in Gdansk.

Prior to sailing, Dirck instructed his brother. "Remember, seamen are tough, and superstitious, so don't get on their wrong side. And never, ever argue with one just to show how smart you are. I won't be there to help you." Dirck was staying behind to oversee the design and construction of his new ship. "And Father doesn't want to have to come to your rescue. He can't take sides, needs to be fair with everyone. Oh, and one last thing—remember to call everything on the ship by its correct name." He looked at Nicolaas's oversized ruffled collar and red beret. "And *never* wear those on the ship."

"Won't need to," Nicolaas said and removed his beret with a flourish. "They're for the girls—not guys."

"Just remember, don't do anything to embarrass Father, or our business."

"Mother already warned me."

Right before sailing, Nicolaas went into the hold and stashed away several kegs of Amsterdam beer, not to drink but to try to sell in Gdansk, and an assortment of household items and small statues, most of which he had taken on consignment from Rijp Dekker.

When Maarten gave the signal for the convoy to get underway, Nicolaas assumed his position at the foresail. A gust of wind tore the rope from his hands—"Damn rope!"—and a sailor had to help him.

"We don't got no ropes on this ship," the seaman said. "There's lines, *only* lines."

"Ja sure, lines."

On Sunday, the convoy was anchored outside of Emden, waiting out a storm in the North Sea. During a pause in the rain, Maarten led everyone in prayer and afterward the men lounged on deck. While the older men took time for contemplation, Nicolaas sat among sailors his age, talking about their favorite subject.

"God created many good things," Nicolaas said," but the very best was *girls*. Me, I like 'em with small waists and big bottoms." He made a lewd thrust of the hips.

"More to hold on to."

"Nee, big breasts!"

"Ja, the bigger the better."

"Nice ass, that's what I love."

"I had a girlfriend with a really nice bottom," Nicolaas said. "Hmm ... I can imagine her right now ... sinking her arse onto the floor and lifting her skirt." He grinned at the guys. "I can't really remember her face—but the bottom—*that* I can't forget!"

Laughs and more banter.

Rykaard and Maarten exchanged looks. Talk of sex and women was standard on ships, but this was Sunday. Intending to put a stop to it, Maarten drew his legs under him and was about to stand, when an older seaman rose and walked to where the young men were seated. He stood over them. They looked warily up at him.

Maarten rose to his feet.

The older guy bent down and said, "You know what I like?" and whispered it.

Nicolaas yelped. The group exploded in laughter. The grinning seaman returned to his spot on the deck, amid chuckles from his peers. Maarten relaxed.

The storm passed, and the fleet continued on. The North Sea supplied its usual quotient of rough seas, but calmed when the convoy reached the northern tip of Denmark and began making its way down the Oresund, the narrow passage separating Sweden and Denmark. There, in the harbor of Helsingor, the ships anchored and the captains went ashore to pay the toll. Maarten explained to Nicolaas the toll was calculated by multiplying the ship's waist (width at the middle of the deck) by the tax rate, and Nicolaas impressed him by doing the arithmetic in his head.

The fleet proceeded southward down the Oresund, skirted the coast of Sweden, and entered the Baltic. From there, it was a straight shot to Gdansk.

Dirck made a second trip to Hoorn to check on his new ship and on returning to Amsterdam found no one home. So he spent a few minutes tasting the soup simmering over the fire before changing clothes for his duties that night on the Night Watch with his militia group.

He had just poured himself a beer and sat down at his desk with paperwork, when the door swung open, sending in a gust of warm wind that scattered the loose pages. His mother and Catrijn walked in, with Konrad Teller right behind. Dirck regarded it as a little odd because Teller usually only visited when his father was home, but he was still in Gdansk with Nicolaas.

Konrad shook his hand, and he and Catrijn bent down to gather the papers, while Betje inquired about the new ship.

"It's nearing completion," Dirck confirmed. "Everything looks good."

"Have you chosen a name yet?" Catrijn asked, aware that Maarten had given Dirck the honor.

"I have a few ideas." Dirck leaned back, crossed his legs, and clasped his hands behind his head. "What do you think of Dirck at Work ... Betje Number One Mother. Or Catrijn the Brave." When Catrijn and Betje told him to stop teasing, he sat up straight. "I'm thinking of something dignified, to reflect that she'll be *my* ship. A new ship, new captain, and a bright future."

"Well, do you have a dignified name in mind?" Catrijn asked.

"How about Amsterdam Ascendant?"

"Ooh, I like that," Catrijn said. Her eyes shifted to Konrad, who had introduced the impressive term, ascendant, into their vocabularies.

Dirck wanted to say: Catrijn, why do you always give Konrad so much credit? Sure he's smart and worldly—but he doesn't know everything! Plus he's old!

Both Catrijn's deference to Konrad and Dirck's apparent annoyance pleased Betje. Things were going as planned. She had invited Konrad to go to the church organ recital today and to come to the house afterward, having sensed Konrad's growing attraction to Catrijn and her possible interest in him.

"I prefer a more personal name," Betje said. "Your father named his ships after his sons. I don't want you to name her after me"—just the thought of her name painted on a hull embarrassed down-to-earth Betje—"but I *do* like Catrijn. Not Catrijn the Brave. Just Catrijn. After all she's like a sister to you. You can save the 'Amsterdam' name for the future. This new ship, it's still a family ship."

"I'm partial to the name Catrijn as well, if I may say so," Konrad interjected. "Family is important."

"Then Catrijn it is."

After supper, Dirck reported for duty to his militia, the Night Watch, whose job was to patrol the dark streets to protect citizens from petty criminals and to keep an eye out for burglaries and fires. He was pleased to learn he had been promoted to sergeant and a new volunteer had been assigned to him. Like him, the new guy was the son of a city councilor with a growing business.

That same evening, Jacques had gone out after telling his uncle he was going to a public bath, which had not surprised Konrad because the two had gone to such places in other cities. A bath was a place for gentlemen to relax, perhaps have a massage, and enjoy stimulating conversation with like-minded men. In Amsterdam, Jacques had heard of a bath with a distinctly different flavor that reflected the Dutch tendency toward bawdiness.

The bath was located in an inn, and after Jacques paid the fee at the door, he undressed, wrapped a cloth around himself and entered the bathing room.

There in front of him was a titillating scene. Nude men and women in large wooden tubs of water were cavorting ... drinking ... eating. One couple was lustily engaged. Very few were washing their bodies in earnest. A shapely naked woman pranced by with a cloth slung over her shoulder and plunged into a recently vacated tub. She shot Jacques a come-hither look.

Jacques's eyes flashed agreement, and he sauntered to the tub, his eyes never leaving hers. Once there, he paused momentarily, worried that someone in the room might know who he was. Oh, who cares? He dropped his cloth.

Admiring his physique, she smiled salaciously, as he climbed into the tub and slid next to her. The waitress delivered two tankards of beer.

Jacques's bath outing turned out to be a lengthy one, first at the bath and later at his bathing companion's house. Sated and tired, he rose from her bed, pulled out a coin and left it bedside, hoping she would not be insulted. When she gave him a sexy kiss, he knew he had done the right thing. After lingering at the door for one last kiss, he stepped outside.

The sky was inky black. No moon. He let his eyes adjust, while groping inside his lantern for the candle ... it was gone. Candles were expensive, and he figured it had been stolen by one of those unsavory characters at the bath. Now he would need to be careful and stick to the most well-lit and active streets. Ahead was a house with faint light leaking through its shutters, and beyond a lively tavern. Then came the dangerous part, the dark narrow lane he would have to sprint through to get to busy Nieuwendijk Straat.

As Jacques passed the tavern, three inebriated, rough looking men came out, and one bumped into him. The man swore at him for getting in his way, but Jacques just kept walking and picked up his pace. When he was ready to turn into the narrow lane, footfalls followed, along with whispers and a gruff "*Hey you!*"

Jacques pushed off on one foot to break into a run—

A strong hand grabbed his shoulder and spun him around, bringing Jacques face to face with a pockmarked brute who snarled, "Gimme that," and snatched his hat. He shoved Jacques to the next man, who clumsily pulled at his cape, and Jacques kneed him in the groin. The man sank to the pavement in agony. Jacques swung his lantern around and bashed it into the head of the man wearing his hat. The third man tackled Jacques and wrestled him to the ground.

Dirck and his Night Watch trainee came around the corner and heard grunts and bodies colliding. Both lifted their lanterns. There on the ground ahead was a man moaning and holding his private parts. Next to him were two men fighting, and a third was standing over them rubbing his head with his hands.

"HALT!" Dirck yelled and ran toward them. "*Halt in the name of the Night Watch!*"

One of the men on the ground scrambled to his feet, and he and the man with an aching head tried to get the third assailant up. When the man fell again, the two fled but not before giving their victim a good kick.

"Stay with them," Dirck told his assistant and chased the two fleeing men while pulling out his whistle. *Tweeeet! Tweeeet!*

Dirck caught up with the slower culprit and grabbed his flapping jerkin. The man stopped abruptly and spun around with one hand flying up to backhand Dirck's face and the other thrusting a knife into his arm. Dirck staggered backward, using his metal lantern as a shield against jabs. When the knife blade stuck in the lantern, Dirck dropped it and slammed his fist into the man's face and followed through with a solid punch to the midsection. The man reeled. Dirck hit him again, and knocked him to the ground. After tying his wrists behind his back with a leather cord and confirming the other assailant was nowhere in sight, Dirck marched his captive back to where he had left the trainee.

There, he made the captive sit next to the trainee's prisoner whose arms and legs were already bound. The prisoner glanced up, and Dirck glimpsed the branding on his forehead. "Not you again!" he said, exasperated, "Won't you ever learn?" Hearing a moan, his eyes shifted to the victim. "Jacques?"

"Dirck," Jacques replied through a grimace and attempted to get up.

"Let me help you." Dirck gripped his friend's hand and elbow and lifted him to his feet.

His voice still shaky, Jacques said, "Thanks, you two saved my life," and then noticed blood oozing from Dirck's upper right arm. "You're bleeding."

Dirck lifted the arm—"Ow!" Until now, pumping adrenaline had concealed the pain. While the trainee wrapped a handkerchief around the gash, Dirck commented:

"You put up a surprisingly good fight, Jacques. *You* against *three*—impressive."

"I guess so," Jacques said while brushing off his cape and trying to regain his dignity. "That knave wanted my cape. There was *no* way I was going to let him take it."

"What are you doing out here this late?"

"Taking a bath."

"Oh ja?" Dirck said, surprised. Ordinarily, people took a bath in their homes once or twice a year, whether they needed one or not. "Where?"

Jacques looked at the trainee and back at Dirck. "I'll tell you all about it later."

When Maarten and Nicolaas returned from Gdansk, Nicolaas raced home ahead of his father, burst through the door, and announced:

"It was an enormous success! I sold everything and have orders for more beer and lots of stuff. I'm a natural salesman and good at the grain business." He grinned at Dirck. "And the crew liked me."

Congratulations went around.

Maarten arrived and confirmed, "We had a good voyage. No mishaps. Our hold is full, and Nicolaas was able to find particularly good quality wheat and rye." He patted his son on the back. "And Nicolaas sold his beer and trinkets—I thought they were a waste of time—but the Poles liked them. The beer could be something we ship in the future, if brewers can produce it in commercial quantities on a regular basis."

When time came for Maarten and his convoy to make their second voyage to Gdansk, Nicolaas surprised everyone by announcing he would go too, for he had already acquired more beer as well as additional products to test on the Poles.

In mid-summer, the convoy returned to Amsterdam, and Nicolaas happily reported he sold all his goods and had orders for more. Again, Maarten was able to sell the Polish grains for a good price, and Pieter's tabulation of the profits confirmed Van der Voort & Sons had sufficient funds to pay for the new ship.

Father and son went to Hoorn, gave the ship a final test run, and Dirck proudly sailed her into Amsterdam's harbor. Sea captains eagerly came aboard to have a look, and the family arrived in a lighter, and so did Uncle Nostrand, Konrad and Jacques. Catrijn was the first to ascend the ship's ladder, and Dirck climbed down to meet her. With a grin, he pointed out the name, Catrijn, emblazoned on the hull.

"Oh!" Catrijn clasped her hands to her breast, "I just love it. The script is so elegant ... the colors perfect," red letters outlined with yellow and black. She reached up and excitedly planted a big kiss on his cheek.

Aboard the *Catrijn*, the sea captains were scrutinizing the rigging and sail configuration and searching for any design innovations. Those who were not seafarers simply marveled at the newness of everything, from the shiny deck to the pristine sails and freshly painted geometric patterns on her side.

That evening during the family's celebratory meal, Catrijn declared:

"I want to go on the maiden voyage of the *Catrijn*. I won't get in the way. I can cook and—"

"Definitely not!" Betje said. "The sea is no place for a young lady, alone, with so many men."

"Dirck will protect me."

"He has work to do." Betje glared at Dirck, as if to say: Don't encourage her!

So the conversation died.

The 1582 sailing season ended well, with good profits and few problems. When the new year came, so did the annual February 1 meeting of the City Council, Maarten's fifth.

In preparation, Maarten again went over the issues family members had asked him to raise. Dirck wanted the sheriff to enforce the 1579 public safety law requiring tavern keepers to hang lamps above their doors after ten o'clock at night. Catrijn petitioned for girls to be admitted to Latin school. Uncharacteristically, Aunt Margaretha had requested nothing. Her previous appeals had been fulfilled with the opening of an orphanage in the former Convent of Saint Lucien, reportedly the first municipal orphanage in Europe. Next year, though, he expected her to make a plea to stop the severe punishments being meted out to wayward juveniles.

None of those concerns, however, was foremost in Maarten's mind. He was worried about the 60,000 seasoned Spanish troops who had marched into the southern provinces last year to supplement the Duke of Parma's army. After wresting many towns from Prince William's control, Parma reportedly was about to challenge the Dutch Republic's blockade of the coastal waterways and Scheldt River in order to stop supplies getting to Calvinist-controlled Antwerp. If Parma succeeded in crushing Antwerp, he might set his sights northward and threaten Amsterdam. All the while, war costs were mounting and the Dutch Republic was in danger of losing its vaunted leader, Prince William of Orange, who had just survived a fifth assassination attempt.

When the time came to leave for the meeting, Maarten put on his new black hat with a wide flat brim, the type that modern Dutchmen were wearing and Konrad Teller always wore. His old beret with a thin brim all round and flaps had finally been retired.

After one last look into the mirror to make sure his hat was level and clothes in order, Maarten opened the door.

Rijp Dekker was standing there with a heavy wooden box in his arms. "Hello, my old friend. I have a gift for you on this important day. Fifth anniversary—am I correct?" Seeing Maarten's eyes narrow mistrustfully, he added, "It's only a little gift, wine," and forced the box into Maarten's arms. "A simple gesture of my appreciation for what you're doing for our fine city." Before a befuddled Maarten could reply, Rijp turned away, saying, "Good luck at your meeting."

Maarten arrived at Town Hall still berating himself for having accepted Rijp's gift. The first item on the council's agenda was expansion of the city to provide direly needed additional housing and warehousing. It would be the first extension of the city's boundaries in nearly a century. The chairman stated the options: expand to the west into farmland, or to the east where the shipyard, river, and submerged land lay. Westward was unquestionably the easiest, so a budget for buying land was approved, and the mayors were instructed to initiate purchases.

The next order of business was war funding. The chairman presented Amsterdam's share of the approved budget for Prince William's army and admiralties and called for a discussion of ways to raise the funds. There were the usual complaints about the high cost of the war, and a few councilors proposed sending men rather than paying more taxes.

"I disagree," Maarten said, "I don't want to send my sons to fight, or yours either. And with our businesses growing, I see no reason to send needed workers off to war. So, for me, the only option is to pay more taxes to let Prince William hire the men he needs. I don't know which tax should be increased, but port duties are fine with me. I can afford them ... business is good." He looked at the other councilors. "We're all making decent profits."

After a few other options were discussed, a motion was passed to increase port duties. The remainder of the meeting was taken up by a myriad of special interest topics, including the ones Maarten raised on behalf of his family. Only Dirck's lantern request generated any interest, and it was approved.

When the 1583 trading season started, Maarten's expectations were running high. Dirck's *Catrijn* had performed well in the previous year, and profits would undoubtedly be excellent this year with two ships in operation and Nicolaas being able to fill part of their holds with beer for export to Gdansk. But on the first voyage, a ship in their convoy sank in a storm, taking some of Van der Voort & Sons' and other merchants' goods to the depths of the Baltic Sea. Summer brought the grounding of another on a Zuider Zee sandbar. Part of its cargo was salvaged, but again a loss was sustained. Adding to Maarten's woes was a bumper crop of Polish grains that flooded Amsterdam's market, depressing prices and profits.

By November, when leaves were flying and winter clouds gathering, Maarten was relieved that the trading season was at last over. Now, with less money in his pocket, he went to the Kalverstraat annual livestock market, where breeders sold their stock before fodder ran out and heads of households acquired them to provide meat for their families for the coming winter months. This year Maarten would be buying a smaller animal than usual, but that could not be helped.

Maarten's arrival at home with his cow marked the beginning of a three-day family festival. Butchering consumed the first day, and preserving the meat the next two. At Betje's direction, half was to be smoked, and half salted.

This year, Betje invited Konrad, who had just returned from England and was bringing the pig that Jacques had purchased. Pieter too was joining them with his small cow because Betje was his only family. He was still a bachelor, not by choice but from a sad string of events in which two fiancées had died. Everyone expected to work hard, including Margaretha, whose efforts would earn her a share of the meat.

The first night's meal of roast beef and omelets was at Konrad's house. Following supper, Konrad brought out more beer and a sack of white clay pipes and tobacco. After explaining that smoking was a new pastime for some Englishmen, he lit a pipe, illustrated its use, and gave it to Maarten.

Maarten tried it, "*Blhhh!*" and passed the pipe back. "Englishmen might like it, but no Dutchman will *ever* consider this a pastime."

"Jacques doesn't care for it either." Konrad offered a pipe to Pieter who refused and then to Dirck who accepted and gamely inhaled, let out a small cough, and continued smoking. Konrad passed a pipe to Nicolaas and was lighting one for himself—

"I'll try it," Margaretha said. She accepted the proffered pipe and without hesitation put it between her lips and, after a brief coughing fit, decided the sensation was not entirely bad. Settling into an almost meditative state, she puffed leisurely and watched as the smoke curled up in graceful tendrils. Soon her smoke joined with the men's to form a silvery haze above their heads.

Konrad sat back and allowed himself to be subsumed under Margaretha's aura of spiritual peace. After two and a half years of knowing her, he was still in awe of her incomparable curiosity, feistiness, and wisdom that only came with age.

Feeling a little sick, Margaretha put down the pipe and turned to Konrad. "How was your trip to England? Successful?"

"Ja. I went there to buy cloth and found exactly what I wanted." Konrad retrieved a bolt of white cloth and rolled it out partway. "This is a sample of what I will be importing from England. We will dye and finish it in the factory we're setting up on Koestraat. Jacques has already leased the building, and I just purchased the necessary machinery."

"You've said your business was a specialty of Antwerp," Margaretha said. "Why don't the English make a specialty of it? They have the cloth."

"It requires a degree of artistry and a particular type of machinery, which they don't have. I suspect they lack capital and trade networks too."

"Skilled labor also," Jacques added. "It's even in short supply in Amsterdam, but I was lucky to find two tradesmen from Antwerp, who had worked in a factory similar to ours."

"Now," Konrad declared, "our factory is ready to go."

Handshakes and congratulations were given, and Jacques poured another round of beer.

"What about England?" Catrijn said. "What do you think of it?"

"England is backward. One of the first things you notice is that the Gregorian calendar hasn't yet been adopted." He laughed. "They seem to think it's a Catholic ploy to take over the country."

Konrad's comment reconfirmed to Maarten there was nothing to like about England or its cowardly queen who had expelled the Sea Beggars. He just had to shake his head at their simple-minded fear of the new calendar of Pope Gregory XII that had nothing to do with Catholics and merely reset the calendar ten days forward to correct for inaccuracies of the old Julian calendar. The Dutch Republic had already adopted the new calendar, which turned January 1 into January 11, and within a few months everyone forgot about it.

"There is another thing that strikes you as soon as you disembark in England," Konrad continued, "Francis Drake's name is on everyone's lips."

"Never heard of him," Nicolaas said.

"He is a national hero and confidant of Queen Elizabeth, though basically just a pirate. Drake's exploits, nonetheless, are dazzling and almost beyond belief." Konrad reached for a map from his desk. "Here, let me show you." On the table, he stretched out the map, which had an ornate perimeter featuring cherubs, two winged female figures and Latin inscriptions.

"I've never seen a map of the entire world before," said map-enthusiast Dirck.

"Me neither," Pieter agreed.

"Look," Catrijn commented, "the map is heart ... shaped." As soon as the word, heart, came out, she regretted saying it. An intelligent person would focus on the map's content, *not* its shape! I hope Konrad doesn't think I'm simple minded.

"Francis Drake," Konrad was explaining, "left England in 1577 with five ships, crossed the Atlantic, and audaciously sailed into Spanish territory." His finger traced Drake's route southward down the coast of South America and around the southern tip. "Only one of his ships, the *Golden Hind*, made it through the Straits of Magellan. The rest sank. Drake sailed up the west coast, raiding Spanish trading posts and ships as he went. They were easy prey, because the king had no garrisons or naval ships to defend them ... never expecting a foreign ship to dare sail into the Pacific Ocean, *his* ocean."

Everyone took turns inspecting the map, and Catrijn read aloud some of the exotic names: "America ... Brasilia ... Cartigora."

"That's not even the most astonishing part," Konrad said and placed his finger on the western side of the Isthmus of Panama. "This is roughly where Drake encountered the enormous Spanish galleons coming from the Orient, laden with gold, silver and gems—and virtually unprotected. Somehow Drake's modest ship was able to attack *two* galleons and relieve them of their treasure. Drake then proceeded to explore the Pacific Ocean, claiming land for England as he went and stopping to make repairs to his *Golden Hind*. Finally, by way around the tip of Africa, he returned home four years after leaving."

"Do you know how Drake was able to capture *two* Spanish galleons?" Dirck asked.

"With a lot of luck," Maarten replied, speaking from experience.

"I defer to the sea captain," Konrad said, bowing his head. "Drake was also lucky to cross paths with the ships in the Pacific, where they're unprotected. Once they're unloaded here," he pointed again to the Isthmus of Panama, "the goods are heavily guarded as they travel overland and then by sea to Spain's fortified colony in the Atlantic. There, they're combined with gold and riches from Spain's American possessions and transported to Spain once a year in a fleet of fifty or more galleons. No one has ever successfully attacked one of those fleets."

"So," Catrijn said with renewed confidence, "Drake just happened to find Spain's Achilles Heel, in the Pacific."

"Now I understand the source of Spain's wealth," Pieter commented.

"Do you know the size of the *Golden Hind*?" Dirck asked.

"About a hundred tons in weight."

"That's the size of *our* ships," Dirck said, amazed and thinking: What a terrific adventure that would be!

Konrad had been particularly lonely while in England. So when invited to dine at the home of a congenial business colleague, he eagerly accepted. There, he met the man's very pretty and recently widowed sister, who charmed him with her knowledge of English literature and ethereal harp playing. Invited again, Konrad was so taken by the soft-spoken woman, her music, and the warmth of family life that he began to contemplate remarrying. After repeated encounters, however, the woman's reticent nature wore on him and his thoughts drifted to Catrijn. Almost from the start, Catrijn had fascinated him with her high ideals, insatiable curiosity about all things, independent streak, and penchant for reciting favorite passages from the classics, many also favored by him, such as Cicero's "A room without books is like a body without a soul." Nonetheless, he had suppressed his attraction to her due to their age difference, seventeen years, and the need to start a business. Now with his enterprise established and fortieth birthday approaching, he resolved to ask Catrijn to marry him.

The day Konrad chose was an unseasonably warm Sunday in late November, perfect for an unhurried stroll after church. It started with a stop along a canal to observe Catrijn's former students skipping stones and them coaxing their teacher to show her skills, which she did admirably. With all the laughter and Konrad showing them up, the time seemed ideal for him to find a quiet spot and segue into the subject of marriage. His plan was to use logic, note their common interests, and avoid getting emotional. Only a cool rational mind could accurately gauge her response and discern whether she loved him or merely liked him, and whether he was making a fool of himself.

"Is something wrong, Konrad?" Catrijn asked, sensing his preoccupation. "Something in your business?"

Konrad stopped, gazed into her eyes, and logic vanished. "I've been a sojourner for so long, lonely beyond belief sometimes, and I'm ... I'm ready to settle down, start a family. Your enthusiasm for life lifts my world-weary soul, and inquisitive mind gives me faith in the future. You stir my passions."

"Oh," Catrijn said softly. Though the proposal was not a complete surprise and she had occasionally fantasized about life with him, now the choice was real and the decision final. Stalling for time, she said, "I always felt I embarrassed myself in front of you. You often seemed distant," which was true anyway.

Konrad was getting a sinking feeling. I've made a fool of myself.

Catrijn was thinking. Is he really right for me? He's so cultured and sophisticated, handsome too ... but not terribly exciting. Is it love I feel? What is love anyway? What if I say no, what will—don't be ridiculous! He's the dream of any intelligent woman. Do you have a better prospect? Dirck fleetingly entered her mind, but her emotions were too jumbled and his intentions unclear and he was essentially her brother anyway, as godmother Betje often reminded her. You need to decide, Catrijn scolded herself. He's waiting. Maybe you should say yes. If you let him get away, you may never get married.

Konrad was searching for ways to salvage his dignity after making such an imprudent proposal.

Catrijn's eyes raised, connected with his, and her lips turned up at the corners.

"You put it so eloquently, Konrad. How can I say nee? I mean—I think that was a proposal. Was it?"

"Ja, of course, it was." He took her into his arms, momentarily looked around, people were watching—Oh, so what!—and kissed her.

Public displays of affection were completely out of character for Konrad, and Catrijn had to suppress a chortle before surrendering to his embrace and the passion of the kiss.

With Catrijn romantic and Konrad rhapsodic, the two sauntered toward home contemplating their momentous commitment.

Catrijn stopped. "Where do we go from here? Is this the start of a courtship?"

"You can be so practical," Konrad said with a chuckle, "yet dreamy at the same time."

"That's *exactly* how I would describe you," she said, confirming to her that they were indeed made for each other.

At the Van der Voort house, Maarten gladly gave his approval and Betje burst into tears. Both declared it was a marriage made in heaven, which is what Dutchmen believed to be true of marriages anyway. Aunt Margaretha gave her blessing and reminded Konrad that Catrijn was not penniless; she owned half of her father's house. After Nicolaas gave her a bear hug, Catrijn looked at Dirck, really wanting his opinion.

Dirck thought he saw uncertainty in her eyes, until he remembered Julius Caesar had said that men willingly believe what they wish. He glanced at all the grinning faces, and a faint smile formed on his face.

"I'm happy," Dirck said, "if you're happy, Catrijn." He kissed her cheek and shook Konrad's hand. "Congratulations."

Relieved, Betje's attention shifted to the wedding. "I guess it's my job to choose the date," she said giddily, for it was her right as godmother, in the absence of Catrijn's mother. "It shouldn't be in May ... bad luck. And *not* on a Sunday ... too solemn a day." She thought more. "December 31, a Saturday, is perfect. Your lives together will start in a brand new year, and the date will bring good luck."

On December 31, 1583, Konrad and Catrijn were married in Nieuwe Kerk, having chosen a religious rather than civil ceremony, both of which were allowed in Amsterdam. By the time Catrijn walked down the aisle in an elegant light green gown with garnet trim, the turmoil of selecting the dress had long been forgotten. Betje had wanted black, a practical choice, for the dress could be used again in the future when in mourning and for her burial. White was out of contention because only poor people wore white.

The reception was held at Maarten's home, and it overflowed with guests. There were neighbors, business associates, Catrijn's current and former students, city officials, and members of the Night Watch. Each shared a drink of brandy with the couple as they sat in the center of the front room, with Catrijn wearing a wreath on her head. Guests brought mostly modest and practical gifts, including a simple pot hanger for the hearth and a trivet to use when the pot was removed, reflecting that hard times still prevailed in Amsterdam. Some read poems, either ones they had composed or well-known verses. Catrijn's former students pooled their money to buy a copy of Plato's treatise on love.

Near midnight the guests finished their dancing and began trickling out, and Jacques and Dirck staggered off to their new residence in the cloth factory, which, though cramped and austere, gave them their first taste of independence.

After the last person had left, Maarten and Betje presented their gift, the deed for Maarten's half of the Hasbrouk house. Catrijn protested that it was too generous, but Maarten argued persuasively it was the least he could do to repay Papa's generosity to him and his family. After a final toast and blubbery kisses from Betje, the newlyweds walked across the street to Konrad's house.

For safekeeping, Catrijn placed the deed and her wedding wreath in the linen cabinet she had inherited from her mother. She imagined her mother doing the same with her wreath on her own wedding night.

Konrad closed the cabinet door and gave his wife a long, tender kiss. "You were captivating today, Catrijn." Taking her hand, he led her to their bedroom, a cozy room above the kitchen he had only recently begun using for sleeping. It was more intimate and private than the bed in the front room and benefited from warmth coming through the floor.

The kitchen fireplace had not been in use, and consequently the air was chilly. Both hurriedly removed their clothes, except for their shirts which everyone wore to bed, and slipped under the covers.

"Oooh," Catrijn purred. The bed was warm. Someone, probably Betje, had placed warmers in it.

Konrad blew out the candle. "My lovely Catrijn." He enveloped her in his arms. "Are you afraid?"

"Nee."

In the morning, Catrijn awoke feeling warm and cozy with her husband by her side. It's nice to be married, she thought dreamily, and be loved. The covers were still up around their necks, and he was sound asleep. She glanced at his face. He looks so contented ... must have found our lovemaking satisfying. She lay there, staring at the ceiling. He was oh so gentle, tender, and gentlemanly. But I wish I'd seen his body. It must be handsome. He never took off his shirt ... or mine. I'd hoped he'd find my body attractive. She closed her eyes and tried to focus on positive thoughts. Betje said it would be very pleasurable, and it *was* ... but not *very*. Somehow, I'd expected more. Shooting stars? Explosions? Oh, I don't know ... maybe I expect too much.

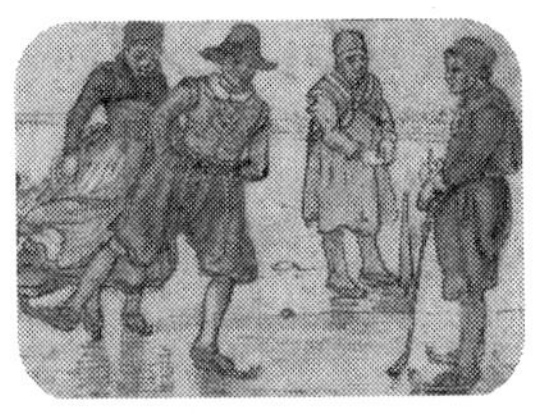

CHAPTER 6

Opportunity and Opportunism – 1584-1590

On February 1, 1584, the annual meeting of the City Council came around again, and Maarten stood in front of the mirror adjusting his large white ruffled collar, a modern addition to his wardrobe. A knock came at the front door. When he opened it, Rijp Dekker was standing there.

"I brought a small gift for you, Maarten," Rijp said with an eager-to-please grin and a heavy box in his hands. "Some sherry to say thanks for the good work you're doing for the city." He thrust it at Maarten.

"Why are you doing this?" Maarten's eyes narrowed. "What do you want?"

"Nothing, nothing at all." Rijp put the box on the stoop. "Just want to thank you for making those important decisions about Amsterdam's future."

What is that supposed to mean? Maarten asked himself, as Rijp strode away. Reluctantly he carried the box indoors and, after inspecting his appearance in the mirror again, headed to the City Council chamber.

The first thing on the council's agenda was expansion of the city, and the chairman reported: "The mayors have been working diligently to buy land on the west side, as instructed, and have successfully negotiated reasonable purchase prices in some cases. These have been with responsible citizens, who have owned their properties for a considerable time and also recognize the benefits of a larger city for all Amsterdammers. They include Beguine Sister Margaretha, Maarten's aunt."

Councilmembers turned to Maarten, nodding their appreciation. Maarten beamed with pride, knowing that the Beguines' reputation as savvy investors as well as humanitarians reflected well on him.

"But," the chairman continued, "further land purchases are stymied by speculators. They're asking exorbitant prices for land they only just purchased."

"Who are they?" one councilor demanded.

"Rijp Dekker and … ."

Maarten was so angered at hearing Rijp's name he didn't even listen to the rest of them.

"It doesn't really matter who they are," the chairman said. "We can't do anything about them anyway. So we'll probably need to abandon the westward expansion and start looking eastward."

"Maybe," the same councilor said, "but I think those of us who know the speculators should first try to talk some sense into them. If the city doesn't buy their land, no one will—not at their prices." He addressed Maarten. "You know Rijp Dekker, don't you? Do you think you can talk sense into him?"

"Nee, he wouldn't listen to me," Maarten said, though he hated to acknowledge even knowing the bastard. He looked from councilman to councilman. "But I'd like to meet the man who *thinks* he can talk sense into Rijp Dekker."

After the laughter died down, the chairman said, "I think that goes for all the speculators. But if anyone wants to talk to them, go right ahead. In the meantime, I propose we give the mayors another month to work on the land purchases. If they can't buy enough at reasonable prices, we should pursue eastward expansion."

"Isn't that going to be far more expensive?" Heer Nostrand said. "The east offers nothing, except sunken land and waterways."

"Compared with the inflated cost of the western land, not necessarily. I've already had the mayors look into it. They say we can create new land by sinking old ships, adding rocks and sand on top, and pumping out water with windmills. That's probably the same way the city was added to a hundred years ago."

"Rocks? They could be the toughest part," Heer Nostrand said. "They're hard to come by and expensive to ship in."

"Then we'll have to get creative. For example, the city collects fines for many reasons: inaccurate weights and measures, stealing. Why can't those fines be paid in rocks? People convicted of a crime would have to pay a fine of rocks, rather than money."

There were guffaws and snorts, but that would be one of the clever methods the city fathers would employ to accomplish their goal.

With the 1584 trading season about to start, Maarten was going over his list of things to do, when a knock came at the door. He answered it and was not happy to see Rijp Dekker standing there.

"I have nothing to say to a land speculator." Maarten started to close the door.

"Wait," Rijp said, wedging his foot inside the doorframe. "I am *not* a speculator—just an *investor*. And I *need* to talk to you."

Rather than risk someone seeing the scoundrel standing on his doorstep and making a scene, Maarten invited him in. "Wait here." He retrieved the box of sherry Rijp had given him prior to the council's annual meeting and pushed it into his hands. "Take this. I know why you gave it to me, and I don't want any more bribes."

"*That* wasn't a bribe," Rijp said indignantly. "If I wanted to bribe you, I wouldn't insult you with *that*." Getting no response from Maarten, other than him pointing toward the door, Rijp said, "Can I sit down? This box is awfully heavy, and I want to talk to you." He plopped into a chair. "Would you like to buy some land? I'm serious. I'm overextended and need to sell."

"Nee."

"Well ... then I need to start selling more of my fine art objects. Could you take some on consignment to sell in Gdansk?"

"Oh, *those* trinkets," Maarten said, dismissive.

"Your son Nicolaas didn't think they were trinkets when he sold 'em."

"I know, but we're still not in the business of shipping and selling trinkets."

"All I ask is this: Consider it and tell me what the shipping costs and commission'll be."

Maarten ushered him out the door and, when Rijp was out of sight, he started to go back inside—

"PRINCE WILLIAM OF ORANGE IS DEAD!" A man was yelling as he ran up the street. "PRINCE WILLIAM ASSASSINATED!" He continued by, and neighbors rushed out of their homes. "PRINCE WILLIAM ASSASSINATED!"

Maarten hurried to Town Hall, where an emergency meeting was convened. By the time he returned home, his front room was full of anxious family members, neighbors and business associates, all wanting to learn what had happened. Maarten confirmed that Prince William of Orange was indeed dead, assassinated in his home by a deranged Catholic. Women began weeping, and men blinked back tears.

Maarten went on to explain that Holland and four other provinces planned to recognize William's son, Prince Maurice, as the new governor of the Dutch Republic. The other two provinces, Friesland and Groningen, would likely choose Prince William's nephew, William Louis of Nassau, who was their native son. Nobody knew how it was going to work, or which of the two would command the Dutch Republic's continuing war against Spain.

"There is other news too." To Konrad and Jacques, Maarten said, "The Duke of Parma has taken control of the Scheldt River and laid siege to Antwerp again. With our ships unable to reach the city and Parma controlling all supply routes, Antwerp is isolated."

"That explains why we haven't received any correspondence from Antwerp for a while. Not from my uncle, or Jacques's cousin."

"After taking Antwerp," Maarten said gravely, "Parma plans to attack the north again."

People in the room gasped.

Realizing his mistake in stating that so bluntly, he tried to assuage their fears. "We should be safe, though, with the big rivers protecting us from an invasion by land. And if Parma sends a fleet into the Zuider Zee, we'll be ready. We're much stronger now than ever before." It was pure bravado, but it calmed everyone.

As people dribbled out of Maarten's house, many confessed to being shocked at the possibility of war resuming in the north. Most of the time Amsterdammers hardly gave a thought to King Philip or Parma because combat had been confined to the south for such a long time and fought by paid soldiers.

After saying goodbye to the last person, Maarten stepped outside and sat down on the bench. Stretching out his legs and leaning his head against the wall, he savored the stillness of the night. Dirck joined him.

"Father," Dirck said, "will you go back to being a Sea Beggar? Help Antwerp, like you did with Haarlem and Leiden?"

"Nee. My job is here to operate a successful business and pay taxes." Maarten rolled his head toward his son. "Do you know Holland pays nearly 60% of the Dutch Republic's budget for the rebellion? And Amsterdam pays most of that because we're the biggest city in Holland?" That elicited the look of surprise from Dirck that he had hoped for. "We're the only thing keeping Prince William's army going in the south. No taxes, no war. And Parma marches or sails right into the northern provinces."

That was not what Dirck wanted to hear. "I was thinking. If I went to Antwerp, maybe we could save it. Stop Parma *before* he comes north."

Maarten looked into his son's expectant eyes and realized that though Dirck always seemed level-headed and mature for his age, underneath he was just a typical twenty-one-year-old with a burning desire to prove his manhood. And war was the most glorious and heroic way to do it, especially a patriotic one.

"You know, Dirck, I was a rebel for ten years. *Ten* years. Had no choice ... couldn't come home. But I'm telling you, it was not fun. Mostly you're bored, sailing around hoping to get a chance to fight Spaniards. And when you *do*, it's just plain terrifying. Blood everywhere, limbs hacked ... friends screaming in pain." Maarten shook his head side to side. "Nee, war is nothing to take lightly."

"Aren't you *ever* going to fight again?"

"Of course I will. I'll fight if Parma crosses those great rivers or sails down the Zuider Zee. We'll all fight, that's for darned sure. But do I relish it? Nee."

"Until then ... we just keep working and paying our taxes?"

"Right."

For the first voyage of the year, Maarten assembled a nine-ship convoy. Dirck sailed the *Catrijn*, assisted by first mate Rykaard Jr., and Maarten commanded the *Nicolaas* with Rykaard Sr. as first mate and Nicolaas aboard. Though Nicolaas had been their exclusive agent in Gdansk for two years, Maarten still liked to go with him at the beginning of each season to help find suitable housing and also assess for himself the status of the grain crop in Poland.

After the usual stop in Emden, the next was made in Sweden to allow several captains to buy timber, including Dirck who had to fill an order from their shipbuilder in Hoorn. In Gdansk, Maarten found lodging for Nicolaas in a small inn, and later he and Nicolaas made the rounds to grain growers and merchants. Pleased that the supply was ample so far and the outlook seemed good, they began purchasing.

As soon as the ships' holds were full, the convoy departed. After a rough patch of weather in the Baltic Sea, it was clear sailing through the Oresund Sound and around the tip of Denmark. In the North Sea, threatening clouds dominated the western sky and streaking rain obscured the horizon. The ships kept on course, hoping to outrun the coming storm.

A squall line marched forward, whipping up the wind and

white caps, and the faster ships surged ahead, including the *Nicolaas*. More heavily loaded, Dirck's *Catrijn* lagged behind.

Maarten lowered some of the *Nicolaas's* sails, trying not to get too far ahead of Dirck's ship.

The sky darkened. Waves grew in height. Showers turned into sheets of rain, and Maarten was losing sight of the *Catrijn* as well as the ships ahead. He and Rykaard discussed what to do and agreed they must press on to avoid being caught in the maw of the storm. It would be exceedingly difficult to sail back to the *Catrijn* anyway, given the wind direction, so all they could do was hope that their sons' combined experience and good judgment, plus luck, would get them through.

Dirck saw his father's *Nicolaas* disappear into a squall. He had lost sight of the other ships as well as the coastline long ago. We're not going to outrun this storm, he concluded, and will have to ride it out. So I need to get some sail down, and fast.

"HAUL DOWN THE MAIN! AND TOPSAIL!" Dirck commanded. Sailors scrambled to their posts.

The seas rose, and gusts battered the remaining sails. A strong gust broadsided the *Catrijn*, knocking her hard to port, and sailors manning the rigging were flung sideways. When the ship righted, they swung back again. One man lost his grip. "*Aaaaaahh!*"

"MAN OVERBOARD!"

Sailors on deck rushed to the gunwale.

"SEE HIM?" Dirck called to them.

"NEE!" A wave washed across the deck, pushing the men back.

The sea continued to build, and wind howled.

"TAKE DOWN THE MIZZEN SAIL!" Dirck yelled and pointed the *Catrijn* into the oncoming swells. When another gust hit, he glanced around ... too many men on deck ... someone else is going to go overboard. Dirck hollered to the boatswain, "GET BELOW!" and pointed to sailors not needed to man the sails, "AND TAKE THEM WITH YOU!" To the men on deck, he ordered, "TIE UP!" Dirck fastened his own tether to the helm, and Rykaard and the seamen found places to secure theirs.

A menacing wave arose in front of them—"HOLD ON!"—and

the *Catrijn* rode up its face and over the top ... and plunged down the backside into a trough. The next wave was more ominous. Up the *Catrijn* rose ... almost to the apex ... the wave broke, tossing the *Catrijn* to starboard and sending her surfing back down its face. Dirck and Rykaard Jr. muscled the tiller, trying in vain to get her under control. The wave crashed over the *Catrijn*, and she heeled sharply. She was righting herself, when ahead Dirck saw another wave cresting. On its face, something seemed to be floating. He squinted through the pelting rain at it and saw logs ... part of a sail ... rigging. The wave's frothy head broke, pushing the debris ahead of it.

A log slammed into the *Catrijn's* hull, and the wave broke over her, sending white water across the deck and seamen tumbling and twisting on their tethers.

Sputtering, the men battled to get up, and the sailor nearest the point of impact edged his way to the gunwale and leaned over.

"WE BEEN HOLED, CAP'N! BY A LOG!"

"ABOVE THE WATER LINE?"

"YES!"

Good, Dirck told himself, we should be able to stay afloat if I can keep her level and the hole above the water. Hope no one is injured below.

The hole had no immediate effect on the way the *Catrijn* handled, giving Dirck hope. He and Rykaard gripped the tiller and steered her through the trough and up the next wave.

The hatch opened, and the boatswain came on deck and fought his way to the helm. "Cap'n, we been holed by a log!"

"How big of a hole?"

"Pretty big," the boatswain said and formed a sizeable circle with his arms. "The log came straight in—right above the water line—and twisted out again when a wave smashed into it. We're working on plugging it, and I got the men pumping and bailing. But we need to lighten up."

Lighten up meant getting rid of cargo, something Dirck was loath to do. He was about to say no, when beneath his feet he felt the *Catrijn* heel and then roll back, as though water might be sloshing back and forth within her. "I agree. We need to lighten up."

The boatswain made his way back to the hatch, and soon men came trudging up with cargo and heaving it overboard.

With much of the cargo cast out, the *Catrijn* rode higher in the water, but every wave that smacked the hull dislodged some of the wood the carpenter and boatswain had worked so furiously to nail over the hole.

With the ship slogging and listing more acutely, Dirck realized his only choice was to take the risk he had been avoiding. He would have to raise the mainsail at least partway to gain speed and put the *Catrijn* on a course where she would heel over to port and the damaged side would rise further out of the water. Overcoming his fear that men might be tossed overboard if they lost control of the unwieldy sail, and the sailcloth itself might shred, he talked it over with first mate Rykaard Jr. before giving the order:

"ALL HANDS! MAINSAIL ONE-HALF, HO!"

As the lines of the sail were loosened, some were caught by the wind and lashed against sailors' bodies. The lines were brought under control, the sail was set, it filled with air, Dirck and Rykaard Jr. leaned into the tiller, and the *Catrijn* turned onto a beam reach course, perpendicular to the wind. Slowly, she heeled over and the damaged side of the hull came further out of the water. Perfect, Dirck thought to himself.

A powerful gust hit. *Riiiiip.* Dirck looked up to see the mainsail tearing. "TAKE IT DOWN!" he ordered. The *Catrijn* leveled, exposing the hole again to oncoming waves.

Crippled and sinking lower in the water, the *Catrijn's* forward motion stalled and she began bobbing helplessly like a cork.

Meanwhile, the other ships had been propelled southward on the intense winds and avoided the full brunt of the storm. Even so, a few suffered torn sails and damaged rigging, but no lives were lost. With the rain stopping and wind subsiding, most were now in sight of each other. They coalesced and waited for the stragglers to show up. All arrived, except for the *Catrijn*, which was nowhere to be seen. The captains agreed to wait a little longer, some using the time to undertake makeshift repairs. Wary of another cloud bank forming in the distance, five of the captains told Maarten that they wanted to press on to Amsterdam, and two others agreed to sail back with him to find the *Catrijn*.

While the rest of the convoy sailed off southward on a freshening wind out of the north, the *Nicolaas* and the two other ships turned windward toward where Maarten had last seen the *Catrijn*.

Beating upwind was excruciatingly slow and nerve-wracking for Maarten and Rykaard, who kept going up the ratline to spell the lookout.

The wind died when they reached the area where Maarten estimated the *Catrijn* should be. He handed the helm to Rykaard and climbed up for a look. There was nothing as far as the eye could see, no ship, no coastline. He came back down, dejected.

The ships drifted on the current, and when a wind from the northeast came, the other two captains rowed themselves to Maarten's ship to inform him they were short on water and eager to take advantage of the good wind direction. They wished the two fathers good luck, and headed south toward Amsterdam.

The two were almost out of sight, when a call came from the lookout.

"*I think I see something.*"

"*A ship?*" Maarten asked.

"*Nee. Things floating in the water.*"

By now Rykaard was scrambling up the ratline. Perched there, he focused hard on the objects and confirmed in a grave voice, "*It's debris, Maarten. Logs ... some sailcloth and bits of rigging. No ship.*" He climbed down and reminded Maarten, "Dirck bought logs in Sweden."

The two fathers stood in silence, fighting tears and unable to acknowledge the obvious.

"It could be from another ship," Maarten rationalized. "Maybe the *Catrijn* was blown way off course and is somewhere out there in the North Sea, or made it to shore and is sheltering in a cove." Though he could not remember seeing any deep coves, he convinced himself they could very well exist because he tended to give wide berth to this shoreline.

By now, the wind was no longer favorable for sailing toward the debris or eastward to scout the coastline, and water was running low. So Maarten said:

"Rykaard, we just have to hope they're safe and will show up later in Amsterdam. They're both capable seamen."

Resigned, Rykaard nodded agreement and put his arm around his old friend.

Maarten steered the *Nicolaas* southward toward Emden and met up with the other two ships. Together, they set off for Amsterdam, with Maarten making a stop in Hoorn to drop off Rykaard to let him report the news to his family.

As soon as Maarten walked through the door, Betje sensed that something was seriously wrong and steeled herself. He delivered the news as factually and optimistically as possible and had to give her time to calm down before calling the family together. When he did, he included Kaatje, whose relationship with Dirck seemed to be on the upswing again. Catrijn arrived, felt the tension in the air, and gripped both godmother Betje's hand and Aunt Margaretha's.

"We lost sight of the *Catrijn* in a major storm," Maarten explained calmly, "and when she didn't meet up with the fleet afterward, Rykaard Sr. and I sailed back with two other ships to look for her. All we saw were some logs in the water and shreds of sail cloth." Catrijn fought back tears, and Kaatje began to cry. "There is no need to panic. The debris and logs could easily have been from another ship. And it's common for ships to be separated from their fleets; I lost sight of my own for almost two weeks during the war. And for captains to take shelter in a cove during a storm or afterward to make repairs. We just have to wait and see, and if they don't return within the month, then we can start worrying."

A few days later, more bad news arrived, this time about Antwerp. Heer Nostrand, a delegate to the Holland assembly, received a communiqué, and he and Maarten went together to Konrad's home.

"I've just learned," Nostrand told Konrad, "Antwerp has fallen. The siege is over. The terms of peace with the Duke of Parma call for Antwerp to be an exclusively Catholic city, and Protestants can either convert or leave. Anyone wanting to leave has two years to sell his property. I'm sorry to be the bearer of such wretched news."

"I'll need to go, and Jacques too," Konrad said. "My uncle will *never* convert, and neither will Jacques's cousin, so we'll have to bring them here to Amsterdam. Since my uncle is in his eighties, there's no time to waste. We'll leave as soon as possible."

"Will you go by ship?" Catrijn asked.

"That would be dangerous," Maarten warned. "Dutch ships have no access to Antwerp anymore."

"Then we'll have to go overland," Konrad said, his shoulders slumping. He was already dreading the arduous hundred-mile journey through war ravaged countryside and involving several major river crossings.

The *Catrijn* had in fact remained afloat after the storm had passed, thanks to sailors manning the pump nonstop and bailing furiously, the boatswain doggedly plugging the hole, and, in Dirck's opinion, an enormous amount of luck. Visibility had improved, and Dirck had seen they were near land and spied a notch in the shoreline. He did his best to steer the faltering ship for it, hoping to find an inlet where repairs could be made.

The notch ended up being the entrance to a cove. As the *Catrijn* entered it, Dirck looked back one last time and saw no other ships.

After Maarten finished selling his grains, he decided to remain in Amsterdam in case Dirck returned, rather than sail the *Nicolaas* on the next voyage to Gdansk. Rykaard agreed to captain the ship with one of his sons serving as first mate and en route would be on the look out for the *Catrijn*.

With Konrad gone and no sign yet of Dirck's ship, Catrijn could barely contain her anxiety. It was Saturday, and, with no tutoring being done on weekends, she had nothing to do but dwell on the unknown. After staying in bed too long and pushing away her half-eaten piece of bread and butter, she pondered what to do. The thought of going to the Van der Voort house, a cheerless place now, held no allure, nor did once again inflicting her moodiness on Aunt Margaretha. What she needed was something productive to do. Recalling that Konrad had mentioned needing a larger factory and knowing that land was being reclaimed on the east side of the city, Catrijn decided to do some reconnoitering for her husband. To boost her spirits, she braided ribbons into her hair, put on her favorite lace cap that formed a heart above her forehead, and wore her pretty moss green outfit. After attaching the money pouch to her waist and positioning it behind the apron, she hooked her basket on one arm and went out the door.

Catrijn first swung by the harbor to look for Dirck's ship, a daily ritual. The visit was fruitless, and she proceeded on to the eastern city gate, Anthonispoort, where thankfully there were no executions or mutilations underway. The place was nonetheless busy, and she stood at a distance to observe the hawkers jostling for customers, most speaking Dutch, but also French, Spanish and a little Hebrew. In their midst, a minstrel was playing, a dice game was about to break out into a fight, and a whore or two with too much face paint and décolletage were strolling around and beckoning passersby. All the while, traffic was entering and exiting the city gate under the watchful eyes of guardsmen who were intercepting incoming undesirables.

Before wading into the crowd to get to the steps leading to the top of the city wall, Catrijn glanced down to make sure the money pouch was inconspicuous and gripped her basket more firmly. She started for the steps.

From behind a boy bumped into her, rolled past, and seized the handle of her basket.

"Hey!" Catrijn yelled and locked her arm around the handle, while shoving the boy away. In a tug of war, the two struggled for possession. Meanwhile, a male accomplice slipped his hand under her apron and snipped the strings of the money pouch. Catrijn felt the tug at her waist at the same time the boy let go of her basket. The boy bolted, and she whipped around to see his accomplice running with her money. She took off after him. "*Thief! Thief!*"

Rijp Dekker, who was not far away, turned.

"*Thief!*" Catrijn ran as fast as she could.

The accomplice banged into a cart, snagged a foot on the spoke of its wheel, went flying, and landed on his belly. Catrijn caught up with him and began smashing her basket into his head while grasping at her pouch. The thief shoved the basket away, hustled to his feet, and started to run—

Rijp arrived and grabbed the thief's arm, swung him around, slammed a fist into his stomach and, when the man doubled over, viciously kneed him in the face. The thief collapsed, and Rijp snatched the pouch and handed it to Catrijn in one gallant move.

Still shaken, Catrijn said, "Th-thanks," her eyes fixed on the bloodied face of the thief and the guardsmen subduing him.

"You all right?" Rijp asked, as he touched Catrijn's elbow and guided her away from the gathering crowd.

"I think so." Looking up, Catrijn realized she knew him. He's the crook who stole the Van der Voort house. "You're Rijp Dekker."

"That's me," he said with a beguiling smile. "Now, can I escort you somewhere?"

"Uh ... nee, thanks," she said and adjusted her cap. His stare was unnerving and leer palpable, and she just wanted to get away. "I'll be all right." She smoothed her apron while scanning the crowd for a familiar face—Uncle Pieter!—and glanced at Rijp one last time. "Thank you."

"My pleasure."

Catrijn walked toward Uncle Pieter, trying to appear as though nothing had happened. He was with a woman, whom he introduced as Floris, and said they had just returned from a stroll along the Amstel. Floris commented that she and Pieter had met while volunteering at the Begijnhof, helping Margaretha in her work with wayward boys. Catrijn liked Floris right away, the calm demeanor and sincere smile ... a good match for Uncle Pieter.

"Anything wrong?" Pieter asked after watching Catrijn repeatedly glance over her shoulder and fidget with her purse. She explained the attempted robbery and her reason for being there, and Pieter suggested they all go to the top of the city wall together, hoping a quieter place would calm her down.

Once there, the three silently took in the view of usable land being created. Old ships had been scuttled, and on top boulders placed to form a base. Men were hard at work spreading rocks and sand, while windmills whirred away pumping out water.

It was all very impressive to Catrijn, but she was having trouble envisioning buildings being constructed on it. Meanwhile, another image—the young boy battling for her basket—kept crowding out other thoughts.

"Uncle Pieter," Catrijn said, "do you think there are more boys roaming the streets and looking for trouble lately?"

"Hmm ... maybe. It has always been an issue, but I guess there *are* more now, with so many refugees arriving. The problem is there's no way to stop them from robbing people."

"And simply branding them," Floris added, "and expelling them from the city doesn't stop the hunger ... or the need to steal."

"Margaretha and the Beguines do what they can, and I'm glad to help," Pieter said. "But they can't fix this all by themselves. These kids need to get off the streets ... have a safe place to stay, be fed and taught a trade. There's a labor shortage, yet these homeless kids and men can't seem to find jobs. Give them shelter and training. That's the answer. It's essentially what your father did for Maarten."

"Ja, it is," Catrijn said, warmed by the mention of her father's goodness. "I think your idea is a good one."

Near Amsterdam's Haarlemspoort gate, Dirck alighted from the fishing boat he had hired to transport him and his crew from Hoorn, where he had left the *Catrijn*. He walked directly to his parent's house.

Maarten heard the front door open, his eyes raised—"*Dirck!*"—and he sprang from his chair. Betje raced in from the kitchen and threw her arms around him, and Maarten enveloped both in his embrace.

"We've been worried sick," Betje said, while mopping tears with the palm of her hand. "Where have you been?"

"It's a long story."

"After the storm passed," Maarten said, "two other captains went back with me to search for you. The wind was coming out of the north, so it took us a long time to get to where we last saw you. Then we spotted logs and debris from a sunken ship and thought the worst had happened."

"One of those logs *holed* the *Catrijn*," Dirck said. "I thought the debris might have come from one of our ships. Did any sink?"

"Nee, but some were pretty battered."

"It's good that they all made it. That was a heck of a storm," Dirck said. "Well, after we were holed, I got rid of the cargo, and then the mainsail ripped. We were taking on water and sinking lower and lower, when the storm started to ebb. We were lucky to survive and to find a cove to make repairs in. It took us a long time to get home because I was forced to sail heeled to port to keep the damaged part of the hull out of the water. And had to be careful not to put too much pressure on the patched sail."

"Is the *Catrijn* in the harbor now?"

"Nee, I left her in Hoorn. Your shipbuilder is careening her to let the hull dry out so he can reinforce the holed area. He said he'll make a new mainsail and cut up the old one for extra foresails. From there, I had a fishing boat bring me and the crew to Amsterdam."

"You look exhausted," Maarten said. "Why don't you go home and get some rest. We can talk later."

Dirck nibbled a few pieces of cheese Betje had offered, before stepping outside.

"*Dirck! You're alive!*" Catrijn called from her window and ran outside. She threw her arms around him, her eyes full of tears. "You can't imagine how worried I was about you."

He hugged her and, embarrassed, stepped back. While wiping a tear from her cheek with his thumb, he said, "I'm all right."

Catrijn composed herself. "If you're going to your home in the factory, I'll walk with you. Give me a minute to get my shawl."

Along the way, Dirck recounted his harrowing tale, and she explained that Konrad and Jacques were in Antwerp and that she was overseeing the factory in their absence.

On arrival, the workers congratulated Dirck on his safe return. While Catrijn inspected the work in process, Dirck hauled his sack up the stairs to the loft he and Jacques shared.

When Catrijn finished, Dirck called down to her, "Want to see, Catrijn?" knowing she had never been to the loft before.

After mounting the steep stairs, Catrijn paused at the top. Her eyes surveyed the dreary space with two straw-filled mattresses bearing unidentifiable stains ... clothes stacked in the corner ... no furniture ... eew, what's in the dirty bowl? It was in stark contrast to the immaculate homes prized by Dutch people. "How can you two live like this?"

"What?" Dirck glanced around and thought the place looked fine. "It's small, but not nearly as cramped as my cabin at sea, or as dank. It even has a window!" Seeing she was unconvinced, he added, "Uh, I guess it'll look better after I straighten up."

Catrijn could not descend fast enough.

The *Nicolaas* returned from Gdansk after stopping first in Hoorn to deliver timber their shipbuilder had ordered and to collect payment. Maarten promptly sold the grain from its hold and eagerly awaited Pieter's tabulation of the profits. They were substantial, but just barely enough to offset the loss incurred from Dirck having tossed the *Catrijn's* cargo overboard during the storm. Pieter proceeded to revise profit estimates for the remainder of the year, taking into account the *Catrijn* being out of commission for the foreseeable future and the bill for repairing her being sizable. The results were grim.

After reviewing Pieter's figures, Maarten sat at his desk, fiddling with the candle and trying to think of ways to increase revenues.

Beer he usually exported to Poland was in short supply, so profits from that weren't going to be much. And Nicolaas had not ordered many specialty items for his Polish customers, so the hold was going to be almost empty when the *Nicolaas* left again for Gdansk. His mind kept coming back to Rijp's request to transport his fine art objects to Gdansk, but the thought of dealing with the crook repulsed him. He decided to solicit other options.

Dirck suggested taking the *Nicolaas* to challenge the Spanish blockade of Antwerp and trade with desperate Protestants, which some sea captains were doing and reaping outsized profits. The excessive risks removed that from consideration. Dirck mentioned another idea, which he presented as more of an observation than an option, expecting his father to also find it unacceptably risky. He told of a Dutch captain who was going to sail to Portugal to sell grain, manufactured goods and weapons to King Philip II. The king reportedly favored Dutch arms and needed foodstuffs for his people because they supposedly grew little grain themselves. The manufactured goods were for his colonies. The king was paying handsomely for such things.

"Why would *any* Dutchman help Spain?" Pieter asked, incredulous. "Especially sell them weapons? Weapons that will be used against *us*." Under no circumstances was Pieter ever going to allow Van der Voort & Sons to do something so utterly immoral.

So together the three men drew up a proposal for Rijp.

Maarten swallowed his pride and knocked on Rijp's door, but not before glancing around to make sure no one saw him there. While waiting, something Margaretha had said entered his consciousness: Dutch merchants would sail through the fires of hell to out-compete someone else. In his case, he was just trying to survive, but could nonetheless feel the flames licking.

"Maarten!" Rijp greeted him affably, suppressing a sneer. Maarten's presence meant he had capitulated.

"I have a proposal for you," Maarten said. "We have space on our outgoing ship next week, and this is the deal: You'll pay for the freight cost and bear the risk of your goods being lost at sea or damaged, just like we do with our own cargo. In Gdansk, Nicolaas will sell your goods on consignment for a 25% fee, based on the price he gets."

"25% is acceptable," Rijp confirmed and started reading the proposal. "My God, Maarten, I can't pay *these* freight charges. They'll bankrupt me." He pleaded, "Can't you reduce them? Maybe use fewer crew to save money ... more sails? I'll bet you can find a way. And don't you have some sort of insurance to reduce the risk?" Insurance was something he had heard about from southern émigrés.

"Insurance?" Maarten shook his head no. He had never heard of it. "We'll spread your goods over several ships, like we do with our own. That's how we reduce risk."

"I'll think about it."

"Fine." Maarten left, very annoyed and vowing next time to charge Rijp double.

Two days later, Rijp again asked Maarten to lower the freight charge, and Maarten refused. With the terms of the deal not negotiable, Rijp signed the contract and reluctantly paid the freight costs upfront, as Maarten had stipulated. Rijp also made sure not to slip in any silver-painted lead coins with his payment, against his usual practice.

The *Nicolaas* sailed off under Rykaard's command with Rijp's goods, which included statues and sea chests containing jewelry, books with beautiful leather covers, a bolt of cloth, and other odds and ends. Dirck was aboard and disembarked in Hoorn to check on repairs to his ship.

Upon returning from Hoorn, Dirck went to his loft for a rest before supper and stretched out on the mattress. He had hoped to catch a little nap, but his mind was still too active, ruminating about the difficulty and likely costs of repairing his ship and hoping she would be ready for the last voyage of the season, which was looking unlikely. Worries about Jacques also crept in, for he had not yet returned from Antwerp. Dirck considered getting up and updating his rutter, but lacking a desk and chair it was too difficult. His eyes rested on the room's dominant feature, a dingy little window. Catrijn's right. How can I live like this? I never realized how dismal this place is. I guess Jacques and I were too busy having fun. When winter sets in, this loft is going to be really depressing. I need to find somewhere else to live.

He found a small house to rent near Nieuwendijk street and purchased a desk, bookshelf, and a table and chairs for it. Betje helped him hire a good cook and stocked his kitchen with utensils and her favorite dry herb mix. For her part, Catrijn decorated a wall in the front room with hand-painted flowers. After a family celebratory meal in the new house, Betje lingered after the others had gone. While she and Dirck finished the last of the beer, she asked:

"Have you seen much of Kaatje lately?"

"On Sunday, at church."

"Did you know she stopped at the house *every* day to ask about you when you hadn't returned with the fleet?"

"That's nice."

Betje looked into his eyes. "Now that you have your own home, you should propose marriage to her—before debonair Jacques or someone else does."

Dirck was astounded not only by her boldness, but also by the use of the impressive word, debonair. He responded with a noncommittal shrug.

"Well, if you don't intend to propose, then *stop* stringing the poor girl along!"

His mother's bluntness startled him, but her description of his treatment of Kaatje resonated. That's *exactly* what I've been doing, keeping Kaatje's hopes up just enough—so I can do what? Have more time to decide? Wait until someone better comes along? Hard to say. But she does love me and she is gorgeous. What man wouldn't want her for himself? Hmm, yet there's something about her that has always put me off ... not sure what. Her perpetual smile? Screechy voice? The fact that I don't have to chase her? She seems willing to wait forever for me. But what if she *does* get tired of waiting? And chooses Jacques or the creepy guy who tied a flower to her doorknocker? Maybe I should marry her.

Betje saw a faint smile cross Dirck's lips and went home a happy woman.

After getting into bed, Dirck continued to think about Kaatje. There are some things I'm not happy about. For one thing, she never challenges what I say. And rarely introduces anything new into our conversations. That's disappointing. Is she just eager to please? Or does she not have opinions of her own? And why isn't she interested in subjects that fascinate me? Like when I gave her my opinion of Poles—that they can be so different from us in some ways, such as their mushy sounding language and odd foods, and so similar in their love for family and reliance on hard work to get through tough times—and she hardly responded. And there's the time I'd hoped we'd have a meaningful discussion after I told her I'd seen an Islamic man give a coin to an old beggar woman, while good Christians just walked by and ignored her. She said he was a nice man ... didn't see the obvious moral contradiction.

Dirck lay there quietly and finally concluded, I can't marry a woman who won't challenge me ... make me a better person. Kaatje's not right for me, and I need to tell her as soon as possible. She'll understand and recognize we'll both be better off. She has many suitors to pick from anyway.

After church on Sunday, he walked Kaatje home by way of the harbor and found a quiet spot where they could lean against a wall and look out at the expansive Ij.

"Nice view, eh?" Dirck said. "I love the sea."

She nodded yes and put her head on his shoulder.

Dirck took a deep breath and turned to face her. "We need to talk."

Kaatje's brow furrowed, surprised by the sudden change in tone.

"We've been seeing each other for several years, and I've been thinking a lot about us lately." He noticed her eyes brighten with anticipation. Oh no, she thinks I'm going to propose marriage. Better get to the point. "We've had some really nice times together, and I feel great affection for you, but ..." His mouth was straining to say, I don't love you, but the harsh statement would not come out.

Kaatje's perpetual smile disappeared.

"What I'm trying to say is ... it has been good, but I think we're not right for each other." When her eyes filled with tears, he took her hands into his. "We're both young." They were twenty-two. "You and I owe it to ourselves to take the time to find a special someone who is perfect for us. You're beautiful and have many suitors. One of them may be right for you."

Dirck watched Kaatje's face fill with anger, cheeks redden ... fists clench—

"I *hate* you, Dirck! I swear I *hate* you with all my heart." She spun around and ran from him with her hand over her mouth, sobbing.

"*Kaatje!*" He took a step ... stopped ... and slumped against the wall, shaking his head. I handled it completely wrong. Humiliated her. Presented it as *my* decision. Why didn't I quit talking long enough to let her say something? And why did I have to say she has many suitors? So patronizing, and stupid!—he slammed the back of his head against the wall—Stupid! Just stupid!

Dirck avoided Kaatje in the coming weeks, hoping her anger would dissipate so he could smooth things over, but his hopes were dashed after every chance encounter resulted in hateful glares. Work became his savior when the *Nicolaas* sailed into the harbor with cargo to be unloaded. The convoy captains reported being plagued by early and persistent ice storms and agreed to cancel the final voyage of the season to Gdansk. Maarten looked on the bright side: prices for the grains were going to soar, and his profits too, given the prospect of no more shipments arriving.

Nicolaas returned with the convoy and went to Rijp's house to pay him for the goods he had sold on consignment. After Rijp thanked him profusely for selling everything and at such high prices, Nicolaas resolved that Van der Voort & Sons should enter the lucrative trade of so-called trinkets themselves.

When a letter came from Hoorn reporting that repairs had been completed on the *Catrijn*, Dirck was elated, until he saw the bill. Pieter reckoned it would consume much of their profits from the recent grain sales.

By the time Dirck brought the *Catrijn* back to Amsterdam, Kaatje's marriage banns had been announced for her betrothal to the brother of Catrijn's former student, who had once tied a flower to the doorknocker of her house. Her great uncle Heer Nostrand and Betje shared their sadness that things had not worked out for Kaatje and Dirck. Maarten concluded it was probably for the best, since Dirck had seemed uncertain about their relationship from the start.

On the first day of October, Konrad and Jacques returned from Antwerp, noticeably thinner and with four wagons, but no uncle or cousin. The cousin had perished in the siege, and the octogenarian uncle had passed away en route to Amsterdam for no apparent reason. He just seemed to have lost the will to live. Konrad embraced his wife as though he never wanted to let go. Though Jacques was as relieved to see Dirck as Dirck was to see him, they nonetheless began their usual verbal sparring.

"When you go to our loft," Dirck said, "you'll see I've moved out."

"Developed a taste for the rich life, eh?"

"Nee, just wanted you to have your own private place to entertain the ladies."

The exchange felt trivial to both in light of their recent experiences, and the conversation died.

Konrad and Jacques's ordeal spilled out during supper at Maarten's house, where Betje served an especially hearty stew for the fatigued men.

"The worst thing for me," Jacques said, "was the devastation: broken dikes, land underwater ... abandoned houses. Almost no food. And listless people and their meagre belongings clogging the roads, mostly traveling northward."

"For me," Konrad said, "the most painful experience was seeing much of beautiful Antwerp ruined. Our family homes were standing, but had been plundered. One warehouse roof had caved in. The factory, though, was strangely intact, and we were able to salvage some equipment and bring it with us. We sold everything else for the best price we could." He seemed exhausted just recounting the trauma.

After the meal, Konrad brought out pipes and tobacco and lit them for the willing, while Maarten refilled the beer glasses. The conversation returned to Antwerp, this time with Konrad reminiscing.

"When I stood in my house, it brought back such memories." He told of happy events and loved ones. "At our warehouse, I could easily envision when it was full, which was almost always. My father had a good eye for opportunities. If he saw well-priced cargo come in—perhaps glassware from Venice, or grain from the north—he'd buy the whole lot. Then he'd wait for the right time to sell, or for the right buyer. Sometimes it took up to a year. He was an exceptional businessman."

"Up to a year?" Dirck said, amazed. "We couldn't possibly hold our grains that long. We *must* sell them right away to have money to buy more grains on the next trip to Gdansk."

"How could your father afford to do that, Konrad?" Catrijn asked.

"Before the revolt, my family had considerable capital in reserve. And Antwerp had a banking and insurance system that provided more flexibility than you have in Amsterdam."

"What exactly is insurance?" Maarten asked.

"Let's say you want to make sure you won't incur a loss if the *Nicolaas* shipwrecks on the next voyage. So you pay a specified amount of money to an insurer for insurance on the *Nicolaas*. If the *Nicolaas* sinks, the insurer reimburses you for its cost."

"Why would an insurer do that? Ships go down all the time."

"Well, there were businessmen, who had so much wealth that they could afford to take chances, even if it meant losing some of it. It's a calculated risk. Not every ship will sink, and hopefully the insurance payments will more than cover the cost of those that do. Of course, the insurer needs to verify the ship's condition and value, and whether the captain is of good repute. It's a business of risks and rewards."

Insurance and banking were something entirely new to Maarten, because neither existed in Amsterdam. And they would not be introduced until the early 1600s.

"Dirck, I almost forgot," Jacques said and left the room. He returned with a roll of paper and said in a voice full of gratitude, "I bought this for you in Antwerp. It's a gift for saving my life."

"No need for a gift," Dirck said, as he unrolled it. "A Waghenaer map. This is very generous of you, Jacques. Thank you."

"I remembered that you admired Waghenaer's maps for their beauty, but didn't find them useful because of the lack of detail. This one seems to be highly detailed. Though you may never get to use it for sailing, because it covers the hostile coast from Holland to Spain, I thought you'd at least find it interesting."

"I certainly do." While examining the map, Dirck's expression changed to one of amazement. "I've never seen a map with so much navigational content." He turned to his father. "It notes shallow areas ... safe directions to enter harbors." His eyes shifted to Jacques. "These are the kinds of notations we sea captains put on our charts and into our rutters."

"Did you notice these symbols, Dirck?" Maarten said. "They're standardized. Here's one for water depth ... another for hidden rocks. What a clever way to provide so much information without cluttering the map with words." They could not know that the symbols invented by mapmaker Lucas Jansz Waghenaer, a retired ship pilot from Enkhuizen, would be used on navigational charts for centuries to come.

As 1584 drew to a close, everyone was relieved that the disastrous year was finally ending and prayed the next one would be better.

It was. Konrad's business flourished, and 1585 ended up being Van der Voort & Sons' most profitable year ever. Grains were of exceptional quality, both ships were in operation the entire year, and Nicolaas successfully filled their holds with a variety of export items he had scoured the city to find, including unique household and decorative items purchased from a wealthy merchant who had fallen on hard times.

On February 1, 1586, Maarten went to his eighth City Council meeting feeling confident in his knowledge of the city's operations and what needed to be done. Today, though, his horizons would be broadened by learning more about issues facing Holland province and the Dutch Republic from Lawyer Johan van Oldenbarnevelt, who had just been appointed Advocate for Holland's government, a newly created position.

Upon arriving, Maarten saw a distinguished-looking man about his own age standing near Uncle Nostrand. Uncle waved him over and introduced Oldenbarnevelt, noting they had something in common, both had helped relieve Haarlem and Leiden during the sieges. The two discussed their war experiences, and the conversation concluded with Oldenbarnevelt inspecting Maarten's partially bitten-off ear with empathy and fascination.

The meeting was called to order, and Oldenbarnevelt was asked to explain the work he would be doing as Holland's Advocate.

"My role will be to support and give direction to the deliberations of Holland's State-General assembly, which sometimes has difficulty reaching consensus because it is a rather large body. As you know, each city sends numerous delegates to it. I will also liaise with the Dutch Republic's States-General assembly and the House of Orange. My work should lead to greater efficiency in the province's work and improve coordination with the Republic's leadership.

"I would like to address the question of Prince William of Orange's successor, now that three years have passed since his death. As you know, Holland province recognizes the prince's son Maurice along with other nearby provinces. Others acknowledge his nephew William Henry. The division in leadership causes concern for many, but I believe it poses no threat to the Dutch Republic. The two men get along well and have evolved a harmonious sharing of responsibilities. Maurice has capabilities as a military commander, like his father, and even shows signs of military genius. William Henry seems destined to handle the affairs of state.

"The important thing, though, is that the House of Orange will continue to be the same unifying force for the Dutch Republic that it was under Prince William."

After approving nods and applause, the Advocate asked, "Are there any questions?"

Maarten raised his hand. "I still hear talk of finding a royal to lead us or help us, which troubles me. I don't see why we need one. What is your opinion?" He spoke candidly, believing all Dutchmen had a duty to speak up on such matters.

"I agree, but some people continue to believe that a relationship with a king or queen gives us legitimacy, or that getting England and France involved will ensure they will help us with the rebellion; but, of course, they'll also expect us to help them if Spain invades them. Others are convinced that only a modern monarch can provide efficient administration. My opinion is that the Dutch Republic can do all that and more—without help from an outside royal."

Maarten was getting a good feeling about Oldenbarnevelt.

Another councilor stood and said, "Now that the Duke of Parma has taken Antwerp and most of the south, do you think he will try to invade the north again?"

"Parma may not have the appetite for a land invasion of the north, knowing how badly the Duke of Alva was defeated at Alkmaar in '73. But a sea invasion is a possibility, despite any lingering memories of Count Bossu's resounding defeat on the Zuider Zee by the Sea Beggars. King Philip is reportedly extremely angry with Queen Elizabeth for helping us try to save Antwerp, and we hear reports that he is building an armada of 130 galleons to vanquish England. After that, the armada is supposed to strike the Dutch Republic."

Some in the audience gasped. Others groaned, knowing that even more taxes would be needed to address the threat. That worried Maarten too, but equally concerning was that cowardly Queen Elizabeth was their first line of defense.

During the church service, Nicolaas saw a buxom girl look at him numerous times. Afterward, he sauntered over and struck up a conversation.

"You're new to our church, aren't you?"

"I just arrived in Amsterdam." The girl lied. She had been in the city for the past half year, but always stood in the back of the church with the family she worked for as a maid. After trying in vain to attract Nicolaas's attention through subtle means, today she had resorted to positioning herself near him and stepping on his foot accidentally.

"My name's Nicolaas van der Voort," he said, while looking her up and down. She's a country girl—Who else would wear those bright red stockings and pointy yellow clogs?—and really young, probably no more than fifteen. She'll be an easy mark.

She showed no recognition of his name, and gave hers as "Griet. From Gelderland." In fact, though, she knew everything about Nicolaas: he was the son of a respected city council member, worked in a family business that owned ships, and had a reputation for his wicked sense of humor and way with the girls. From the first day she laid eyes on him, she found his mischievous grin, joy of life, and moneyed family irresistible.

After a little small talk, Nicolaas found her and her throaty voice alluring. "I'll be ice skating on the Ij this afternoon. Perhaps I'll see you there, Miss Griet from Gelderland."

"Perhaps," she said nonchalantly, but considered it a date.

Merry skaters, looking roly-poly in their multiple layers of clothes, already covered the Ij when Nicolaas and the family arrived. He sat down with Catrijn and Dirck to put on their blades. While Betje remained in her armchair sled, Maarten lashed on his.

Konrad and Jacques, who were newcomers to the sport and opted to watch for now, guided Margaretha to a seat on a rowboat frozen to the ice. Together, they took in the lively scene of skaters, ice fishermen, and horse-drawn sleds. A ball came flying at Konrad, he ducked, and it landed behind him.

A worried-looking young man carrying an L-shaped stick came to retrieve it. "I'm sorry, sir."

"What game are you playing?"

"It's called Kolf, sir." He held out the stick. "Do you want to try?" Konrad accepted it, and he instructed. "Stand like this. Now hit it to my friend."

Maarten stumbled as he stood up, drawing laughs, and pushed Betje's sled onto the ice. Dirck, the best skater, zipped off and with hands behind his back followed alongside his mother. Seeing Catrijn and Nicolaas clasp hands and move off tentatively, he began gliding in broad circles around them, until they regained their old form and sped up, intending to out-skate him.

Griet was sauntering along the edge of the Ij with her skates slung jauntily over her shoulder and spotted Nicolaas. He was holding hands with a sophisticated young woman, laughing, and swerving and weaving across the ice. Her ego deflated. Urgently, she searched for a familiar male face. Putting on his skates was the butcher's helper, who regularly flirted with her.

"Hi. Great day for skating, eh?" Griet said, as she settled down next to him to attach her blades.

"Ja," he said and looked up. "Oh, Hi!"

Griet stood up, pretended to lose her balance—the butcher's helper eagerly caught her—and she giggled. Arm in arm, they stepped onto the ice. Discreetly, she edged them toward Nicolaas.

"Griet!" Nicolaas exclaimed and swung Catrijn around. The two skidded to a stop in front of Griet and her companion.

"Whew!" Catrijn said with a laugh. "You and Dirck are getting too wild for me."

"Catrijn, this is Griet from Gelderland," Nicolaas said, and added with a smirk, "She won't reveal her last name ... *very* mysterious." He turned to Griet. "This is Catrijn, officially my aunt, uh, by adoption, but actually more like my sister."

"Hi," Griet said. "My last name isn't mysterious at all. It's Strijker."

"So your father is an iron worker," Catrijn said, for *strijker* meant that.

"Oh, uh ... ja. Ja." The question flustered Griet for she never knew who her father was.

When Griet made no attempt to introduce her friend, Catrijn

tried to smooth over the awkwardness with a smile to both. "Well, I must be going. I need a rest." She took Nicolaas's hand.

As soon as the pair left, Griet excused herself from the butcher's helper, feigning a sore ankle, and slowly made her way to the edge of the ice, hoping Nicolaas would catch up with her. And he did.

Nicolaas dazzled Griet with his skating until the winter sun dipped low in the sky. They left together, and in a narrow lane out of public view Nicolaas stopped. Placing his hands on her shoulders, he said, "Griet from Gelderland, I'm glad we met. We could have so much fun together." He pulled her close. "I have the most incredible urge to kiss you." His groin pushed gently against hers.

After the initial shock of his tongue entering her mouth, Griet found herself giving in to the sensuous feeling. It was unlike anything she had experienced before ... extraordinarily erotic. Her hips started moving in rhythm with his—

Griet came to her senses and pulled back.

"Don't you like it?" Nicolaas's eyes connected with hers. "I know you do." He tried to resume—

"N-nee. I'd better be going." Griet tugged at her jacket. "I *must* go."

Seeing it was useless to try again, Nicolaas walked Griet to the house where she worked and lived.

Nicolaas's presence in the street saying goodbye to Griet was observed by Griet's employer from an upstairs window and created a conundrum for her. She had an obligation to protect the girl's reputation and in doing so prevent a scandal for herself, yet she did not want to squash any opportunity the penniless orphan might have with this young man from a respectable family. The employer decided to let the relationship run its course, as long as Griet did nothing overtly stupid.

From Nicolaas's way of thinking, the first encounter had been a tantalizing taste of things to come. He resolved to pursue Griet until she succumbed. How long that took would be his challenge.

Betje was waiting in line at the fishmonger's stand at the Damrak, when she spotted Catrijn buying vegetables across the way. Her eyes immediately went to Catrijn's flat belly. Why hasn't she become pregnant after four years of marriage? Betje had been giving that a lot of thought lately and was coming to the conclusion that Konrad's advanced age, forty-four, was the source of the problem.

The fishmonger finished with her customer and asked Betje. "What would you like, my good lady?"

"I'm not sure," Betje said, though she knew exactly what she wanted. "What do you recommend?" She was testing the knowledge of this seller, a newcomer and possible replacement for her favorite fishmonger, who had died recently.

"Well, I have nice herring," the woman said and reached into a barrel and plucked out a brined fish. "Plump, eh?" She put it back, and her hand passed over the stack of salted herring and stopped at the pile of fresh fish. "These just came in. I recommend the fresh bream ... they're the best."

Betje inspected the fishes' translucent eyes and shimmering skin. "Very nice."

"And I'd suggest you cook them with lots of pepper. You look to me to be a bit of a chilly type—probably phlegmatic." She gave a look that said: Am I right?

"I guess I am a little chilly," Betje replied and pulled her shawl a little higher around her shoulders. "But I don't know about phlegmatic. What's that?"

"It's one of them four humors: phlegm, bile, blood, and black bile," the fishmonger explained. Seeing confusion in Betje's eyes, she cautioned, "You need to beware of them, 'cause they control your health. You balance them in your body, and *you* control what happens to you."

Betje was skilled at reading omens, something she considered to be an excellent tool for *divining* the future. But omens could not *control* the future. If the fishmonger knew how to do that, Betje wanted to learn. She drew closer and listened intently.

"The four humors are part of the order of things ... four points of the compass, four seasons of the year, and four elements: water, fire, earth, and air." She added boastfully, "I've made a study of it, so's I can advise my customers."

Wow! Betje thought to herself.

"Like I was saying, today you look pale, if you don't mind me saying so. It means your phlegm is out of balance—you know, like on a balance scale?—so you should eat some hot, dry foods to bring it back in balance."

Betje was catching on to the principle. "Fish are cold and watery, so I shouldn't eat them unless I cook them in pepper. Makes sense."

"Now, if you come next week and your cheeks are red, it means you have too much blood. You're too hot, see? I'd tell you to eat the fish without pepper. Or if you and the mister was havin' trouble with the you-know-what"—she winked and jabbed her elbow into an invisible person—"I'd urge you two to stand outside in a hot, dry wind."

"How did you learn all this?"

"I always like to learn somethin' new. My sister cleans house for a physician, a real smart man from the south, Italy I think." To her, Italy was an exotic place that abounded with new ideas. "He told her about Galen—he's an ancient guy who figured out the humors. I liked what I heared and bought meself a little pamphlet to educate meself." She wiped her hand on her apron and pulled a wrinkled booklet from inside her bodice.

Betje scanned the pages, and her eyes lit up. "Where can I find this physician?"

When Betje arrived at the physician's house, the sun was directly overhead. She peered into the open upper part of the door. The interior was completely black, and she waited for her eyes to adjust.

"May I help you?" came a voice from within the void.

Betje's vision brightened, and she saw a distinguished man rise from his chair and walk toward her. "I, uh, I'm sorry, I didn't see you there."

"May I help you?"

Betje explained she was seeking advice—not for herself, mind you, she was perfectly healthy and never had need of physicians—but for a gentleman with a young wife.

The physician invited her in and made an informed, snap assessment of Betje: sanguine and phlegmatic, which accounted for her ruddy complexion and slow-witted, confused speech.

"You say this gentleman is elderly, has a young wife, and no children?" the physician queried.

"Ja." Betje watched the physician examine several books from his prodigious collection and was duly impressed. Books were a sign of intelligence, and so many books hinted at genius.

"I think," Betje added, "the gentleman is probably phlegmatic, because he is calm and not easily irritated."

The physician's eyebrows shot up. Perhaps I underestimated this woman. She clearly knows something about the humors. He scrutinized Betje again, particularly her eyes, and revised his diagnosis: she's a melancholy type ... lots of black bile ... and enigmatic.

He selected a book and began leafing through it. "This is a complicated matter, not just involving the humors. There are many factors to consider."

Betje was already turning the coins over and over in her hand and hoping this wouldn't take too long. She had brought what remained of her food budget for the week, and it wasn't much.

"From the information you've given me," the physician said, as he closed the book, "the gentleman in question is dominated by the dry humors, which is characteristic of a man of intelligence and advanced age. I will write down my advice so you may take it with you." When finished, he also delivered it orally.

"Your gentleman should stop eating turnips, because they're too dry and cold for a man with a young wife. To conserve his youth, he should drink broth consisting of cinnamon, cloves, cardamom, saffron, sugar, juice from an orange, minerals ... and alcohol. To increase the functioning of his nether parts, he should eat dry, hot foods seasoned with considerable amounts of pepper. He would benefit from walking briskly, occasionally getting angry, and avoiding conjugal bliss on humid days."

Betje was flabbergasted.

"Though I normally don't give such advice to women, I suggest his young wife eat as much cloves as possible to increase the forces of Venus. In fact, both should eat more cloves."

Betje's head was reeling. This was powerful information. How could she ever thank him enough? The bill shocked her back to reality, and she left his office saying, "I'll bring the final payment next week, I promise."

In the comfort of her own kitchen, Betje read the physician's instructions, and her euphoria dissipated. Nearly all the ingredients were completely out of reach—expensive and rare. The only one she might be able to afford was pepper, and, if exceedingly lucky, maybe cloves. Pepper and cloves will have to do, she told herself, resigned. But how will I influence what Konrad and Catrijn eat? And when they have conjugal bliss? She stared at the small pots of home remedies on her shelf, an oil/soap/lead unguent and dry rye/herb mixture. Why couldn't the physician recommend something I already have?

Konrad opened the door to his house, and the unmistakable aroma of Betje's *speculaas koekjes* wafted out. Though he normally liked those tasty spice cookies, he intensely disliked Betje's. He found the plate of offending cookies sitting on the table between Catrijn and Margaretha.

"Why does Betje keep bringing these?" Konrad asked, as he sat down.

"I don't know," Catrijn said and offered him a slice of the peach she and her aunt were sharing. "She has always baked *speculaas koekjes*. So does every other Dutch housewife, especially on Saint Nicolaas Day." She shrugged. "She might be baking them more often because Maarten, Uncle Pieter and the guys like them so much."

Margaretha tasted one of the *speculaas koekjes*. "Eew, she never baked anything like *this* before—way too much pepper and cloves. She must have lost her touch."

"Maybe she can't get all the spices she usually uses." Catrijn stared at the plate. "I don't care for them either, so I think we should give them to Nicolaas. He ate the whole plateful last time."

"That's fine with me." Konrad took another piece of peach.

"I remember the time," Margaretha reminisced, "when spices were more available. I never cared much for cooking or spices, but I did enjoy sniffing each one at the market. There was cinnamon … I think from China. And nutmeg … not certain where it's from."

"Did your family trade in spices, Konrad?" Catrijn asked.

"Nee. Spices were a secretive monopoly of the Portuguese crown, and only a few Antwerp merchants had trading privileges. My family never did."

Hearing the church bells chime noon, Konrad said to Margaretha, "I almost forgot. Catrijn and I have to leave to meet Maarten. He's going to show us land for a possible new house. Would you care to come?"

"Nee, you go ahead. I have things to do at the Begijnhof, but I'd like to hear what you learn from him."

The two headed to the west side of the city, where the mayors had finally acquired enough land to allow 450 feet to be added to Amsterdam for a chiefly residential neighborhood. While they strolled, Catrijn envisioned a nice quiet home, far from noisy Nieuwendijk street. Konrad was pleased just being able to afford a brand new home, which in large part was due to profits from Nicolaas selling the fine cloth produced in his factory to customers in Gdansk. Along the way, Catrijn noted that stories were being added to many buildings and commented that Amsterdam was undergoing an upward *and* outward expansion. At the edge of the city, they joined Dirck who also was considering a new house for himself.

Maarten was walking briskly, aware he was late. In the distance, he saw the kids and felt a surge of pride at how well they had turned out. Catrijn was married to the perfect man for her, and their relationship seemed to be one of pure harmony. Dirck had still not found that special someone. After Kaatje, he had had several girlfriends, but none seemed to work out. According to Betje, he was too picky. Maarten wasn't sure why.

"I'm sorry I'm late," Maarten said. "Just as I was leaving, Uncle Nostrand came to tell me some important news. England has defeated King Philip's massive armada. I thought it was impossible ... never had much regard for Queen Elizabeth—"

"We know," Catrijn said with a chuckle.

"I guess my grudge against her was pretty obvious," Maarten admitted, "but she really *did* make it tough for us Sea Beggars when she kicked us out of Dover. Maybe I was wrong, maybe she's not a coward. But she wasn't the one who commanded the English ships against the Spanish Armada either. Her friend Walter Raleigh was. And *his* skill and small maneuverable ships won the battle, as well as a lucky shift in the wind that sent his fireboats straight into the Spanish galleons."

"That sounds similar to the Sea Beggar victory in the Zuider Zee, except for the fireboats," Dirck commented.

"Ja, that was another unlikely victory," Maarten said and savored the Sea Beggars' remarkable achievement for a moment. "Is everyone ready to go up?" he asked and led the way to the stairs.

From the top of the city wall, Maarten pointed to a deep trench being dug. "That will be the new moat. And next to it, a new city wall will be constructed." His hand patted the one they stood on. "This old one will be torn down, and the old moat will become a canal called the Singel. It'll be lined with streets and lots that can be purchased."

Maarten gave them time to envision the transformation, before continuing.

"If you decide to buy a lot, you'll need to meet the city's building requirements: a solid foundation with deep pilings, and brick—no wood—for the house."

"Seems reasonable," Dirck said, and Konrad agreed.

"*And* you will have to pay for paving the street with cobble stones and lining the canal with bricks." Seeing the disappointment on their faces, Maarten countered with, "It's the only way the city can afford all this expansion."

Catrijn and Konrad remained at the wall, and Dirck and Maarten left for home.

"What are your thoughts, Dirck?" Maarten said, as they walked along. "Do you think you'll build a new house?"

"Not sure. I'm having second thoughts about investing so much money in a house, especially since I'm hardly ever home. I think I'd be better off buying a new ship."

"That's why I'm not building a new house. Your mother likes ours, which is fine with me."

A little further along, Dirck said, "I've been thinking. With this news of the Spanish fleet being destroyed, maybe now is a good time to go south to trade. You're familiar with La Rochelle from your Sea Beggar days, and, as you've always said, they have good wine and plentiful salt. Nicolaas tells me the Poles are always asking for both."

"Not a bad idea. We should stop by Uncle's house to ask his opinion." Uncle Nostrand was privy to international news in his capacity as delegate to the Holland provincial government and from his regular contact with well-informed Advocate Oldenbarnevelt.

They found Uncle at home and at his desk. He confirmed that La Rochelle was still a Huguenot (French Calvinist) stronghold and also that fewer Spanish ships were being spotted along the southern coasts. Enthused, Dirck went home to consult his maps.

When Maarten arrived at his home, the intoxicating aroma of *speculaas koekjes* greeted him. He sampled one and found it to be as delicious as ever, despite Margaretha having complained that Betje was putting too much pepper and cloves in them lately. "Mm, mm. I love your *speculaas koekjes,*" he said and patted his wife's rump.

After supper, Maarten went into the front room and sat down at the table with a beer and a book that Catrijn had lent him. Betje joined him and started scrubbing the table top.

Maarten shifted his eyes from the book to Betje and wished she applied less effort to housework and more to conversing with him. Sometimes he needed someone to talk things over with or get another opinion, like now when he was reading an intriguing new book and contemplating starting to trade in La Rochelle. Having observed Konrad and Catrijn interact, he had come to realize they had a way of discussing matters that resulted in a better decision than either one could have come up with alone. It was as though one person's idea plus the other's idea did not equal two—they equaled three, or at least a third better one.

"Maarten," Betje said, "did the kids seem happy to you today?"

"Ja."

The answer filled Betje with joy, and her attention shifted to her treasured copper candle holder and could not resist removing the little spot marring it. Maarten thought and thought about ways to get Betje interested in topics of conversation other than family. Betje polished and polished trying to eradicate the spot.

Maarten's eyes met hers, and, when Betje smiled contentedly at him, he concluded that he was never going to change her. She was happy with who she was: a very good wife and mother, a terrific cook, and a thorough, though obsessive, housekeeper. For that he had to be thankful. Maarten placed his hand on hers, winked, and gave his look of desire. With a tilt of her head and glance out of the corner of her eye—which said, You devil you!—Betje replied with a beckoning grin.

It took another year for Maarten and Dirck to organize a La Rochelle foray, owing to Gdansk trade obligations and the need to persuade other captains to form a convoy with them.

When the February 1 annual meeting of the City Council rolled around, Maarten was in good spirits about the upcoming La Rochelle trip and also the meeting. This time he would not have to raise Catrijn's request for girls to be admitted to Latin school, for she seemed to have abandoned the notion after facing rejection numerous times. On the war front too, things were looking up. Not only had England's defeat of the Spanish armada averted an invasion by sea, but chances of a land one seemed nonexistent because King Philip II was rumored to be withdrawing his troops from the Dutch Republic's southern border. It was said they would be redeployed to the French border because a Huguenot was about to ascend the throne of France.

On an additional bright note, all of Aunt Margaretha's harangues about the need to help wayward children and fallen women were finally bearing fruit. Dr. Sebastian Egbertszoon, with whom Margaretha, Pieter and other concerned citizens had been consulting, had just proposed an imaginative way of dealing with the problem: Instead of just punishing people for their wrongdoings, find the reasons behind their misbehavior and treat those. It was called rehabilitation.

Based on Maarten's own experience as an orphan on the path to waywardness, he thought the idea made sense. The City Council agreed and passed a resolution endorsing it. The mayors were tasked with determining how to put Dr. Egbertszoon's proposition into practice.

His city council obligation fulfilled, Maarten began preparing for the first trading voyage to La Rochelle. He and Dirck were going to sail the *Catrijn*, and Rykaard Sr. and Jr., the *Nicolaas*. All that remained was to wait for the Ij to become navigable.

When the usual date to commence sailing passed, Amsterdam's sea captains gathered daily at the harbor to speculate when the ice might disappear. Most attributed the frustratingly slow rate of melt to the unusually cold winter and the vicissitudes of weather. No one suspected the phenomenon heralded the start of a decade-long, mini ice age.

The wait was especially annoying for Nicolaas, for he was eager to leave Amsterdam after having failed to seduce Griet and given up on the chase. In Gdansk, he faced better prospects.

When the ice at last cleared and the fleet was ready to depart, Betje prepared *speculaas koekjes* for her men and the crew, and also made some for Konrad and Catrijn. As soon as both batches came out of the oven, Nicolaas showed up.

"Do I smell *speculaas koekjes?*" Nicolaas said *speculaas koekjes* in the singsong way that always charmed his mother. He went straight to the pans.

"*Nee,* not those!" Betje said, "They're for Catrijn and Konrad," and directed him to the other pan.

"What's the difference? They're all *speculaas koekjes*." Again, saying it singsong.

"They're *not* the same. I add special ingredients to yours," she said, fibbing and smiling lovingly.

After being in Gdansk for only a few months, Nicolaas returned to Amsterdam to fill a special order from a well-to-do Polish man who favored statuary and Amsterdam's fine cloth.

A few days later, Griet noticed him walking ahead of her on Warmoesstraat. She ducked into a side street and ran past Oude Kerk to get ahead of him. After tugging a piece of hair from under her cap and letting it dangle immodestly, she sauntered onto Warmoesstraat and almost bumped into him.

"Griet! Griet from Gelderland. How're you doing?"

"Oh, Nicolaas, I didn't see you there. I thought you were in Gdansk."

"I was, but had to return to buy goods for an important client. I've already bought loads of fantastic stuff." She seemed impressed, so he asked, "Want to see it? I have it all stored at my brother's house. I'm on my way there now."

"Ja, that'd be fun."

When Nicolaas opened the door of the house, Griet peered in. "Is your brother at home?"

"He's at sea ... won't be home for awhile." Nicolaas followed her inside and closed the door. "Tell me, Griet, how've you been?"

"Me? Good. And you?"

"A bit lonely. I've missed you."

She smiled demurely.

"Look at all this," Nicolaas said, waving his hand in an arc around the room.

Griet marveled at the collection of candelabra, tapestries, and bolts of shimmering cloth, things she had never seen before. "Your family must be rich."

"Ja," he said, without a trace of modesty.

"Buying and selling these things must be *really* hard work."

"Not for me; it comes easy to me. But my brother? He has to work hard. All he does is work, work, work, same as my father ... very *boring*." Nicolaas sat down on the edge of the desk. "You wouldn't like them." He picked up a stick from the floor and began twirling it in his fingers. It whirled faster and faster, and terror filled his face, as if it were alive and dangerously out of control.

Griet giggled. "That's what I like about you, Nicolaas. Always fun and *unpredicable*."

"Unpredic*table* ... and I am." With the stick still twirling, he added, "My brother used to be fun too. We did all sorts of crazy things when we were kids." He chuckled. "You know those out-houses sitting over the canals? Well, Dirck and I used to throw stones into the canal every time old man Jacobs went into one. The water'd splash up on his arse. We'd hear him curse, and we'd laugh until we cried. But you wouldn't know Dirck was so much fun then—now he's just *boring*. When he's not at sea, he stays home and goes on the Night Watch—but, other than that, he's just—"

"*Boring*," Griet said, matching Nicolaas's refrain. She burst out laughing.

"Griet from Gelderland, you're a lot of fun."

"And you're the *funnest*, most *unusualist* guy I ever met."

"I don't understand why we don't see each other more often." Nicolaas ran his fingers under her cap until curls came cascading down. "Your hair is beautiful." He pressed a lock to his nose and smelled it sensuously. "You're irresistible." He pulled her gently toward him ... and kissed her.

Griet surrendered completely, letting his lips devour hers and hands roam her body. She had already resolved to do whatever was necessary *not* to lose him again. By the time his hand was at work under her skirt, she was simmering with passion. Lustily, she hiked up the skirt and wrapped a leg around him.

By mid-season, Maarten and Dirck had confirmed that La Rochelle was a safe and lucrative trading destination, having encountered no problems at sea and finding strong markets for La Rochelle's wine and salt in both Amsterdam and Gdansk. To adequately exploit the trade and also continue to ply the Gdansk-Amsterdam route, however, Van der Voort & Sons would need additional ships. So when returning from La Rochelle, father and son stopped in Hoorn to talk with their shipbuilder. They purchased a ship under construction and ordered a second one. The first was to be Dirck's, and he named her *Amsterdam Ascendant*. The other was for Nicolaas to name, and he would later choose *Nicolaas II*. Dirck remained in Hoorn to work out the details of the ships' designs, while Maarten went on to Amsterdam with the *Catrijn* and her cargo.

After Dirck concluded his work with the shipbuilder, he caught a ride on a fishing boat to Amsterdam and went to his parents' house. There he found his father and Konrad huddled over a desk, so deep in conversation they failed to notice him. His mother greeted him with a kiss and hug and excitedly told him that Catrijn was pregnant.

Konrad and Maarten rose to shake Dirck's hand, and he congratulated Konrad on the upcoming birth of his first child.

"You two both looked so serious when I came in," Dirck commented. "What were you talking about?"

"Livorno," Betje answered, "wherever that is."

"It's in Italy," Maarten said. "Have a seat, Dirck. You should be part of this discussion."

Konrad explained, "Your father and I have been working on an opportunity proposed by my cousin Lodewyk, who lives in Livorno. He sent a letter asking me to ship grains and other foodstuffs to him because there is a famine underway, which he expects to last a good while because of persistent crop failures. If I did, he said, 'We will both get rich.' I take his statement seriously, insofar as Lodewyk is not given to making extravagant claims."

"Konrad and I have tentatively agreed," Maarten said, "to jointly finance sending a fleet to Livorno. Pieter and Jacques have already prepared some estimates and confirm the profit potential is good—very good, indeed." He glanced at Konrad. "We've also talked about starting to stockpile grain and dried fish to sell there."

"That happened awfully fast," Dirck said, a bit overwhelmed. "But it *does* sound like a great opportunity."

"We've been waiting for you to get here," Maarten said, "to help with the logistics: the ships and when to go."

"Well ... as you know, our ships are already committed for the remainder of the season, and next year too," Dirck said, thinking aloud. "I suppose we could send the two new ones to Livorno next year instead of to La Rochelle. But we'd have to store all the stock-piled grain and dried fish over the winter—wait a minute. Where exactly is Livorno?"

Konrad unrolled the map he had brought. "Here it is, between Genoa and Rome."

"Livorno is a *long* way away. None of us has ever sailed those waters." Dirck studied the map. "And we'd have to figure out how to navigate safely around Spain."

"You'd need to hire a pilot," Maarten said.

"And we'd need extra cannons and arms aboard." Dirck rubbed his chin, thoughtful. "We may have to hire some ships and captains because we'd want a sizable fleet, for safety."

The door opened, and Catrijn and Margaretha walked in.

"You all seem so intense," Margaretha commented. "What are you talking about?"

"I bet it's Livorno," Catrijn said and briefly told her aunt of Lodewyk's letter and the tentative plan.

"Where exactly is Livorno?" Margaretha asked, and Dirck pointed it out on the map. "Ah, ja." Margaretha's finger glided over the names of various towns nearby and rested on Assisi. She turned to Konrad. "Why Livorno? Why did your cousin settle there?"

"After Jacques and I left Naples, Lodewyk moved to Livorno because the Medici family was developing it as a seaport for Florence and offering asylum to refugees. Protestants like Lodewyk came, as well as Catholics from England, and also Jews and Moors from Spain and Portugal."

"So," Margaretha asked, "are the details of this venture settled?"

"Not yet," Maarten replied. "We're not sure which ships we'll have available to send, and when. We have commitments in La Rochelle and Gdansk for next season. Obviously, we can't buy or build an extra fleet just for this project."

"Isn't it much warmer in Livorno?" Margaretha asked, and Konrad nodded yes. "Then why not take your fleet there for winter, after you've finished the trading season here? And bring the ships back in spring."

Dirck gaped at her. "Aunt Margaretha, you're a genius!"

Why didn't I think of that? Maarten asked himself.

On the following Sunday when everyone gathered at Maarten and Betje's house for the traditional after-church meal, Margaretha arrived in high spirits and announced:

"I've decided to go with you to Livorno. I've always wanted to make a pilgrimage to Assisi, for Saint Francis, and this will be my only chance."

The response was overwhelmingly negative, except for Maarten and Uncle Nostrand who knew that arguing with her was pointless.

"What's the worst that can happen? I die at age 74 at sea, rather than at home? It doesn't matter where I am when the good Lord decides to take me. Besides, Saint Francis said that death is our sister and nothing to be afraid of."

"I should go with you," Catrijn said, "I've always wanted to see the birthplace of Latin," and implored Konrad, "*We* should go.

"Absolutely not!" Betje stared at Catrijn as though she was crazy.

"You're pregnant," Konrad said.

~

Griet stood demurely in the street, while her employer knocked on the Van der Voort front door.

Betje answered and was surprised to see a woman whom she had seen in church but never spoken to. And now the woman had a scowl on her face. "Oh ... hello," Betje said and searched her mind for the woman's name, "Frau Brinker."

"Frau Van der Voort, you and I have a problem: your son Nicolaas and my maid Griet." She nodded toward the girl behind her. "I'd like to talk with you—in private."

"But wh ... please come in." Betje motioned to Griet to come along also and remembered where she had seen the girl before—in church flirting with Nicolaas.

"Frau van der Voort, I'll come right to the point. Griet is pregnant, and Nicolaas is the father. I'm sorry to be blunt, but immediate action is necessary."

"Wh-what? That can't be. Nicolaas was gone for over *four* months, in Gdansk, and only just returned."

"Oh, this happened *well* before that."

Griet placed her hands over her belly to reveal a well-formed mound.

"I've seen Nicolaas and Griet together myself," Frau Brinker said, "but only in public places. Griet tells me that Nicolaas took her to your other son's house."

"My son Dirck's house? Well, ja, he does rent a house, but ..." Betje realized she'd better choose her words carefully in case the girl was lying. "I'll have to speak to Nicolaas, of course. But a girl, an unwed one—Who's to say?—perhaps she's spread her favors to other unsuspecting boys."

Griet glared at Betje, barely controlling herself.

Frau Brinker was indignant. "Frau van der Voort! I take my duties as Griet's employer *very* seriously. She's an orphan, from Gelderland—I'm her only protector. I can assure you, she has *not* spread her favors, because I would have known. This case with Nicolaas was unique. He had an empty house in which to seduce her."

Betje stood up. "I'm sure you understand, I must first talk to my son, in private, before I can respond."

"I thank you for your time. Griet and I shall await your response at my house."

When Maarten returned home, Betje met him at the door. "I have fresh beer, Maarten. Do you want some?"

Betje served the beer and sat down next to him, all the while going over in her mind how she would broach the subject calmly and unemotionally.

Maarten stretched out his legs and noticed his wife's pensiveness. "You look like you have something on your mind, Betje."

"Nicolaas made a girl pregnant," Betje blurted out.

Maarten bolted straight up in his chair and slammed the tankard on the table. "I always expected he'd do something *really* stupid someday!"

"I knew you'd be upset."

Maarten stewed for a minute, gathered his wits and leaned back into the chair. "Who is she?"

Betje related the facts, and the two vented about their mischievous son and the loose morals of today's youth. Maarten drew in a deep breath ... memories of his own youthful indiscretions entered his mind. He exhaled forcefully.

At this point, Betje still wanted to tell Frau Brinker to go stick her head in a bucket, but even she knew that wasn't going to happen. "What do you think we should do?"

Maarten sighed again. "Well, I think we should be prepared if he denies it or refuses to marry her. Then we'd probably have to pay for her to leave town quietly."

The front door opened, and in walked Nicolaas. "Hi, Mother! I'm home."

"Sit down," Maarten said sternly.

Maarten lodged the charges against him, and Nicolaas seemed mildly surprised, but did not deny it.

"What do you have to say for yourself?"

Nicolaas mulled it over. It probably *is* my child ... maybe I should marry her. The sex is really good, and she's downright raunchy sometimes. But do I want a kid? Not really. When visions of Dirck and himself as kids came to mind, and Catrijn too, he concluded, kids can be fun.

A wedding was hastily arranged. Griet's only demand was she be given a pair of leather shoes (she only had wooden clogs) and a nice gold ring with cupids engraved on it. Her request for a dramatic rose-colored robe was rejected as too extravagant. Instead,

Betje chose a black dress for the usual practical reasons: it could be worn again during times of mourning and ultimately for her own burial. Griet's only consolation was that at least the dress was new.

Wanting to squash any suspicions about the timing of the wedding, Betje happily spread a rumor that it had been in the offing way before Nicolaas had left for Gdansk. The married couple took up residence in the Van der Voort home so Betje could help Griet during her pregnancy and afterward with the baby.

While Betje was cleaning the front room shortly after the couple moved in, she overheard Nicolaas in the kitchen comforting Griet about her morning sickness. Aw, Betje thought to herself, isn't he considerate? Things are going to work out fine.

"Maybe you should eat some of Mother's *speculaas koekjes*," Nicolaas said, singsong as usual. "Catrijn said they helped settle her stomach." He leaned closer and whispered, "Actually, Mother bakes special *speculaas koekjes* for me, but I like the ones she makes for Catrijn and Konrad better—more spicy. I always go over there and eat theirs."

Betje nearly passed out on hearing that and had to sit down. While furiously fanning herself, she pleaded: Dear Lord please don't send me *straight* to hell!

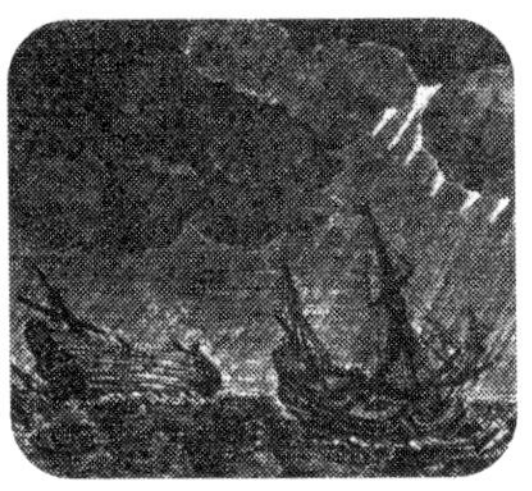

CHAPTER 7

Voyage to Italy – 1590-1591

At the end of the 1590 northern trading season, Van der Voort & Sons scrambled to turn around their ships to start the long voyage to Livorno before winter set in. Maarten was convinced he had done everything possible to conceal the mission from competitors. Grains and dried fish had been stockpiled in Hoorn to avoid arousing suspicion in Amsterdam, and the additional hired ships and captains were from Hoorn. Even Margaretha had already gone there, under the guise of visiting a friend.

As Dirck stood in the front room gathering maps, Maarten issued last-minute instructions. "If you see any Spanish ships, try to outrun them. Let the admiralty's ships do the attacking, if they're sailing with you." Uncle had asked Holland's Advocate Oldenbarnevelt to request an admiralty escort along the French coast for them. "And don't even think of trying to take a prize. Just keep your eye on the *real* prize—Livorno."

Nicolaas advised his brother on goods to purchase, and Betje pressed a shiny new Saint Nicolaas medal into his hand. "This will protect you." Dirck put it into his pocket next to the well-worn one.

Maarten went alone to the harbor to see them off, concerned that the family's presence would draw too much attention to their departure. At the Schreierstoren, he remained until the ships were out of sight. While uttering, "God speed," he again marveled that his son was actually going all the way to Livorno. To Maarten, north-south trade had always meant Gdansk-Amsterdam-Antwerp, and Dirck substituting La Rochelle had been logical, given the inaccessibility of Antwerp. But a Mediterranean terminus was something he would have never imagined in his wildest dreams.

"Dear Lord, what have I done?" Margaretha lamented and covered her mouth, hoping to avoid vomiting again.

"Look, Aunt Margaretha," Dirck said, "there's La Rochelle." He added with a wink, "*Now* you can get a good meal *and* practice your French."

"I don't care about food," Margaretha said, feeling too sick to appreciate his humor. "I don't care about French. I just want to get on terra firma. That's what keeps me going. That and Assisi ... and Saint Francis's fortitude. Lord, give me his strength!"

In the harbor, a Dutch admiralty fleet was riding at anchor, and Dirck later learned they would escort his fleet to the Portuguese border, as requested by Holland's Advocate Oldenbarnevelt. After reprovisioning his ships and hiring a skilled pilot for the next leg of the journey, Dirck stood on deck and gave the signal to get underway. It was a glorious day with sunlight dancing on the gentle waves.

After the ships were on a steady course, Dirck handed the helm to his first mate Rykaard Jr., retrieved his Waghaener map, and joined Jacques and Margaretha at the rail. "I want to see how accurate this map is." The three began comparing the coastline to the features shown on the map, and by the time the fleet was turning away from shore to cross the Bay of Biscay, all agreed that it was indeed very accurate. "Thanks again, Jacques, for giving me this valuable map."

"My pleasure," Jacques said and left to find a place to take a nap in the sun.

Margaretha rested her arms on the rail. "I love the sea when it's like this. I know it won't last, and I've decided not to complain when it changes, because Saint Francis said that storms and rain are our brother and are necessary to sustain us." She sighed. "I so look forward to reaching Livorno and making a pilgrimage to Assisi to see Saint Francis's grave."

Dirck was pleased to see his aunt again at peace with the sea, but the mention of Saint Francis raised a nagging question for him. "Aunt Margaretha, isn't Saint Francis the founder of the Franciscan Minor Friar order, the one that operated the Inquisition? Does that bother you?"

"Ja, it greatly saddens me that good friars can so easily be corrupted by an evil king. But their brutal misdeeds take nothing away from the good works of Saint Francis and his *true* disciples."

"Hmm ... Father said that some Sea Beggars were corrupted in the same way by cruel leaders." He watched his aunt acknowledge his comment and then stare at the sea and drift into one of those mystical meditations his father had spoken of.

After the fleet cleared the northwest coast of Spain and was approaching the Portuguese border, the admiralty ships turned back to French waters, and the pilot instructed Dirck's captains to give wide berth to the coast. For a few days, the Dutch ships sailed within sight of each other in relatively calm seas, until a storm rolled in and scattered the fleet. After it cleared, Dirck nervously scanned the ocean but had difficulty seeing any ships in the still rough seas, so he sent a lookout up the mast.

"I SEE ONE, PORT SIDE!" the lookout called from his perch. "ANOTHER TO STARBOARD." Later, he confirmed, "I SEE MOST OF THE FLEET."

Good, Dirck thought, relieved.

"SOMETHING OFF THE BOW."

"ONE OF OURS?"

"JUST A DOT. CAN'T TELL!" Later, he reported, "THERE ARE TWO DOTS!"

The pilot came on deck and stared at the dots. As the sea calmed and they came into better view, he concluded: "Not ours ... too big. Probably Portuguese, or possibly Spanish."

Over the coming hour, the wind shifted, abated, and shifted again. The two mystery ships were visible now.

"They're *Nao*—Portuguese great ships," the pilot confirmed, "most likely returning from the East Indies with spices."

"They're *huge*," Dirck commented. "Could be twelve-hundred tons. And they have such high prows and sterns."

"They're a carrack design," the pilot explained. "The Portuguese improved on the Venetian and Genoan carracks, and made them larger. They are enormous ... probably have three or four decks, a poop and forecastle." He observed them again. "They're sailing sluggishly. Must be fully loaded."

"Are they heavily armed? Should we be concerned?"

"Nee, not as heavily as you'd expect. They don't like to carry the extra weight of armaments, and instead prefer additional cargo—often far more than is safe." The pilot checked the *Amsterdam Ascendant's* sails, which were billowing, and the sea. "Don't worry. We're in a current that should take us out of their path, especially on this freshening wind."

Meanwhile, Jacques's mind was on the spice trade. "Uncle Konrad says the Portuguese have a complete monopoly on pepper and most spices."

Dirck had never before heard the word monopoly, but guessed its meaning from the Latin word *monopolium*—right or exclusive sale—and silently thanked his father for insisting he complete Latin school.

"He says," Jacques continued, "the Portuguese control the source of spices in the East, *and* prices in Europe. There's no other competition, except for an occasional overland spice caravan that comes through Egypt."

"Wouldn't it be a feat to take one of those *Naos* as a prize?" Dirck speculated.

"Having the monopoly would be better yet."

"Now there's a thought," Dirck said. "Next time, I'll have to set my sights higher."

—~—

Meanwhile in Amsterdam, Betje took charge of Catrijn's pregnancy and did everything that custom dictated, including making her fast during the final month, which forced the starving mother-to-be to scavenge the kitchen whenever alone in the house.

When Catrijn's labor started, Betje lit a candle and was pleased that it burned with a blue flame, a sure sign no evil spirits were present.

On November 21, 1590, a healthy girl was born and named Jaane after Catrijn's mother, and time-honored rituals went into motion. The midwife gave the baby first to grandmother Betje. She sneaked a speck of salt onto the baby's tongue to ward away evil before passing her to Godmother Griet. Each gave the midwife a tip. While Catrijn ate buttered bread and ewe's cheese, the midwife cleaned and dressed Jaane before handing her to Konrad and saying, "Here is your child. May Our Lord grant you much happiness through her, or else may He call her back to Him soon." Konrad gave her a tip and proudly donned a quilted satin hat with feathers.

To the front door, Betje lovingly attached a lace-trimmed wooden placard, to which she had added a piece of white paper to signify a girl had been born. Later she saw to the proper burial of the afterbirth in the backyard, while Catrijn's maid went out to spread word of the birth.

Soon the scent of the traditional drink for the occasion—a hot caudle consisting of wine, bread, sugar, and spices—wafted through the house. It was ready just in time for the arrival of well-wishers.

Betje then turned her attention to Griet, who was approaching the final months of her pregnancy, and to baking *speculaas koekjes* with copious amounts of cloves and pepper for recently married Pieter and Floris.

Dirck's fleet sailed along the coasts of Portugal and Spain without incident, passed through the Strait of Gibraltar, also known as the Pillars of Hercules according to the pilot, and entered the Mediterranean. In seas varying from glassy to roiling, the ships threaded their way through the Balearic Islands, rounded the tip of Corsica and at last sighted Livorno. Dirck passed the helm of the *Amsterdam Ascendant* to the pilot, who led the fleet between the fortified outer islands and into the harbor. While the ships were anchoring, the sun slowly sank in the west and cast its orangey brilliance on Livorno's imposing Fortress Vecchia.

In the morning, Dirck, his captains and Margaretha went ashore. Lodewyk and his sons were waiting at the dock, and Jacques made the introductions and mentioned that Margaretha wanted to make a pilgrimage to Assisi.

The first order of business was for Dirck to inform port officials of the purpose and length of the fleet's intended stay, and, afterward, allow them to inspect the holds. Lodewyk's sons went along and translated for him. Meanwhile, Lodewyk walked with Jacques and Margaretha to his house where they were going to stay. En route, a gentleman cheerily called out, *"Lorenzo, Ciao!"*

"Ciao, Giovanni!" Lodewyk called back and tipped his plumed hat.

"Lorenzo?" Jacques questioned, having never heard him called that previously.

"I've found it is better to fit in, than to resist. People like Lorenzo better than Lodewyk. So what can I do?" Lodewyk shrugged his shoulders and threw up his hands in a very un-Netherlandic way. "Besides, I like Lorenzo. More lyrical, no?"

"Si," Margaretha agreed with a sly grin, for she was already finding this Lodewyk/Lorenzo fellow in his colorful and ultra-stylish clothes to be both intriguing and charming. He was similar in appearance to Konrad Teller, but possessed a unique and appealing quality—panache—which set him apart.

Dirck and Lodewyk's sons completed their work and arrived at Lodewyk's home in time for a sumptuous late afternoon lunch. During the leisurely meal, Lodewyk revealed the sad news of his wife's recent passing. Condolences followed, but he seemed not to want to dwell on his loss and instead peppered Jacques with questions.

"How is Konrad doing? Is he happy?"

"Very. He and Catrijn are a compatible couple." Jacques looked to Margaretha for confirmation, and she nodded agreement. "Their first child is probably being born right now."

"Do you have a painting of Catrijn? I want to see this woman who captured my cousin's heart."

Jacques said he did not, and Lodewyk instructed him: "Next time you come, you must bring a portrait of Konrad, Catrijn and the newborn. There's nothing more important than family."

"Here, here," Margaretha said and raised her glass.

After all the toasting, talking, and eating ended, it was too late to do anything else, and Lodewyk proclaimed, "Tomorrow we work."

In the morning, Lodewyk boarded Dirck's ships and particularly liked the quality of the rye and wheat, saying that Polish grains were the best in Europe and would fetch high prices. The dried fish also met with his approval, but the Dutch Republic flags flying on many of the ships did not.

"You shouldn't fly those," Lodewyk warned Dirck. "Spanish ships won't hesitate to seize any vessel with a Dutch Republic flag. You were truly fortunate not to encounter any on your journey here, but on your way home you may not be so lucky."

"What else would we fly?"

"You'd do better with a flag of the Netherlands or even Spain. I know, I know, you don't want to lie about your proud Dutch Republic origins. But I advise you to get other flags and documents—you never know when they'll come in handy. And don't forget that your Dutch Republic is still under King Philip's domain, until he agrees to let you go. So in a way, a Spanish flag would be legitimate since you're bringing goods from an Antwerper in Amsterdam to an Antwerper in Livorno."

"You're probably right," Dirck said. "I've also heard that Corsair pirates, from Africa, harass ships at sea. Do we need to worry about them too?"

"Corsairs go after ships carrying gold, arms, and other high-value goods, which they can easily identify by the abundance of cannons aboard." Lodewyk glanced at the Dutch fleet. "You have few, so they'd know you carry bulk goods and probably leave you alone—unless they wanted your ship, or men. They always need more ships and slaves."

The next day began the process of transferring cargo to Lodewyk's warehouses and Lodewyk and his sons contacting prospective buyers. On the fourth day, Lodewyk offered to take Margaretha on a tour of Livorno.

"Aren't you too busy?" Margaretha asked.

"Nee, my sons and your captains are quite capable of doing their work without me, and I've already sent word to my buyers, many of whom live outside Livorno. When they start arriving in a few days, I'll be busy. Until then, I want to enjoy your company and show you our lovely city."

Lodewyk took her for a stroll, wending his way down sun drenched streets, up densely shaded ones, and along canals, and pointing out churches that seemed modest to Margaretha, compared to Amsterdam's masterpieces, and residences that were more regal than any she had ever seen. He noted where the Arno River came into the city. In front of a massive red-brick bastion under construction, he halted.

"This will defend the northeastern approach to the city and is truly a modern marvel. There are underground passageways that allow troops to move quickly and stealthily to where an attack is occurring." He noticed Margaretha's eyes going blank. "Shall we go on?"

"Margaretha, tell me about the Beguines. What do they do? Pray all day? In a remote cloister?"

"Heavens nee," Margaretha said with a chortle. "We do pray, but we're too busy to pray *all* day. Our Begijnhof is in the heart of Amsterdam, and everyday we're out in the city working with needy children and women in distress ... destitute ones or those with illegitimate pregnancies."

"My, I thought Catholic nuns mostly led quiet lives of contemplation."

"We're not nuns. We're Beguines. There is a difference. We come with our own money, own our homes, and are free to leave whenever we want. There are no lifetime vows like nuns take."

"Hmm, how does one become a Beguine?"

"Choose to be a Beguine and agree not to marry, be chaste, and live a modest life. There is an eighteen-month trial period, and after that it takes a few more years to be accepted into our sisterhood. But you can still leave at anytime, perhaps to get married, or simply if you decide a Beguine's life is no longer for you."

"Hmm, very interesting."

As they neared home, several men passed by and Lodewyk returned their "*Ciao!*"

"Lorenzo," Margaretha said, "I can't help but notice you dress and act more like an Italian than a Netherlander."

"It's true," Lorenzo said with a smile. "It seems I've adopted many of their traits over the years. Most of them good ... but unfortunately a few bad ones too." His mood changed, as though something unpleasant had entered his mind. "I'm not as virtuous as my cousin, Konrad, I'm sorry to say."

The next day, Lorenzo stopped by his house to tell Margaretha he had arranged for his eldest son Giovanni to take her to Assisi, where he had business to conduct. Lorenzo promised to give her more details after supper.

By the time supper was over and others were disappearing upstairs to their bedrooms, Margaretha was fatigued and wished she too could go to bed. Nevertheless, she accepted Lorenzo's enthusiastic offer to go with him to the rooftop terrace and take in the fresh air and full moon.

A table and two chairs awaited them, and Lorenzo brought a bottle of wine and two glasses, as well as a woolen throw. After wrapping the throw around Margaretha and asking whether she was comfortable, Lorenzo poured the wine, made small talk about the weather and the brilliance of the moon, and took a sizable gulp from his glass.

"Margaretha, I have a big favor to ask of you when you go to Assisi." He pulled a letter from within his cape. "I'd like you to deliver this to my daughter Maria and bring her back to Livorno with you. Maria lives with the Poor Clares in their convent in Assisi.

She hates her life—though they seem to treat her well—and has been sending more letters than usual, begging me to bring her here."

"So why haven't you brought her back by now? She must be free to leave the Poor Clares because you said she *lives* with them, which I assume means she hasn't taken her vows."

Lorenzo's eyes closed momentarily, and, when they opened, Margaretha saw tears glistening.

"Maria is illegitimate. And an illegitimate child doesn't have many options for leading a normal life in Italy, especially one from a Calvinist father and prominent Catholic mother." His eyes took on a distant look. "We do things we shouldn't; we don't know why. Passion? A few moments of pleasure? Love? But the child, beautiful Maria, is the one who suffers. Her mother can't acknowledge her and chose to place her with the Poor Clares. I'm the only one who visits and keeps up her spirits. I also pay for her to have the best life possible there."

"What will Maria do here in Livorno?"

"Nothing. That's the problem. Men from good Catholic families wouldn't marry her, and I doubt a good Calvinist would either. There is no life for her here. But you can give her a new one in Amsterdam. From what you've told me, she can live in the Begijnhof with you while she decides what to do. I will send her money, and my cousin Konrad will embrace her as family."

"Well ... I'm not—I don't know what to say. I'll have to think about it."

While the moon slowly made its way across the sky, the two talked further about Maria's plight, and in the end Margaretha agreed.

En route to Assisi, Margaretha enjoyed the rolling landscape, which was wearing its winter colors and dotted with dramatic hill towns, while Giovanni regaled her with grisly tales of town rivalries and perfidy. Along the way, he also confessed to having only recently learned of Maria and that he had visited her just once with his father. Yet when they arrived at the Poor Clare cloister, Maria treated him like a brother she had known forever.

Margaretha found Maria to be a courteous, attractive,

well-mannered and well-read young woman, much as Lorenzo and Giovanni had described her. Also that she looked more Italian than Dutch with her sun-kissed complexion and lustrous dark hair. Neither, though, had mentioned she had a curvaceous body, too much natural sensuality for her own good, and was completely inexperienced in life. Margaretha knew she had a *big* job on her hands.

Margaretha gave the letter to Maria, and Maria cried joyously and asked only one question: How soon can we leave? When Margaretha went with Maria to her room to collect her belongings, Margaretha discovered a new meaning of the word *modest*. The Begijnhof was modest, but the Poor Clares' accommodations made the Begijnhof look absolutely luxurious.

With a box under her arm, which contained all her worldly possessions—books, sewing needles, quill pens and ink—Maria raced out of the cloister.

The three arrived at Lodewyk's house to find no one at home, except for the servants who were waiting with gift boxes of new clothes for Maria from her father. A flood of tears was unleashed as well as a request to try them on immediately. Maids carried them upstairs to the bedroom, and Maria, astounded by the splendor of the room, wandered around touching the heavy drapes, silk bedspread, and carved wood. Turning to the clothes, Maria quickly disrobed and, rejecting the maid's help, put on every single garment before deciding to wear the prettiest underwear, softest leather shoes, and an elegant dark green velvet dress. Completing the outfit was a hat with a black lace veil, which could be raised or lowered.

After beholding herself in the mirror, twirling around, and smiling contentedly, Maria said to the maid, "Burn these, please," and pointed to the pile of Poor Clare clothes on the floor.

"Nee!" Margaretha said. "We'll keep them." She was thinking a nun-like habit might come in handy on the voyage to discourage unwanted advances.

When Maria and Margaretha made their entrance downstairs,

the men were sipping wine in the dining room while a musician played a lute.

"*Bellissima!*" Lodewyk rushed to Maria, kissed both cheeks, and escorted her into the dining room. Giovanni offered his arm to Margaretha.

Dirck saw Maria come through the door—Geez!—and went to greet her.

Seeing Dirck take a step, Jacques spun around—Wow!—and followed the mass movement toward the stunning young lady.

Lodewyk announced that Maria was his daughter, shocking some of his sons, and that she was moving to Amsterdam. He introduced her to the half-brothers first, and each embraced her, bringing tears to her eyes. He presented Jacques, saying he was a relative of his cousin, Konrad, but not her blood relative. All the while, Maria blushed, flustered by the attention.

Jacques gallantly kissed her hand. "È un onore conoscerti, signorina. Tu porti il sole ai miei occhi."

Maria looked as though she might swoon.

Next came Dirck. Following Jacques's lead, he kissed Maria's hand and said, "*Signorina*," mispronouncing it.

She smiled and blushed again.

The meal commenced and attention focused on Maria, with her half-brothers wanting to know more about her. What did she do at the Poor Clares? Did she read? Draw? Sculpt? Have a garden? Unaccustomed to the fast-flowing discussions that prevailed at Lodewyk's table, Maria answered every question thoughtfully and with brevity. Soon it became evident she was not skilled in the fine art of social intercourse, and the conversation shifted to Margaretha.

"Did you have a rewarding pilgrimage to Assisi?" Lodewyk inquired.

"What are your impressions?" one of his sons asked.

"Everything about Assisi was inspiring, from kneeling at Saint Francis's tomb beneath the sublime frescoes depicting his humble and humanitarian life, to visiting the tomb of his companion, Saint Claire, founder of the Poor Clare order. But the most exciting part was when wild boars charged our coach and our horses took off.

Giovanni yelled, 'Hold on!' and pulled and pulled on the reins. Then he stood up—Giovanni actually stood up. More amazing, he jumped onto one of the horses! It was a hair-raising ride, until he finally brought the horses to a halt." She laughed. "And we lived!"

Grinning, Giovanni rose and took a bow. Their companions burst into applause.

The conversation moved on, and Margaretha sat back, sipping wine and observing the interplay of personalities. Lodewyk and his sons were growing ever more voluble and their hand gestures increasingly demonstrative. The musician played on, though could barely be heard. Jacques was angling for Maria's attention, and she was stealing furtive glances at Dirck. Margaretha suspected Maria had the misimpression that Dirck was a kindred spirit because he rarely spoke, not knowing his silence was rooted in language. He did not understand or speak Italian.

After dessert, Margaretha and Maria retired, and the men disbursed. Dirck brought a bottle of wine to where Jacques had sat down and refilled their glasses.

"Jacques, you said something in Italian when you were introduced to Maria that she seemed to like. What was it?"

Jacques repeated it, his finger waving in the air to the flow of the words, as if they were music. "It means: It is an honor to meet you mademoiselle. You are sunshine to my eyes."

"Nice. Can you teach me that?"

"Of course not," Jacques said with a laugh. "You have to develop your *own* lines."

In the coming week, preparations for departure were made. Provisions were purchased, and goods to sell in the north were loaded, chiefly wine, olive oil, and leather and sundry goods. Jacques's brocades and colony of silk worms also went into the hold. On the *Amsterdam Ascendant*, Aunt Margaretha's walled-off portion of Dirck's cabin was enlarged to accommodate Maria. With much less space for the men, Dirck informed Jacques that he would be traveling aboard Rykaard's ship along with the pilot. Jacques protested, but Dirck said there simply was no room for him, though his wry smile belied his pleasure in putting distance between Jacques and Maria.

At the farewell meal, gifts were exchanged. Lodewyk gave Dirck a stylish hat whose soft brim sloped down on one side and was adorned with a plucky feather. He said, with a coy smile, "I hope you will remember me by this," but in fact his goal was to help Dirck realize how utterly artless his somber flat-brimmed hat and beret with ear flaps tucked inside were.

In turn, Dirck presented Lodewyk with a map of the Netherlands, depicted as a bellicose lion. "I hope this gift will remind you of your family and friends at home." The Leo map, as it was known, was fast becoming an icon of the nascent Dutch Republic, and Dirck was lucky to have found two of them to purchase, the other being a gift for his father.

Jacques made the most of his last evening with Maria, charming her with clever comments and humorous asides.

When the fleet set sail, Dirck gave a final wave to Livorno, confident that he would return to trade again and again. Profits from the sale of his foodstuffs had been so good he had been able to buy huge quantities of goods to sell in the north and also have money left over, which was now safely stored in his strongbox. Beside him stood Maria, who was not the least bit interested in returning to Italy, except perhaps to see her father. When Dirck glanced her way, she smiled up at him with hope in her eyes.

Homeward bound, Dirck steered the *Amsterdam Ascendant* through the outer fortress islands and around Corsica. With every tack and shift of the sails, he began noticing men bumping into each other and lines slipping from hands, leaving sails to flap. The wind was not especially strong, the sea was relatively calm, but Maria was on deck, and the men were mesmerized. Dirck ordered the carpenter to construct makeshift chairs on the rear deck for the women and erect a canvas barrier to conceal them. In time the novelty of Maria's presence diminished, and the rhythm of sea life resumed.

The fleet successfully navigated its way back through the Strait of Gibraltar and into the Atlantic Ocean. Off the coast of Portugal, storm clouds formed on the horizon. They coalesced and grew taller, and the Dutchmen were treated to a brilliant display of lightning. There were oohs and aahs, as flashes of light exploded and danced through the cloud bank. It was a heavenly sight that went on for hours.

Then the cloud bank started marching toward them, and the rumble of distant thunder intensified.

Dirck ordered the women into the cabin and the men to secure everything on deck and to haul in the sails, except for a small one. That sail plus the rudder would hopefully allow the *Amsterdam Ascendant* to track through the massive swells that were on their way.

The storm advanced, pushing wind ahead of it. Gusts snatched lines from hands, and sails flew loose and rap-rap-rapped. The sea grew turbulent and washed across the deck. Sensing that the storm was going to be ferocious, Dirck sent the men below to ride it out. After closing their hatch securely, he, the carpenter and first mate Rykaard Jr. sloshed across the deck to the captain's cabin. Dirck opened the door. Margaretha and Maria were huddled together and staring wide-eyed at him.

"Rykaard's going to stay with you," Dirck said to the women, "You'll be safe."

Before stepping into the cabin, Rykaard paused. "Dirck, are you *sure* you don't want my help?"

"Nee, you're too valuable. If anything happens to me, you'll need to take over." Dirck grinned at the carpenter, who was tall and muscular. "Anyway, I need his strength to help muscle the tiller, plus he knows how to make repairs."

The carpenter forced a confident look and followed Dirck to the helm, and they lashed themselves to it.

Lightning was flaring all around, and thunder clapped in close succession—Flash—CRACK—Flash—CRACK. Swells were becoming massive.

"*We're in for it now, cap'n!*" The carpenter's bulging eyes were fixed straight ahead.

Dirck turned and saw a wave exploding over the bow. "*Hold on!*"

A wall of water smashed into them and exited over the gunwale.

Coughing and sputtering, the two scrambled to their feet and prepared for the next onslaught.

The storm raged on, with waves smashing into the hull, seemingly from every direction. The *Amsterdam Ascendant* pitched and yawed violently. Amid the din of the storm, Dirck heard a *creeeak* coming from the center of the deck. While blinking water from his eyes, he watched with alarm as the longboat broke loose, torqued sideways, scraped along the deck—crashed into the mast—and skidded toward the starboard gunwale. A final push from a wave washing across the deck shoved the longboat through the gunwale and into the raging sea, taking rigging with it.

Creeeak ... CRASH. A tremor ran through the ship.

"Saint Francis give us courage," Margaretha prayed and pulled Maria tighter to her.

"Heavenly Jesus—don't let me die—not *now!*"

On one of Amsterdam's coldest days of winter, Griet gave birth to a boy. Nicolaas had already decided on a name, Rolfe, because it sounded robust and manly and utterly unlike his own, which people readily turned into a silly pun about Saint Nicolaas or jovial Sinterklaas.

While Nicolaas waited outside the birthing room, the midwife passed the newborn first to grandmother Betje and then to godmother Catrijn, and both pronounced him to be adorable.

Adorable? Nicolaas thought to himself. I don't want my boy to be adorable! Just saying the word made his lips turn down in disgust. He burst in.

"You shouldn't be in here!" the midwife said.

"Just let me see him."

The blanket was pulled back—Nicolaas was aghast. His son wasn't adorable at all. He wasn't even cute. He was coated with stuff, and his face was red and grimacing.

"We have to bathe him," the midwife said. "Go!"

In the hallway, Nicolaas paced to the sound of splashing water and an occasional tiny cry of protest. Finally the midwife emerged and placed Rolfe in his arms.

Nicolaas stared at the little face, clean now and angelic, and touched the soft cheek. "Hello there little Rolfe." Nicolaas cleared his throat and changed his voice into a deeper one. "I mean *Rolfe*." Rolfe's eyes popped open and his adorable pink lips puckered and smacked, convincing Nicolaas the little guy was trying to talk to him. Rolfe's fists rose and legs kicked rambunctiously, confirming he was surely going to be feisty and strong and live up to his name. He tweaked his son's chin. The tyke seemed to giggle. "Oh boy, are we going to have fun, *Rolfe*."

"Oh!" The midwife said, startled at hearing Rolfe said in such a gruff voice.

Nicolaas looked at her. "It's time for a drink. Where's the caudle? And my hat?"

Dirck watched in horror as the mainmast snapped and slammed onto the deck, just missing him. Along with it came a shower of broken spars, smacking his head and flattening him to the deck. The rain-soaked sail fell hard against his body. Pinned there and dazed, he feebly pushed the canvas up. A wave swamped the sail, pressing it against his face. Gasping for breath, he shoved at the unyielding cloth. The wave retreated and the pressure on the sail diminished, and he frantically gulped in air. Another wall of water forced down the canvas. His breath spent, he lost consciousness.

Waves continued to batter the ship.

As soon as Rykaard Jr. felt the energy of the storm lessen, he told the women not to move and tried to open the cabin door. Debris was blocking it, but he was able to force it open a crack. "*Dirck!*" he called out. Getting no response, he threw his body against the door until it opened enough to squeeze out. There before him lay devastation. The longboat was gone. The broken mainmast lay atop the helm, rocking as the ship heaved and rolled. A tangle of canvas and lines covered the rear half of the ship and hung over the side.

"*Dirck!*" Rykaard climbed onto the mast. "*Dirck!*"

A faint voice filtered through the dense fog in Dirck's head. It came again, and he tried to float toward the sound. The haze in his head began thinning. Gradually he became aware of his body.

"*Dirck!* Are you here?"

Dirck's eyes opened ... everything was fuzzy.

Rykaard was scrambling along the edge of the canvas and looking under.

To his right, Dirck saw daylight. Wriggling, he moved toward it and grasped the edge of the sail—

"Dirck!" Rykaard exclaimed and gripped his hand, then his shoulders and pulled him out.

"Where ... carpenter?" Dirck asked in a slow, confused voice. "What ... "

Seeing his stupor, Rykaard warned, "Don't move. I'll find him," and climbed over the mast to search on the other side.

Dirck rested on his haunches and stared at the deck, his head gradually clearing. A puff of wind carried faint voices:

"Cap'n!" "Help!"

The men! Dirck clambered toward the hatch and shoved away debris. The men pushed it open. Dirck looked in and asked:

"Everyone ... right?"

"Think so," the boatswain said, as he emerged. "Dirck, you got a nasty gash there. Are *you* all right?"

Still lightheaded, Dirck slowly moved his hand to his head, and blood oozed between his fingers.

"Sit down, Dirck," Rykaard said and began helping men out of the hold. "Anyone hurt?"

"Gonna puke," a seaman said and ran to the gunwale.

The next was grimacing. "My arm, think it's broken."

Alert now, Dirck wiped the blood from his eye and joined Rykaard, "Where's the carpenter?"

"Dead," Rykaard said, "crushed by the mast. Must of died instantly."

Men kept coming up from below. A seasoned sailor with a huge toothless grin proclaimed, "Damn! What a wild ride!"

Another was shaking badly and said nothing.

"Holy hell … hope I never see another one like that!"

Margaretha appeared in the cabin doorway. "May we come out?"

Dirck answered yes, and Margaretha began walking around inspecting the injured. "Let me help," she said to the man with a broken arm and turned to Maria. "Get some cloth … my extra head scarf will do."

Margaretha used the cloth to tie a splint to the man's arm, and went on to Dirck and forced him to sit down so she could bandage his head. All the while, his eyes were scanning the sea. In the distance, he saw the *Nicolaas II* and was pleased that her sails were mostly intact. Several other ships of the fleet were following behind.

Meanwhile, Rykaard ordered a contingent of men to haul up the sail and rigging dragging in the water and assigned sailors to gather pieces of timber. He then took Dirck to the carpenter's body, and together they prepared it for burial at sea.

When the *Nicolaas II* came into hailing distance, Rykaard Sr. scanned the deck of the *Amsterdam Ascendant* and was relieved to see his son waving at him. He shouted to Dirck, "*Ahoy! Everyone all right?*"

"*The carpenter was killed when the mast fell on him,*" Dirck called back. "*Some men are injured, but none real serious.*"

"*Dirck, can we help?*"

"*That's Lisbon over there!*" the pilot said, pointing and looking worried.

Dirck swung around to see a large town nestled below undulating hills and a harbor full of ships.

"The Portuguese will come sooner or later to see what we're up to," the pilot called out.

Dirck glanced around the deck. *"Well … there's no way I can make enough repairs to sail away before they do."*

"*What do you want to do?*" Rykaard Sr. asked.

"*We can't do anything, except wait,*" Dirck replied with a tone of resignation. "*But I want you to take the fleet and continue on. There's no point in you getting caught up in this.*"

Rykaard Sr. did not protest. "*Do you want me to take your aunt and the girl?*"

"*Absolutely not!*" Margaretha said, "*I'm staying with Dirck and his men,*" believing she was their only protection because the Portuguese would never dare harm someone they thought was a nun. "*And Maria stays with me!*" There was no way she would let a vulnerable young woman sail, unprotected, all the way back to Amsterdam with so many men.

Rykaard Sr. set the fleet on a course toward open water.

After Dirck oversaw the burial of the carpenter at sea, work resumed on deck, and Margaretha went into the cabin with Maria. Dirck did a final check of the ship, making sure no Dutch Republic flags were on display.

Two Portuguese naval vessels arrived after pieces of broken mast and spars had been stacked and lashed neatly together, as well as torn pieces of sailcloth.

Margaretha positioned herself prominently on deck, with Maria behind her looking demure yet haughty like a noblewoman, as Margaretha had instructed. Maria wore her best clothes and the hat with the black veil down. Dirck gave a tug to his hat, the one with a feather and brim that slouched to one side.

The Portuguese officer came aboard with a detachment of armed men and walked directly toward Dirck.

Margaretha stepped in his path and boldly addressed him in French and then in broken Spanish (she did not speak Portuguese). "I am Sister Margaretha. We have just come from Livorno and are on a very important mission to deliver Senorita Maria della Papallo Delgado," a name she made up, "to Antwerp in the Netherlands to his Most Excellency Senor Francesco Louis Diego Penaranda," another made-up name that hopefully sounded important. "Senor Penaranda hired this captain," she nodded toward Dirck, "to take us there. We request your assistance to make repairs so we can resume our journey as soon as possible. Senor Penaranda will be most unhappy otherwise, as will his commander, the Duke of Parma."

The Portuguese captain gave a graceful and deferential bow to Maria. "Senorita, it is an honor."

Dirck was dumbfounded and humbled, for he had just witnessed a deeply religious and selfless Beguine risk the fires of hell by telling a whopper of a lie, just to save him and his men.

When the Portuguese captain turned to him, Dirck used fragments of Latin, Italian, and French, plus a profusion of gesturing to explain how he intended to rig a temporary mast and attach a salvaged sail to get the ship to Lisbon.

Escorted by the two Portuguese ships, the *Amsterdam Ascendant* limped into a small harbor not far from Lisbon. Dirck noticed how little protection it afforded from incoming Atlantic swells and hoped another storm would not hit. A shipwright came aboard to determine the materials required and to quote a price, which Dirck quickly learned was not negotiable. The work began promptly and went smoothly, though Dirck did complain more than once that he would rather be in Lisbon's harbor where prices were undoubtedly lower, the water calmer, and where he would have a chance to see a *Nao* ship up close.

Margaretha reminded Dirck to count his lucky stars instead of complain. In Lisbon, their ruse was likely to be exposed when someone invited Senorita Maria della Papallo Delgado ashore to dine with important Portuguese personages. And heaven forbid anyone came aboard to meet her and saw the tiny, austere cabin she occupied with a Beguine *and* the captain.

Dirck did, however, take the opportunity to record details of the harbor and coastline on his Waghenaer map.

After the repairs were made, the Portuguese officer came aboard one last time. He brought a man introduced as the customs inspector, who reviewed Dirck's manifest and delivered the bill for port duties. It could be paid in silver, gold, or goods. If not paid, the cargo would be seized.

Dirck wanted to object to the outrageous amount—40% of the estimated cargo value—but Margaretha advised him to go to his strongbox instead.

While sailing northward, Dirck tried several times to thank Aunt Margaretha for saving him and his men and to tell her how humbled he was by her selfless act. She always responded matter-of-factly, "desperate times require desperate actions, and I did it for all of us," and refused to discuss it. He thought he saw remorse in her eyes, though, which saddened him.

The *Amsterdam Ascendant* called in at La Rochelle, and Dirck found a letter waiting for him from Rykaard Sr., which had been written nearly four weeks earlier.

> Dear Dirck,
> We leave today. All is well. I wish you a safe voyage to Amsterdam.
>
> Your faithful friend,
> Rykaard Sr.

Maria observed Dirck reading the letter. Worried, she asked Margaretha, "È la lettera da una donna?" Is the letter from a woman?

"*No, da un capitano di mare.*" Margaretha responded. No, it is from a sea captain.

Dirck pointed to himself with a grin—"*Capitano di mare*?"—assuming they were talking about him, for Aunt Margaretha had told him that it was his title, captain of the sea.

"Nee, nee." Margaretha shook her head and laughed. "Maria asked if the letter was from a woman, a *donna,* assuming the elegant script was written by a female. I told her it was from a sea captain, but didn't say it was Rykaard, because she probably wouldn't believe that such a rugged man could write so beautifully and might think I was trying to conceal that you had a lady friend."

Maria understood not a word and smiled sweetly at Dirck.

While the *Amsterdam Ascendant* was being provisioned and a replacement longboat brought aboard, Dirck gave the women a tour of La Rochelle. Maria took in the scene without saying a word, from the half-timbered houses to the French language, which she had never heard before. Her only comment came when they visited the Calvinist church.

"*Perché non ci sono belle finestre, statue o affreschi in questa chiesa?*" Why are there no beautiful windows, statues, or frescoes in this church?

Margaretha's first instinct was to say—They were violently

ripped out by intolerant Calvinist zealots, who believed their reformed version of Christianity was better!—which made her cringe. She always refrained from disparaging others' beliefs and could only attribute it to her heightened appreciation of Catholicism after having been in Italy and probably lingering anger at Amsterdam's Calvinists for trying to convert the boarded-up Holy Place Church into a lowly and unholy storage warehouse. They might have succeeded, if not for Maarten persuading the city council to object to it. After reining in her emotions, Margaretha answered Maria's question with equanimity:

"Maria, I will let Dirck explain the lack of decorations to you."

"We Calvinists believe that graven images and statues of saints aren't necessary. And they should never be prayed to," Dirck said, assuming that Maria wanted to have an informed discussion about Calvinism versus Catholicism. Margaretha continued translating between the two.

"*I Santi non sono necessari? No Saint Claire? No Saint Francis?*" Saints aren't necessary? Not Saint Clare? Not Saint Francis?

"Nee, um, they were invented by popes, not God," Dirck said.

Maria glared at him, incredulous. "*Che cosa?*" What?

"Those saints are not in the Bible. I've read it. Have—" Dirck stopped, realizing this conversation was not endearing him to her, and turned to Aunt Margaretha with pleading eyes. "Maybe Konrad should explain this."

"Dirck has a good idea," Margaretha said and gave him a wink. "Your Uncle Konrad can explain this better. You have much to learn, and there will be ample time in the future. Today, we should enjoy being on terra firma, and Dirck doubtlessly has additional interesting things to show you."

"Would you like to sample some French cheese?" Dirck asked with a beguiling smile, "and wine too?"

Rykaard had informed Maarten of the *Amsterdam Ascendant*'s damage and of Maria being aboard, so when the ship was spotted in the harbor, the entire family assembled quayside at the Damrak to welcome them home. Catrijn, holding her newborn, waved excitedly at Aunt Margaretha, as the lighter glided to the dock, and Nicolaas held his Rolfe aloft for all to see.

Margaretha was the first to disembark, and the babies were placed in her arms. With teary eyes she nuzzled each in turn.

Jacques was at hand to help Maria alight, and Catrijn was disbelieving that the young woman, whom Rykaard had described as a "former nun," was in fact an exotic beauty with an aptitude for fashion. Her green dress was stunning and so was the matching hat, whose veil she lifted to exchange cheek kisses with Jacques and Konrad. Catrijn noticed that Dirck's eyes were on Maria, as he disembarked, and saw her glance back to meet his gaze.

As soon as Dirck was on land, Nicolaas brought Rolfe to him. "Surprise! This is *my Rolfe*, your godson, and this is my wife Griet."

"You've been busy," Dirck said and greeted Griet, while Nicolaas passed the infant to him, who almost immediately started squirming. "He's just like his father, already on the go."

Catrijn arrived, bussed Dirck's cheek, and placed Jaane in the curve of his other arm. "This is Jaane, your goddaughter."

Jaane's alert eyes connected with his, and Dirck cooed to her angelic but rather plain face. Feeling his plumed hat fly off his head, he turned. "Hey!"

Grinning at him was Nicolaas with the hat sitting rakishly over one eye. Catrijn snatched it and examined the feather—"Very stylish"—before returning it to Dirck's head.

In the coming weeks, Konrad took to heart Lodewyk's request for a portrait, and he and Catrijn hired an elderly journeyman painter. They also offered to pay for portraits of other family members, and only Margaretha declined.

Prior to the sittings, the portraitist instructed everyone on how to dress—in Calvinist black—but granted an exception for Maria, whose green dress he hoped to capture in exacting detail, especially the nap and shimmer of the velvet. He stipulated that no one look at his portrait before it was finished.

In his studio, the artist posed each subject in a setting full of symbols. The bible showed religious devotion, and skull and hourglass illustrated the transience of life. For men, he included a business ledger and coins representing hard work and productivity. For women, there was a broom and ball of thread to show domesticity.

Griet and Nicolaas were the first to sit for their portrait because he was leaving shortly for Gdansk. For the same reason, Dirck was next, and he wore his feathered hat and brought a few of his maps, which the artist placed in the background.

Maria came with Jacques, who would serve as her interpreter. She remained afterward, while Jacques sat for his portrait.

When Catrijn and Konrad's turn came, they arrived with books, maps, and paintings, and Catrijn requested that the broom be removed if there was not enough space to display everything. The painter reluctantly complied and also allowed her to hold both Jaane and a book in her lap. During the sitting, the artist felt he had not captured baby Jaane's face accurately, and asked them to return.

After the second session, Griet stopped by to ask how it had gone and whether Catrijn had sneaked a peek at her painting.

"I did," Catrijn admitted sheepishly. "I'll bet you did too. What do you think?"

"I took a look and don't like it. Too stiff. No sense of humor, and doesn't show that Nicolaas is *unpredicable*—"

"Unpredic*Table*."

"There's no twinkle in his eyes. And you wouldn't even know we like each other." Griet did not mention her other complaint: the painter had failed to capture her sexiness.

"Ours is a bit stilted, but portraits are supposed to reflect the seriousness of life."

"Why not show people doing normal things?" Griet said. "Couples laughing—or the husband leering at his wife's breasts? Maybe a baby giggling, and the mother snuggling him. What's wrong with that?"

Catrijn laughed. "You have a point." She found the idea of depicting families informally so intriguing that she shared it with Konrad, who also thought it had validity. Neither, however, knew of a painter who portrayed people that way, and in all likelihood none ever would.

By early summer, the portraitist finished his work and dramatically unveiled the paintings all at once to the entire family, his face beaming with pride. It was easy to identify who was who in each portrait, but there was a stern sameness to all the faces. No hint of a smile or real expression in the eyes. The babies too were depicted similarly and looked like diminutive adults. In some cases, the details of the clothing had been transformed. Dirck's feathered hat had been changed into a flat-brimmed Calvinist one, and Konrad's stylish ruffled collar had been rendered smaller. The artist did achieve moderate success, though, in capturing the texture of Maria's velvet dress.

"I think they're wonderful," Betje exclaimed.

Griet and Nicolaas saw nothing remotely wonderful about them and thought the painter had failed to capture even a hint of their personalities.

"They're all reasonable likenesses," Konrad said in faint praise and paid the artist.

The paintings went to their respective homes and found prominent places on walls, except for Griet and Nicolaas's. Theirs was stored in the attic and would only see the light of day when Konrad and Catrijn came for a visit.

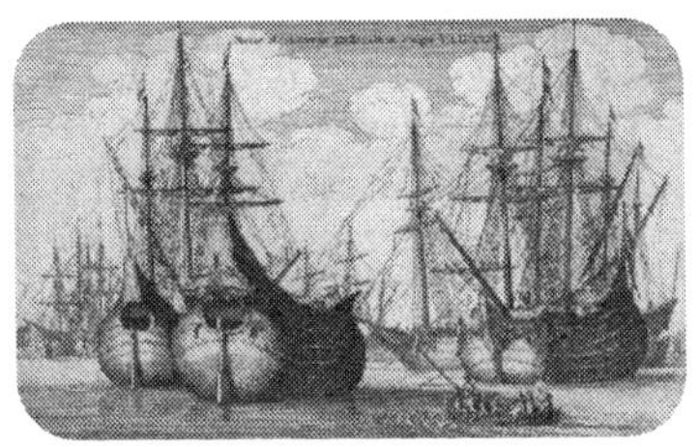

FLUYT SHIPS

CHAPTER 8

Transitions to Other Realms – 1591-1593

Maria was having difficulty comprehending the appeal of Calvinism, despite Uncle Konrad explaining its tenets and Jacques trying to convince her that Protestantism was a purer form of Christianity because there were no priests intervening between the believer and God. Dirck thought the key to her understanding was the Bible, which Maria had never read, and planned to buy one for her in Latin, a language both could read.

Though Aunt Margaretha remained impartial, she had come to believe Maria could not be swayed by logical arguments. Her beliefs, like Margaretha's, were imbued with mystical elements: chanting and achieving an almost trance-like state, and taking comfort from the Begijnhof's treasured relics and saintly art. Maria would remain a Catholic, of that Margaretha was confident, but whether she would join the Beguine sisterhood was still in doubt.

Catrijn suggested that Maria might benefit from attending a Reformed Church service with the family, and she did so on Sunday. While in church, Catrijn tried to gauge her reaction and was surprised when Maria closed her eyes during hymns, hummed, and sometimes mouthed familiar Dutch words. Singing! That's the way she's going to learn *both* Dutch and Calvinism, she concluded. I'll ask Jacques to start singing hymns with her; he has a good voice.

After the service, Konrad and Jacques asked Maria whether she had any questions. She shook her head no, and her satisfied smile indicated she had enjoyed it.

A new pastor, Petrus Plancius, had officiated at the service, and afterward the congregants lined up outside the church to introduce themselves to him. When the family's turn came, Konrad stepped forward.

"Konrad Teller!" the pastor said, "I haven't seen you in years."

Konrad shook the pastor's hand, while trying to recall where they had previously met. The man's serious gaze and long nose were vaguely familiar, but not his name.

"I fear you don't remember me," the pastor said, dejected. "We met when we were exiles and I was studying theology. I was known as Pieter Platevoet then."

"Of course, ja, Pieter."

"I Latinized Pieter Platevoet to Petrus Plancius because it's a more refined name for my maps. I'm a cartographer too, and right now I'm working on a series of biblical maps."

"I'd like to see those maps when they're finished," Konrad said and went on to introduce his family. The pastor offered to give Maria religious instruction, if an interpreter could be provided, and Jacques volunteered. In turn, Konrad promised to invite Plancius to supper, but not before he and Catrijn had moved into their new house on the Singel canal in autumn. By that time, his seafaring in-laws would also be home, and he assured Plancius that he would have much in common with fellow exile Maarten and his map-collector son, Dirck.

Maria went to Aunt Catrijn's house for a chat and found Griet there as well, both embroidering. Though the day was warm, Maria wore a cape closed tightly around her neck.

"*Ciao*," Maria said and exchanged cheek kisses. Still wearing her cape, she sat down. After inspecting their needlework, she crossed her hands in her lap, and grinned at the two of them.

"Something up?" Griet asked, but Maria did not understand.

"She means," Catrijn said in Italian, "Has anything happened? You look happy."

Maria removed her cape, revealing her elegant green dress beneath. "I leave Begijnhof."

Catrijn translated for Griet, who asked, "Why?" and Maria did not reply.

"Did you tell Aunt Margaretha?" Catrijn asked, and Maria nodded yes. "Will you leave the Catholic church, become Calvinist?"

"Nee, I am Catholic."

"Then why are you leaving?"

Reticent, Maria stared at her hands.

"Are you thinking of getting married?" Griet asked, and Catrijn repeated it in Italian.

Maria meekly nodded yes. "Men like me. Jacques, Dirck ... men in church. I know. I see."

Catrijn translated for Griet.

Griet scowled, envisioning young men lining up after church to leer at available women such as Maria, with the most ardent ogler being Nicolaas—the bastard!

"But who is right?" Maria asked. "How ..."

"You want to know *who* to choose?" Catrijn said. "*How* to choose?"

Maria nodded affirmatively.

"With men, you must follow your heart."

"Maria," Griet said, leaning forward and coming face to face with her, "don't be in a big hurry to get married. It's *not* wonderful, like you think," and waited for Catrijn's translation.

With a disapproving frown, Catrijn shook her head, and her eyes questioned: Why would you say such a thing?

Maria stared at the two, perplexed.

"Maria," Catrijn said, continuing in Italian, "what does *your* heart tell you? Who do you love?"

"I confuse. I like Dirck, but too … too? I like Jacques … passion. More Italian, no?"

"Dirck is very Dutch, and Jacques isn't. Jacques speaks Italian too. But only *you* can decide which one is best for you." Catrijn said and added, "While you decide, you can live here with Uncle Konrad and me as long as you want after leaving the Begijnhof."

Maria's eyes beamed gratitude. "Thank you."

When Rolfe and Jaane awoke from their naps, Maria left the room to see them, and Catrijn glared at Griet.

"I wish you wouldn't discourage Maria about men," Catrijn whispered. "This is all new to her. She's completely inexperienced."

"That's the problem, too innocent *and* too sexy. She's going to get hurt if she doesn't wise up."

"Since when did you decide to dislike men?"

"I've always been realistic, and just want to help her," Griet defended herself, while thinking, You're so innocent, Catrijn. You don't know the ways of men, never had to fend for yourself, always had someone looking out for you.

"You look so angry. Why?"

"I am *not* angry," Griet insisted and, in fact she was not. She was *livid*, because Nicolaas was in Gdansk having a love affair. Her intuition told her so, and loose comments by his shipmates had confirmed it.

The 1591 northern trading season was coming to an end, and Nicolaas was packing up the last of his belongings in Gdansk and looking forward to being reunited with Griet and little rambunctious Rolfe, whom he missed dearly.

Helga put her arms around him and rested her head on his back. "I'm going to miss you."

Nicolaas patted her arm and pulled away, not wanting to encourage his housekeeper's growing obsession with him. He resumed packing and nonchalantly said, "After I leave, you should return to Gotland. Your family must miss you."

"Won't you be back soon?"

"Probably not. Maybe not even next season. I've found a good Polish agent to take over for me." He was lying.

Helga snuggled against his back again, pressing her ample breasts into it.

"Well," Nicolaas said, "time to go," and hoped she would not ask again to go with him.

Outside, Nicolaas gave Helga a peck on the cheek and repeated, "You should go home." When she tried to kiss him, he turned and walked away, waving a goodbye. Whew, he thought to himself, I'm glad that's over. Next time, I'm going to hire someone who *believes* me when I say I'm not looking for a permanent relationship. Down the street, he saw Dirck standing on the corner, waiting for him.

"Hard to say goodbye sometimes, eh?" Dirck said wryly.

"Ja, I guess so. You know how it is, these housekeepers miss home and latch on to you, for company."

"Sure."

"Dirck, do you mind if I sail with Rykaard Jr.? We've got a mean dice game going, and I want to win back some money."

"Nee, go ahead."

A smirk formed on Nicolaas's lips. There was no dice rivalry with Rykaard—he was a lousy dice player. He merely wanted to avoid Dirck's inevitable moralizing during their days and nights together aboard the same ship.

The convoy left Gdansk on a brisk wind and proceeded without incident through the Baltic Sea and around the northern tip of Denmark. The unforgiving North Sea delivered its customary quotient of foul weather and scattered the ships. Once in the Zuider Zee, some came within sight of each other and, as nightfall approached, prepared to anchor together.

Nicolaas was standing at the bow checking water depths, when Rykaard Jr.'s order came, "*Prepare to come about!*" The sails started coming down and the ship slowed.

"*Make ready the anchor!*"

Men came to the bow and began lifting the heavy anchor, and Nicolaas hoisted himself onto the gunwale to get out of their way.

He lost his balance, fell forward, and landed on all fours. One hand touched down in the center of the coiled anchor line.

"*Drop anchor!*"

The anchor went over the side, and instantly the rope uncoiled, with Nicolaas's hand trapped within.

Nicolaas felt his arm and body lurch—Snap! Blood spurted. "*AAAH!*" Nicolaas rolled on the deck, thrashing and holding his arm. "My hand! AAAH ... my hand!"

"My God!" The anchorman was aghast at the sight of the missing hand. "*Get the cap'n!*" He tore off his shirt and bent down—"Don't move, Nicolaas. Stop movin'!"—and wound it tightly around the arm, just above the stump.

Rykaard Jr. arrived just as Nicolaas passed out. "Good Lord!"

"We gotta burn it, cap'n!" the anchorman said, his eyes wild. "Gotta stop the bleedin'!"

"Get the cook," Rykaard said, "Hurry!" The cook, with his supply of herbs and knives, was the doctor in residence, administering home remedies to sick crewmen and performing surgery when necessary.

Rykaard raised Nicolaas's head and tried to pour brandy into his mouth. "Nicolaas. Nicolaas! Drink this!"

Nicolaas's head rolled ... his eyes slowly opened.

"Drink!" Rykaard demanded. "You drink all the time. Now, when you need to, you don't! Come on man, *drink!*"

Nicolaas guzzled most of the bottle.

The cook arrived with a pot of hot coals and assured Nicolaas, "You're gonna be all right," and shoved a piece of wood between his teeth. "Chomp down on this." The cook took a deep breath and grabbed Nicolaas's arm—"Get ready!"—and pressed the stump into the pot.

"AAAOOOWW." Nicolaas passed out again.

One man ran to the side of the ship and vomited. The nauseating smell of burning flesh lingered for several minutes until the wind swept it away.

In Amsterdam, Nicolaas was brought to the Van der Voort house on a stretcher and carried to his bed. Griet and Betje were in near hysterics at the sight of the missing hand. Rykaard Jr. calmly told Maarten what had happened.

Betje sat down beside Nicolaas's bed and gently applied her home remedies to the grisly stump, pausing every time he cried out in pain. She also closely watched his upper arm for any signs of redness and checked his forehead for fever because those were the real dangers for which she had no treatment, except to call a surgeon to bleed him. Betje waited and watched, and, when she had to leave his side, Griet and Catrijn rotated in and out of the bedside chair.

Nicolaas slept for lengthy periods, or pretended to while contemplating life without the hand he did everything with, including writing. His despondency drew sympathetic words, gentle strokes to his forehead, tankards full of beer, and copious amounts of *speculaas koekjes.*

Reveling in all the attention, Nicolaas remained in bed as the wound healed. No signs of infection surfaced.

When Betje noticed her son reach out and lustily tweak his wife's breast, she suspected his continuing gloominess might be an act. And seeing him give Griet and Rolfe the beaver hats he had brought as gifts and then clownishly prance around with one on his head, Betje knew the time had come for Nicolaas to go to church with her.

The two went to Oude Kerk, formerly Saint Nicolaas Church, and once inside Betje fell to her knees. "Thank you, God, for sparing my son's life. I don't deserve Your blessings, but please heal him so he can be of service to You and his family." Tears streamed down her cheeks.

Seeing his mother praying earnestly—not for herself, but for him—moved Nicolaas deeply. So much so that when they left the church, he waited patiently while she took scrapings from the stonework around the door, placed them in a small leather pouch, hung it around his neck, and said, "These holy grains will protect you."

Feeling strangely soothed and disbelieving that he had felt no urge to poke fun at her superstitions, he said, "Mother, I'm going to stay here a few minutes." After watching her leave and standing there for a while, the feeling of tranquility dissipated, and Nicolaas headed for his favorite ale house near the harbor.

A shaft of sunlight broke through the clouds and illuminated the street in front of him ... spread in his direction, bathed him in a warm glow, and then vanished. He stopped. Maybe this is a sign, like Mother looks for. Lifting his stump, he questioned, Did God do this to me for a reason? His other hand went to the pouch and gave it a squeeze, and he pivoted. I'm going home, where I belong, and I'm going to stop drinking so much and having sex with housekeepers.

After Konrad and Catrijn moved into their new house on the Singel canal, they were eager to show it off and chose to host the family's traditional Saint Maarten's Day meal on the eleventh of November. Konrad invited Pastor Petrus Plancius, telling him that he and fellow exile Maarten would have much to talk about and that Dirck was bringing newly purchased maps.

Plancius accepted the invitation at his wife's insistence, even though he abhorred Saint Maarten celebrations or any other saint-day event, believing they were useless contrivances of the Catholic church. He did look forward, however, to bringing his new biblical map that had just been printed.

When the Planciuses arrived, the air was filled with the aroma of roasting fowl and Catrijn was lighting the candles on the table while observing Aunt Margaretha recite a funny poem to Jaane. She and her aunt were hoping a little humor would erase Jaane's frown lines, which seemed to go along with her squinting. Rolfe, who Betje was babysitting, was crawling around until Maarten grabbed him by the back of his shirt and deposited him on his wife's lap. Jacques sat in the corner talking with Maria, in Italian, and Dirck was gulping down another glass of wine.

Konrad made the introductions and gave a tour of the house, mentioning that the front room had been made larger to accommodate both his office and Catrijn's ever-growing number of students.

He also noted that a hook with ropes and a pulley system to hoist up goods had been installed outside the third-floor window, and said he greatly admired this clever Dutch invention. The interior had not yet been painted the soft colors the couple desired; nonetheless, its elegant simplicity was evident. Lacking in ostentation or extravagance, the home was quintessentially Dutch.

While drinks were being served, Griet came through the front door with a smirk on her face. Nicolaas followed, wearing a big grin and a beret perched rakishly on his head, and proceeded to strut around saying "Hello" while inclining his head toward each person.

"You're so naughty!" Catrijn said after noticing that attached to his hat was a ribald pin shaped like a winged penis in flight. Muffling a giggle, she averted her eyes and gave a reproving push to his shoulder,

"I just bought it at the market," Nicolaas said, pleased with himself. Seeing disapproval in his father's eyes, he promptly removed the hat. "There were loads of fun things for sale for Saint Nicolaas day too." He took out wooden blocks and a toy soldier he had purchased for the upcoming holiday—"Rolfe's going to love them"—and passed them around.

The maid brought in the roast and placed it on the table, and the feasting began. Afterward, Betje served *speculaas koekjes,* and Margaretha commented they smelled even better than usual.

"That's because of the cinnamon," Betje said while passing the plate around, "you don't see cinnamon in the market very often."

"Spices come from the infidels," Plancius warned, "buying them helps *their* cause and drains money from good Christian purposes—money that will never return."

"I-I never thought of spices that way," Betje said, puzzled.

"Surely, you can't mean that?" Maarten said. "We buy spices and cheese and bread every day. Food is food. We can't worry about whether it comes from a holy source or not. Dirck goes to Livorno to sell Calvinist-made cheese and Catholic-grown grains to mostly Catholics, but also to some Protestants, Jews ... and maybe an infidel or two."

"It's just a cautionary note," Plancius said, "but in the end it is in God's hands."

Maarten stared at him, wondering: What's in God's hands?

"Pieter—I mean Petrus," Konrad intervened. "Why don't you show us your new map."

"With pleasure." Plancius unrolled his approximately eleven-by-fifteen-inch map on Konrad's desk. Heads bumped together to get a look.

At the center of the map was the Mediterranean Sea with a handsome three-masted Dutch ship bearing the Republic's orange-white-blue-striped flag. Landmasses bore the names of communities and empires existing during the time of Jesus Christ, and around the edges were fifteen illustrations of biblical stories. Plancius noted his innovation, inscriptions in both Latin and Dutch, which drew accolades.

Konrad pointed to one of the biblical scenes. "This must be the stoning of Steven."

Judgment Day caught Betje's eye, with the dead rising and angels helping the righteous heavenward. She flinched at the sight of the devil's demonic helpers dragging the sinners into flames.

Nicolaas snickered at naked bodies in the Judgment Day scene and poked Griet to share his irreverence.

"This must be Paul's voyage to Rome and his shipwreck," Catrijn observed and turned to Dirck. "That was your favorite bible story when we were kids."

"Ja, I thought it was a great adventure story, even though Paul was a prisoner."

"Acts, Chapter 27," minister Petrus Plancius said and began reciting, " ' ... and when it was determined we should sail into Italy, they delivered Paul and certain other prisoners unto one named Julius ... ' "

Maarten noticed Rolfe crawling toward the kitchen and leaned over, grasped him by the shirt, and handed the wriggling boy to Griet.

" ' ... and when we had sailed over the sea of Cilicia and Pamphylia, we came to Myra, a city of Lycia—' "

"Myra?" Betje said, "Saint Nicolaas was born there, wasn't he?"

"Saints are for papists." Plancius's voice was full of disdain. "Calvinists shouldn't perpetuate such superstitious beliefs."

"But Saint Nicolaas is ... Amsterdam's ... patron ..."

"I *myself* rather like Saint Nicolaas," Nicolaas joked. "But really, what harm does it do? Kids love Sinter Klaus and try to be good to get presents."

Before Plancius could respond, Konrad said, "Dirck, why don't you show us the maps you brought."

Dirck retrieved a stack of maps, noting, "These are by map-maker Mercator."

"I know Gerardus Mercator," Plancius boasted, "an excellent cartographer."

"Maps are getting to be a family ritual," Catrijn remarked and sat down on the floor to help Dirck arrange the eighteen sheets into a large square.

"These maps are strange," Nicolaas said. "Lines on maps are usually curved, not straight."

"I agree," Dirck said. "I bought them because I was told the straight longitudinal lines will be useful for navigating over long distances, but I don't see how."

"They're supposed to," Plancius explained, "correct for problems of compass bearings and curvature of the earth. A sea captain can simply plot a straight line and then follow it." Seeing Dirck's questioning expression, Plancius added, "I'll explain it to you later."

Griet stared at the maps, unable to make any sense of them, except they matched her intuitive sense that the world was flat. "Where do we live on these maps?"

"Amsterdam is here," Konrad said with a finger point.

"And Livorno?" Maria asked, and Jacques showed her.

"Where do spices come from?"

"The East Indies." Konrad circled the area of India, Southeast Asia, and China. "The Portuguese reach the Indies by sailing around Africa." His finger traced the route.

"I wonder why," Griet said, "because going this way looks

shorter." She drew an imaginary line from Amsterdam to the Arctic, across the North Pole, and down to China.

"That route may be shorter," Maarten said, "but the Arctic is too frozen to sail—"

"I'm sorry, Maarten, I must disagree," Plancius said. "It is *not* frozen all the time. Cartographers from England and German states, *including* Gerardus Mercator, have told me the Arctic thaws for five months during summer, when the sun shines continuously. Though the rays are weak, they give enough warmth to melt *all* the ice and allow men to live there and grow grass for animals. So it *is* possible to sail across the Arctic and directly down to the East Indies."

"Nee," Maarten said, his head turning side to side. "I cannot agree. I've sailed north many times and talked to sea captains from far north ports in Norway and Muscovy. And they *all* say their ports are ice-free for only a few months in summer. And when they leave their ports and sail north, they see giant islands of ice. If they're lucky enough to avoid crashing into an ice island and keep sailing north, they see nothing but *solid* ice ... and there is no way to sail through it."

"I'm sorry, Maarten, but you are wrong."

"Have you ever sailed in the north?"

"Nee, but I have it on good authority that sailing through the Arctic *can* be done."

"Well, I think my wife's tired," Maarten said and rose to his feet, "and I myself have a busy day tomorrow." Maarten indeed had work to do on Dirck's upcoming departure for Livorno, but in truth he simply wanted to get away from sanctimonious and know-it-all Petrus Plancius, who had also proven himself to be unpatriotic and hypocritical by changing his name. To Maarten's way of thinking, there could be no justification for changing a perfectly good Netherlandic name to a Latin one. If Dutch is good enough for the map, then a Dutch name is good enough for the mapmaker. As Maarten walked out the door with Betje, he was still grumbling about Plancius's rude comments to his wife about cinnamon and Saint Nicolaas day, a holiday all Amsterdammers observed and enjoyed.

When the time came for Dirck and Jacques to make their second voyage to Livorno in late autumn 1591, the family said their farewells at the Damrak. Aunt Margaretha embraced Dirck and whispered, "Remember the Italian words I taught you and be sure to practice."

"I pray for you, Dirck," Maria said, straining to make the Dutch words understandable. She looked as though she might kiss him on the cheek, but blushed instead. To Jacques, she said in Italian, "Please give this to my father," and handed him a letter. As their lighter departed, she fluttered her embroidered handkerchief at them.

"*Don't forget to go to Pisa!*" Catrijn called out, reminding them of the unusual leaning tower she had read about. After a vigorous wave goodbye, she started toward home and saw Maria lingering dockside, dabbing tears. Who's she crying for? Catrijn wondered. I hope it's not Dirck. She's not right for him ... way too boring and not at all interested in things that fascinate him. She never even touched the books Konrad gave her, avoids discussing anything of importance, and is only interested in needlework and babies. Was she always like this? Or is it possible that being cloistered away robbed her of curiosity?

After the fleet was well underway and in calm waters, Dirck had time to relax, and Maria promptly came to mind. She favors me over Jacques, I can tell. There's a better than even chance I'll marry her. His eyes shifted to Jacques, who was sitting with his writing desk propped on his knees, twirling a quill pen, and staring off with a smile on his face. He's writing again ... probably love letters, in Italian! That's his *big* advantage. I *must* learn to speak and write Italian. If I practice a little every day, I should be pretty fluent by the time we get to Livorno. Then I won't need *him* to translate for me.

During their stop in La Rochelle, Dirck noticed Jacques was distant and uncommunicative, and remembered that their chess games while at sea had taken on a combative dimension. If Jacques keeps this up, he lamented, I'm afraid our friendship will be lost.

In Livorno, Dirck addressed the customs agent in Italian, explaining the purpose of their visit and goods they carried. Faced with the agent's look of incomprehension, he repeated himself and fumbled to find other words that might be better understood. When the agent threw up his hands, Jacques stepped forward. A similar thing happened when Dirck tried to josh with dockworkers. As the misunderstandings mounted, Dirck realized he needed help. So after lunch one day when everyone except Lodewyk had departed for a siesta, he remained at the table casually sipping his wine.

"Lodewyk, I'd like to ask a favor. Can you recommend a *private* tutor to help me master Italian, because I'm not making much progress on my own."

"I know the *perfect* tutor for you," Lodewyk replied without hesitation, "my son Giovanni. His pronunciation and grammar are excellent, as good as any paid tutor. And I know he'd feel honored if asked to help you."

That evening with a bottle of wine tucked under his arm, Giovanni escorted Dirck to the roof terrace. He began with Italian words for familiar objects—bottle, table, chair, ship—which Dirck mastered quickly. He fared less well with pronouns. Beyond the familiar *I*, Dirck had never before used *you* or *he* because it was easier to use a person's proper name instead. By the time Giovanni introduced the objective and possessive cases of pronouns—him, me, his, mine—far too much wine had been consumed. Dirck slurred his way through them and remembered little.

After a lesson in verbs—to go, see, say—Dirck was able to create sentences. His first was to Lodewyk. "I go ship." The question, Which ship? brought consternation, for he had not yet learned the word *which*. Despite some successes, Dirck fell again into a pattern of failing to comprehend queries especially from fast speakers, forgetting and bungling words, and mispronouncing almost everything.

Verb tenses and conjugations provoked despair for both teacher and student, and the following day Dirck ducked out of the house early, strode with his head down as if in deep thought to avoid making eye contact with passers-by, and went straight to his Dutch compatriots for some *real* conversation.

Giovanni changed tactics and started teaching Dirck complete sentences that could be memorized and repeated until some semblance of lyrical Italian was achieved. Using them along with considerable hand gesturing and facial expressions, Dirck began breezing through simple conversations for which he had stock questions and replies at the ready. People began to think he spoke Italian and initiated open-ended conversations, which left Dirck apologizing, "I'm sorry, I speak Italian only a little," a handy phrase from Giovanni. With that, his progress plateaued.

Lodewyk sensed a hint of defeatism in normally confident Dirck, especially when he was trying to keep up with fast-paced conversations at the dining table. So in passing, Lodewyk asked:

"How are your Italian lessons coming along, Dirck?"

"I've become fairly proficient at reading Italian under Giovanni's patient tutelage, and my knowledge of Latin helps me derive the meaning of unknown words. Writing, though, is coming slowly because I haven't yet grasped grammar and syntax. Conversational Italian?" He sighed. "I've come to believe that for some reason I lack the ability to comprehend spoken words and correctly pronounce them."

"Don't be too hard on yourself" Lodewyk said and put his arm around Dirck's shoulder. "Let's walk." Out the door they went and down the street, and to each passing person Lodewyk paused and chatted. At the harbor, he asked Dirck, "Do you think I speak Italian well?"

"Certainly."

"I don't. I speak with a heavy Dutch accent and my grammar is only passable. Like you, I don't have a talent for languages and take no pleasure in mastering them. My cousin Konrad—he's different. Loves the intricacies of languages and practices until he gets the accent and cadence perfect. Me? I learn only the essentials and rely on my other abilities, which your Aunt Margaretha described as my 'wit and panache,' if I remember correctly. So don't worry, because you have many other gifts: an open mind, diverse interests, business aptitude ... seafaring skills." He rested his hand on Dirck's shoulder. "If you lived here and *needed* to speak Italian to survive, you'd learn. But you don't, so you'll probably just stumble along, making do with sentences Giovanni teaches you. There's nothing wrong with that."

"I suppose you're right, but I do *still* hope to improve." Dirck smiled and put out his hand to shake. "Thank you for being honest about your own language skills—I never would have guessed it—and for your encouragement."

Italian lessons came to a halt when preparations for departure took precedence, and withing a week Dirck was exiting the harbor with his fleet. Taking one last glance at the city, he bid a silent farewell: *Arrivederci,* Livorno. I won't miss you one bit, or the chance to make a fool of myself every time I walk your streets trying to speak Italian.

Once the fleet was on a steady course, he thought of home and the pleasure of seeing family again, and Maria. He imagined her rushing up to greet him, pouty lips turned up at the corners and eyes sultry, and him reaching out and loosening her braided tresses and them cascading down around her shoulders, and his hand sliding to her breast—he let out a little laugh. It was truly wishful thinking, because to date Maria had not yet allowed him to kiss her, let alone touch her voluptuous body.

Jacques heard the titter and turned to Dirck, his eyes inquiring.

"I was just reliving some of my blunders while trying to speak Italian." He grinned. "I need to practice more."

"Good luck."

In Amsterdam, the sight of Maria walking along the Damrak fueled the men's competitive spirits as they alighted from their rowboat. Jacques called out to her. She turned, waved, and went straight to Dirck.

"Welcome home, Dirck. You were away a long time," she said in impeccable Dutch, repeating phrases she had mastered through repetition.

She's speaking Dutch! An elated Dirck responded in his practiced Italian, "Hello, I am happy to see you."

Maria switched to Italian, thinking Dirck had learned it. "How was your voyage? Is my father well? Did he send a letter for me? I'm dreaming of seeing him again, and next time I want to go to Livorno with you."

Dirck's brow furrowed, for she was speaking so fast that he could only decipher a few words: father, family, letter.

"I have a letter for you," Dirck said in Dutch, "from your father." He pulled it from his pouch, and continued to speak in Dutch, "Your father and everyone else is well, and all send their love and asked that you come next year to visit."

Maria feigned understanding, though her vacuous eyes indicated otherwise.

Jacques stepped forward and said in Italian, "Ah, there you are my lovely friend, Maria," and swept her hand to his lips and kissed it sensuously.

Flustered, Maria looked from Jacques to Dirck.

Jacques went on to report to her, in Italian, the news from Livorno.

The family arrived. Betje called out, "Dirck!" and tearfully pressed her cheek to his. Maarten and Pieter shook his hand, and Nicolaas gave the usual bear hug.

Catrijn kissed his cheek. "Tell me about your trip. Did you go to Pisa?" She leaned back against a barrel, ready to hear every last detail.

Dirck tore his eyes away from Jacques and Maria and focused on her. "Everything went well. No major problems. I bought a new map; I'll show it to you later. We didn't go to Pisa, but I did travel into the countryside a bit."

"What was it like?"

"Hilly. The day I traveled, the hills were clear but fog had settled in the valleys. We never see that here; our land is so flat that fog hangs uniformly over everything. The trees were unusual too: tall, thin, and lonely looking. People who live in the country are different as well. In Livorno, everyone is hardworking and purposeful, like us. But in the country, people don't seem to work. It is said that the well-off are proud of doing nothing, and the poor have nothing to do."

"Hmm, people don't seem to work?" Catrijn mulled over the alien notion, trying to make sense of it. "I remember you saying that Lodewyk's sons and their families live with him. Do all Italian families live in one house, all generations together?"

"The ones I met did. Of course, that's the opposite of what we do here." In Amsterdam, young couples formed their own households after marrying.

"Maybe not all members of a family *need* to work," Catrijn speculated, "if at least someone in the household does—"

"Catrijn. You're always trying to figure things out. Your mind never stops." His head was turning side to side in feigned disbelief, but in fact that particular quirk of her nature and her curious mind had always charmed him.

No sooner had the cargo from Livorno been unloaded, than Dirck and Maarten had to get their ships ready to sail northward. Though Dirck was not happy about leaving Maria alone with Jacques for the entire northern sailing season, there was nothing he could do about it. He was a sea captain, by choice, and had obligations, so he went to work arranging for the replacement of worn-out sails, repair of damaged timber, and the repainting of hulls. Meanwhile Nicolaas organized goods to be sent and readied himself for the months-long stay in Gdansk. While final preparations were being made, a letter arrived for Maarten bearing Rykaard's elegant script:

Dear Maarten,

When Dirck stops in Hoorn to pick up me and my sons, please come with him. Pieter Jansz Liorne has been working on a new ship and wants you to see it. You'll both find it very interesting.

Your faithful friend and fellow Sea Beggar,

Rykaard

Father and son were well-acquainted with the fine work of Pieter Jansz Liorne, because he had built most of their ships. They also knew that Rykaard would not have taken the time to write if the ship had not been special.

In Hoorn, Nicolaas helped Rykaard and his sons stow their things aboard the ships, while Maarten and Dirck went to the shipyard. Right off, they could see that the new ship was indeed different from theirs. The hull was fuller, and the sails notably reconfigured. Gone from the main mast was the upright sail that swung side to side, and in its place were two rectangular sails suspended from horizontal spars.

Pieter Liorne appeared on deck, waved and came down. He shook the men's hands and asked:

"What do you think?"

"Pretty interesting," Maarten said. "I like the bigger hull and extra cargo she'll carry. But I'd worry the extra weight could be a problem out there." His head tilted toward the shallow Zuider Zee.

"Don't worry. She won't ride any lower in the water than your current ships, even with extra cargo, because I made her of pine to reduce her weight. Pine is *much* lighter than oak, which I usually use."

Dirck inspected the hull, knocking on it and running his hand across the surface.

"Tell me about those new square sails," Maarten said. "I've never sailed a ship rigged like this."

"Square sails give more power and should be easy to handle because I did a couple of things: put two smaller sails on each mast, instead of one large one ... and added extra block and tackle." Liorne smiled and nodded toward the sails. "You'll be happy to see they can be reefed," made smaller, "without difficulty when the wind picks up."

"Sounds good," Maarten said. "But you'd have to show me how to handle them, and I'd have to train my crew."

"It won't take long for you to learn, and your crew will have no trouble either. In fact, I believe this ship is so efficient she can be managed, fully rigged, with less than *half* your usual crew."

"*Half?*" Maarten and Dirck said, nearly in unison.

"Maybe even less, once I've tweaked her." Liorne turned to Dirck. "Here's something you'll like. I made templates of the frame, so the next ship I build will be identical to this one. You've been bothered in the past that I never build two ships exactly the same. This'll solve the problem."

"Templates should allow you to construct ships faster too," Dirck commented, and Liorne agreed.

"Oh, and one more thing," Liorne said, "I've modified the stern," and led them to the back of the ship. "You'll notice I made the rudder much bigger and stronger. That's to counterbalance the tendency of such a wide ship with powerful sails to drift sideways."

"You seem to have thought of everything," Dirck said, "I'm impressed." He exchanged glances with his father, and Maarten's knowing nod told him they were both thinking the same thing: If this ship carries more cargo *and* can be operated with less crew, we'll be able to undercut every other merchant shipper's cost in Amsterdam. And with a fleet of them, we'll outcompete everyone in Holland *and* even Europe!

"If she handles as well as you say, Pieter," Maarten said, "we'll buy her *and* order an entire fleet. When can I sail her?"

"In a couple months."

"Good, I'll come as soon as you let me know she's ready." Maarten added with a wink, "And don't show her to any other captains." But he was not overly concerned because sea captains tended to be conservative about ships, and most would be wary of risking their limited capital on an unproven design.

"It's a deal," Pieter Jansz Liorne said and shook both men's hands.

"By the way, do you have a name for this ship?" Dirck asked.

"My wife calls her a fluyt," Liorne said, his hands forming the shape of a fluyt, a wineglass. "She thinks it's shaped like one, and I guess that's as good a name as any."

Maarten returned to Amsterdam with fluyts foremost on his mind.

Dirck had little time to reflect on the fluyt, because as soon as he sailed his *Amsterdam Ascendant* out of Hoorn to join the fleet bound for Gdansk, blustery weather closed in on the Zuider Zee and later unrelenting squalls battered them in the North Sea. It was not until the wind died and the sea became glassy off the coast of Denmark that the tired crew had a chance to hang out their bedding to dry and stretch out on the deck for a rest.

Dirck found a sunny spot on top of his cabin, and Nicolaas joined him and lay down, exhausted from sea sickness that had plagued him the entire route.

"Feeling better?" Dirck asked, and his brother nodded yes, before closing his eyes. Dirck put his hands behind his head and observed the men repairing a sail that had torn before it could be taken down, which made him wonder how the fluyt would have performed in recent conditions. Was Pieter Liorne right? Could those sails possibly be handled with *half* the usual crew? It seemed unlikely, and Dirck hoped his father would test the fluyt in a variety of conditions.

Nicolaas opened his eyes and rolled his head to face Dirck. "I've been thinking about Maria."

Dirck's eyebrows raised.

"I can see she's waiting for you to propose marriage, and I understand why you might want to—she's so sexy. But I want to know how that would work. I mean, Maria still can't speak Dutch, and Jacques says your Italian stinks. She wouldn't get your jokes—not that you're such a great joke teller—and wouldn't be able to discuss your precious books. Catrijn says Maria isn't interested in reading, doesn't like new things." Nicolaas paused to gauge Dirck's reaction, which was not negative. "I'm saying this because I'm married and know a thing or two. And you're my big brother and I want you to be happy." He finished with, "Nee offense taken, I hope."

"None taken," Dirck said sincerely.

Nicolaas watched as Dirck's brow furrowed, which meant he was mulling it over.

"Well, I've certainly had misgivings," Dirck confessed. "But I kept telling myself things'll get better. I'll learn Italian. She'll learn Dutch. She'll take an interest in things I like. I even gave her copies of Marcus Aurelius and the Bible in Latin, which she can read, but she keeps putting me off when I try to talk about them. I'd hoped to learn what fascinates her, but haven't. I want to share everything with my wife, and now I see that won't be possible with her."

Nicolaas was about to make a glib remark about there being women in every port and Dirck will find someone else, but stopped himself. It wasn't appropriate. Instead, he lay quietly and observed his brother. When Dirck's pursed lips relaxed into a slight smile, Nicolaas sensed his brother might be more relieved than sad about letting Maria go.

Dirck's convoy returned from Gdansk as the sun was setting over Amsterdam. It was too late to do anything more than haul in the sails and set anchors, so most of the captains and crew went ashore to sleep in their own beds, intending to return at daybreak to unload their ships.

By the time Dirck disembarked at the Damrak, darkness had fallen and there was little chance of running into Maria, a big relief. He had already devised a plan for letting her know his decision—recede subtly from the competition and let Jacques's deft repertoire woo her into marriage—even though he considered it a cowardly ploy and dreaded doing it. His preference was a direct approach, but that was not an option after the disastrous results with Kaatje.

On his way home, Dirck stopped by his parent's house, and right away Betje started quizzing him. "Did the voyage go well? Was Nicolaas seasick? Was he able to rent a nice house in Gdansk?"

After answering the questions to her satisfaction, Dirck said, "Father, did you get a chance to test the fluyt?"

"Ja, I did. She was easy to maneuver and efficient to sail. I tested her with Liorne several times, in both good and bad conditions, *and* with only *ten* sailors. Of course, they were all trained by Liorne, but still ... *just* ten."

"Ten? That's hard to imagine," Dirck commented. Their ships required twenty-five to thirty.

"The combination of rectangular sails and small lateens, and the way Liorne rigged them, made all the difference. They're easier to raise and lower, and reposition, than ours. He made the upper rectangles bigger to give speed. And positioned the lower ones high enough above the deck to give a clear line of sight the whole length of the ship—from stern, to bow, and the sea ahead. Oh, and something else. The waist," width at the widest part of the deck, "is the same as our ships. I measured it myself."

"I wouldn't have guessed it." Then the implication dawned on Dirck. "That means the tolls in the Oresund will be the same, even though she'll carry more cargo." Tolls were calculated on the waist dimension. "These fluyts are going to be *real* money savers."

Maarten's head was going up and down in agreement. "That's why I bought her without talking to you first. I plan to take our best sailors to Hoorn soon, so Liorne can train them, and then I'll sail her to Gdansk when the convoy goes again."

"Good. And I think we should order a whole fleet."

"I did that too. I knew you'd approve," Maarten said with a smile. "But now, you and I need to figure out how to pay for them. Pieter and I looked at the books. We can pay for the first fluyt ourselves, with reserves and future profits, but not a *whole* fleet."

"Hmm. What about Konrad? And those wealthy exiles he knows from Antwerp? Maybe they'll lend us money."

"It's a possibility," Maarten said, thoughtful. "I can talk to Uncle Nostrand too."

"This might sound crazy," Dirck added, "but maybe we should go into business with Liorne, so we can make money from building fluyts for others. Liorne will be deluged with orders after everyone sees how efficient ours are, and he'll need capital and business expertise to organize and operate a large shipyard. We're the logical ones to do it. We've done business with Liorne for years, and we trust each other."

"Clever idea, Dirck."

"And Konrad and those other men might be *more* willing to lend money for our fleet, if they know they'll also have the opportunity to invest in a fluyt-building business that will be a monopoly. Liorne won't have competitors for a long time because he's so secretive about his designs, and it'll take a while for others to figure out everything, especially those templates that'll make construction fast and cheap."

"That's probably right," Maarten said. "We can talk to Pieter tomorrow and get him to prepare some cost estimates. And when I go to Hoorn to get the fluyt ready to sail, I'll broach the subject with Liorne, if the time feels right."

While Dirck was ferrying grains from the *Amsterdam Ascendant* to the Damrak, he saw Maria for the first time. She waved and met him quayside. With eyes bright, she greeted him, "I miss you," in less than perfect Dutch. He replied in Dutch, with less enthusiasm than usual, but she did not notice. He vowed to be less subtle the next time.

Maarten had no difficulty obtaining commitments from Uncle Nostrand and one of Konrad's colleagues to lend money for the fleet. Konrad had declined, saying he needed to conserve capital for expansion of his silk business, but would like to invest in the shipbuilding venture. Jacques asked to be counted in for the fluyt shipyard too. So Maarten, together with Dirck and Pieter, began crafting a proposal for Pieter Jansz Liorne.

In the morning, they were putting final touches on it when Betje returned home from the market. She looked over Maarten's shoulder and asked, "Hmm, something to do with the fluyt?"

"Yep, you wouldn't believe all the great ideas we have."

"Good," Betje said and raised her basket, "because I bought something special for tonight hoping we'd have a reason to celebrate." That earned an approving look from Maarten, and she went into the kitchen, humming.

The men made a final read of the proposal, and later Maarten and Pieter went out to do some business, leaving Dirck behind.

Betje returned to the front room. "Dirck, would you like some beer?" He nodded yes, and she brought in two mugs and sat down opposite him.

Sensing she wanted to talk, Dirck kept his eyes down and tried to complete his rutter entries.

"I noticed Maria and Jacques in church together on Sunday."

"Ja."

"Aren't you worried they're spending so much time together?"

"Nee," Dirck said, without emotion. Seeing the shocked look on her face, he put down the quill pen and wiped his fingers. "I know you're disappointed that I'm not married and hoped Maria would be the one. For a while, it seemed that way. But she's not."

"Language is the problem," Betje said knowingly. "I can see that." She squeezed his hand and gave a consoling look.

Dirck returned to his work.

"While you were at sea, Kaatje's husband died."

"I'm sorry to hear that," Dirck said, barely raising his head.

"She asked about you the last time I saw her."

He put down the quill. "Mother, I'm not desperate to get married. I'm willing to wait for the right woman to come along. Besides, I'm at sea most of the time."

"Things'll work out fine, I'm sure."

"I'm sure too." The statement came out sounding dismissive and glib, and he felt obliged to make amends. "Mother, I know you're trying to help and want the best for me." His eyes connected with hers. "And I appreciate it."

"Well, I'll let you get back to work." Betje patted his hand and stood. From the kitchen, she paused to look back at him. He's such a good boy, always has been.

By the time Betje came back into the front room, Dirck had already gone out. The stew was simmering and the *speculaas koekjes* baking, so she decided to take a break and sit next to the front window to see what was going on in the street. The first person to walk by was Heer Nostrand; he tipped his hat and pointed toward the leaden sky that was growing ever darker. Betje waved to him and studied the greenish gray clouds with ominously dark undersides. A large raindrop hit the window, then another. Passersby quickened their pace. A deluge broke loose, and Betje squinted to see through the rain-streaked window. People were turning into blurs. An indistinct brown figure went by, and Betje thought it might be Pastor Plancius leaning into the wind. A black blotch zipped past—Betje gasped and jumped back—it looked like a witch on a broomstick.

CRACK. A clap of thunder brought her to her senses, and she remembered that the front door was open.

Betje rushed to the door. Lightning flashed, illuminating the street and revealing a small white form in the middle of it. "My God! It's a child!" A toddler had wandered outside, fallen down, and was trying to get up.

CRACK. Another clap of thunder. A horse neighed. Betje saw a vendor down the street trying to control his spooked mare. "*Whoa!* The horse was rearing up, lifting the front of the cart. "*Whoa!*"

CRACK. The horse bolted.

Betje ran out the door and into the street with arms outstretched.

The horse bore down, its cart careening behind and the man giving chase. "*Whoa!*"

Betje slipped—saw the horse's flared nostrils—pushed the child toward the gutter, and fell face down.

The horse galloped directly over Betje, its front hooves clearing her, and rear ones just grazing her back. The cart, bouncing wildly, flew into the air. Its front wheels banged onto the pavement on the other side of Betje, missing her completely. A rear wheel made a direct hit, bashing her head.

The cart bumped along on two wheels, slid sideways, and crashed into a house. The vendor caught up with the horse and desperately grabbed at its reins, as the horse thrashed and leaped.

The man of the house threw open his door. "*What's going on?*"

"*Help the woman!*" the street vendor yelled and pointed to Betje, while pulling on the reins. "*Whoa!*"

The man saw a screaming child and a woman lying face down in a blood-stained puddle of water. He ran to the woman and knelt down beside her. "Betje?"

Betje's eyes flickered open. She groaned.

"I'll get you inside, Betje. Just lie still." He searched up and down the street. "HELP! HELP!"

By now the mother had come to retrieve her hysterical toddler and joined in, "HELP!"

Neighbors came out and carried Betje into her house. One

ran to the warehouse to get Maarten, Dirck and Pieter. Another to Griet's house, and one to Catrijn's.

Maarten arrived breathless and saw a trail of blood leading from the door to his bed, where a neighbor was wrapping Betje's head. Soaking wet people were standing around looking distraught and helpless.

Maarten went to his wife and touched her face. "Betje."

Her eyes opened. "Maarten ... I'm done ... *gasp* ... am I ..."

"What did you say?" Maarten leaned closer.

Catrijn and Konrad burst through the door, along with minister Petrus Plancius. Maria followed. Dirck and Griet were not far behind. Pieter could not be found.

Plancius stepped forward to offer spiritual help.

Betje's hand grasped Plancius's sleeve. "Am I ... "

Plancius leaned closer. "What?"

"Am I ... going ... to ... heaven?"

"Only God knows," Plancius said. "It's in His hands—"

"Of course, you are!" Maarten said and stroked her head.

"Nee ..." Betje's eyes filled with fear. If the minister didn't know whether she was going to heaven, it could only mean she wasn't. God's finally punishing me ... for failing all His tests. I'll never see my father or mother again. A vision of them in heaven appeared. Betje reached out to touch them, but they vanished. "Oooh ..." She collapsed, and died.

Maarten gaped at his wife's face, frozen in anguish.

Plancius placed his hand on Maarten's shoulder—

Maarten pushed the hand away and glared at Plancius. "How could you say *that* to her? She was a *good,* God-fearing woman. Of course she's going to heaven!"

"Leading a good life and fearing God will not get you into heaven, Maarten," Plancius said with conviction. "Only God knows who will enter His kingdom. And good works cannot change the outcome."

"Rubbish! God does *not* send good people to hell!"

A collective gasp arose in the room.

Plancius's smug confidence enraged Maarten. "Get out! Get

out of my house!" He grabbed Plancius's arm and started dragging him toward the door, and Dirck had to pry the pastor from his grip.

Maarten returned to Betje. "You're going to heaven, Betje," he said and stroked her face, "God is good. He knows you're a good person. He's waiting for ..." He collapsed on her chest, sobbing.

Later, Maarten prepared Betje's body for burial, bathing it and putting on her wedding dress, and was disturbed that all his tender caresses could not remove the angst from her face. Finished, he closed the drape around the bed and, after wiping tears on his sleeve, lay down beside her and fell asleep.

The family returned in the evening to prepare the house for the vigil, which they agreed should be for two days to accommodate the expected large number of mourners to pay their respects. Extra furniture was removed, and pictures and mirrors turned toward the wall. A death notice was written and people hired to read it at various locations around the city.

The task of finding a suitable minister for the funeral fell to Dirck, and he expected to have to travel to Haarlem or Utrecht to find one. The few he knew of were uninspiring, poorly trained, highly conservative, and prone to religiosity. Dirck was fortunate to hear of a new pastor, Jacobus Arminius, recently arrived in Amsterdam. He was well-educated, had a calm temperament, and exhibited no hint of rigid piety. Though only in his early thirties, not much older than Dirck himself, Arminius had already completed studies at the illustrious University of Leiden, University of Padua, and in John Calvin's city of Geneva. Dirck liked him right away.

At the funeral, Pastor Arminius spoke glowingly about the humanity of those who sacrificed themselves for others. Betje had given her life to save a child, not unlike Jesus had given his own for our salvation. He read Betje's favorite biblical passages and paraphrased Matthew 5:12, the Beatitudes: "Her reward shall be great in heaven."

Dirck barely had time to mourn when notified that the convoy would set off for Gdansk the following week. Maarten was not up to the task of going to Hoorn to get the fluyt ready and decided to delay its maiden voyage until next year, 1593, when additional fluyts would be completed and the shipbuilding venture would be underway.

Dirck departed with a profound hollowness in his being.

For Jacques, Dirck's leaving came at an opportune time. He had been courting Maria with such ardor, and she utterly accepting, that he was confident she would say yes when he proposed marriage in a few weeks. The impending wedding would be a fait accompli by the time Dirck came back.

In the weeks following the funeral, sympathetic people regularly stopped by Maarten's house to console him, and he was not surprised when another knock came at the door. Standing there with an earthen cooking pot in her hands was the widow of an old acquaintance who had died several weeks earlier.

"Ah, Frau ter Williger ... how kind of you." Maarten reached for the pot. "You shouldn't be carrying such a heavy thing. Let me take it."

"A man needs his strength, so I brought you some stew," Letje ter Williger said without making eye contact. "I'm sorry about Betje, your loving wife and my dear friend, God rest her soul."

A smile of appreciation formed on Maarten's lips, and he invited her to come in.

She glanced up and down the street with worried eyes.

"Perhaps you'd like to sit here for a while." Maarten motioned toward the bench in front of the house.

Letje ter Williger sat down, her feet barely touching the ground, and folded her hands.

Maarten balanced the pot on his lap and said, "Hmm, this smells delicious." Letje nodded appreciatively, and Maarten added, "I'm sorry for the passing of your husband. He was a good man." Actually, Maarten thought the death of senile old ter Williger was a blessing.

"I'm accustomed to cooking for two," Letje said. "I'd be happy to bring meals to you." Letje saw Maarten's head move slightly and interpreted it to mean yes. As abruptly as she had blurted out her offer, she stood and said goodbye.

Letje was out of sight when Pastor Arminius showed up and sat down. Maarten explained how the pot had come to be resting on his lap, and both agreed that people were indeed charitable when a fellow man was in need. Arminius again offered his condolences and waited for Maarten to take the lead in the conversation.

Maarten was not about to bare his soul to this young pastor or anyone else about his relationship with his wife and the loss he felt, so the two sat in silence.

"Heer van der Voort," Arminius finally said, "it seems you and I have something in common. Your son said you were adopted by a very generous man, Heer Hasbrouk, after your parents died. I too was adopted by such a man when mine died. And after my adoptive father passed on, another kindhearted man took his place and provided for my education. Both of us have been blessed by the generosity of others."

"Ja, we have." Maarten glanced at the pastor's face and saw the same compassion and humanity that had shone in Papa's. He smiled down at the pot, warmed by the memory and the goodness of people.

Arminius leaned back and rested his head against the wall.

"Pastor," Maarten said, "I'm confused about something Heer Plancius said when my wife was dying: 'Only God knows if Betje will go to heaven.' Why *wouldn't* God reward her sacrifice with a place in heaven?"

"Heer van der Voort, Calvin tells us God elected certain people for salvation prior to Adam's fall and only He knows who will achieve salvation in His grand scheme."

"I'm not as learned as you, Pastor, but I do read the Bible, God's own words. And nowhere do I read of God condemning to hell someone who lives a godly life, like my wife, just because she was chosen to go there long before Adam lived ..." Maarten felt he was getting emotional, so he paused and looked off into the distance where clouds were darkening. "What I'm saying is," Maarten resumed, "I didn't realize we were doomed to heaven or hell no matter what we did. I always thought God was fair, and loving. He'd smite my enemies and reward me in heaven, if I did as He asked. A fair and loving God wouldn't condemn Betje to hell, would he?"

"To me, God is both fair and loving, but God is also unfathomable, as Calvin said. So nee, I don't have an answer for you. Nevertheless, God commands us to lead virtuous lives regardless of whether or not we're chosen to enter the kingdom of heaven."

Maarten could not conceal his disappointment with Arminius's pathetic answer. It was basically what Plancius had said and did nothing to sooth his anger and confusion.

"I will stop by tomorrow, Heer van der Voort, and we'll talk again." Arminius stood, shook Maarten's hand, and walked away feeling unsettled. He too was beginning to have questions along the line of Maarten's: Why would God endow man with the ability to think and make choices, if He didn't expect man to use those abilities? And why wouldn't man's choices in life, like Betje's selfless act to save a child, help attain a place in heaven?

A miserable drizzle started, capping a dreary day and mirroring the moods of both men.

Having received word that Dirck's convoy was entering Gdansk harbor, Nicolaas hurried to the dock, eager for news from home, especially about Rolfe and how things had gone with Maria. He paced back and forth impatiently until Dirck came ashore and then smothered him in a bear hug.

Dirck tried to match Nicolaas's enthusiasm, but dreaded telling him about the death of their mother.

"Is something wrong?" Nicolaas asked, sensing tenseness in his brother.

"Let's go to your place, where we can talk."

"Something *is* wrong." His mind was racing—Oh God, no, please don't let anything be wrong with Rolfe!—and he demanded, "Nee, tell me *now*."

"All right." Dirck's eyes met his. "I'm sorry to have to tell you ..."

Nicolaas was only half listening, convinced that something had happened to Rolfe and afraid to learn the truth. He heard the word mother. "Mother? You said Mother died?" His eyes widened in disbelief.

"Ja. She died saving a child." Dirck expected a flood of tears, for he knew that Nicolaas and their mother had a special relationship, though she never showed any favoritism toward him. Early on, she was proud when people complimented her on his bright blue eyes, shock of golden red hair, and infectious laughter. Later, she indulged in his silly jokes and antics and came to count on them to brighten her day. For his part, Nicolaas reveled in playing up to his mother and seeing her laugh.

The reality was sinking in, and Nicolaas blinked back tears. "You say she was saving a child?"

Dirck explained the circumstances, which seemed to comfort his brother.

"Did she get a nice burial. Lots of people?"

Dirck nodded yes.

"That's good. She deserved it."

Jacques considered himself fortunate when he spotted Dirck walking briskly toward his house, pulling his sea chest on a cart. He was salty and disheveled, obviously had just returned from Gdansk and was eager to get home. Good, Jacques thought, he probably hasn't spoken with anyone yet. He waited around the corner, until Dirck went into his house, before knocking on the door.

"Jacques." Dirck wiped his hand on his breeches and put it out to shake. "Come in."

"I heard that your convoy had returned and wanted to stop by to see how you're doing, with the loss of your mother and you having to leave right away. I know how devastated I was when my sister died and had to escape from Antwerp with Uncle Konrad very soon after."

"Ja, I'm sad but doing fine. Thanks." Dirck motioned for them to sit down. "I wish I had beer to offer you."

"I happen to have some sherry." Jacques pulled a flask from within his doublet, and said sheepishly, "I don't usually carry a flask, but it's a gift from my uncle." Dirck produced two glasses, and Jacques raised his. "To happier days."

"Here, here." Dirck gulped his down and leaned back, tired. "Nicolaas asked me to tell you that he sold your entire shipment of cloth for the price you wanted."

"Nicolaas is a gifted salesman." Jacques moved his chair forward. "Dirck, I want to be the first to tell you about something that happened while you were gone. Maria and I spent considerable time together, and I asked her to marry me. She said ja." He braced for an angry response and possibly being tossed out and never spoken to again.

"You won out" Dirck said with equanimity. "Actually, I'm not really surprised. You two are perfect for each other, and I could see I had an uphill battle."

"Well." Jacques was momentarily stunned. "That's very gracious of you, but I *do* think it was a difficult decision for her ... could have gone either way. I got lucky."

"Ja, you did. You're a lucky man." Dirck took another swig of sherry. "When's the big day?"

"In two weeks. We set the date for when you'd be in town."

"Thanks. I'll look forward to it."

The couple were married in a civil ceremony, because Maria had decided not to convert to Calvinism. A few months later, the two sailed with the fleet to Livorno for another celebration with Lodewyk.

The 1593 northern sailing season was well underway by the time Van der Voort & Sons' new fleet of fluyts were ready for their maiden voyage to Gdansk. Maarten had tested each one, trained the crews, and acquainted Dirck, Rykaard and their other captains with the ship's capabilities and quirks. The fluyt-building shipyard in partnership with Pieter Jansz Liorne also was nearly ready. Financing had been secured, land acquired, sawmills set up, and pine timber was being stockpiled. Now, all that remained was for Maarten to take orders from interested sea captains and then let Liorne do his work.

When the fluyts sailed out of Hoorn's harbor to rendezvous with the convoy coming from Amsterdam, they drew stares. As the convoy made its way northward in the Zuider Zee, all eyes were on them to see whether they scraped bottom—they did not—and whether so few crew could actually handle those new sails—they did. The final test came at the Oresund. When the fluyts paid no more than the usual toll, the other captains waited in line to inspect the intriguing new ships and to ultimately place orders.

The arrival of the fluyts in Gdansk drew further attention, and Maarten and Rykaard remained onboard to field questions and give tours. Dirck and Nicolaas were left with overseeing the unloading of the ships, and that evening Dirck went to the tiny house Nicolaas had rented for the season. There, he met Tatiana, a skinny Russian with unhappy eyes. Though she was utterly unlike Nicolaas's previous housekeepers, he seemed mesmerized by her. Each night after supper, Dirck observed the two sitting close together, deep in conversation. As far as Dirck could tell, Tatiana was dispensing wisdom about life, most of it dark and maudlin. After hearing "Life is misery" several times, he decided to move to a boarding house on the excuse that the place was too small for three.

When the convoy was ready to depart, Nicolaas informed his father that he wanted to return to Amsterdam, even though the season had not yet ended. The reasons he gave were he had already arranged grain purchases for the final voyages and, more importantly, had a newfound sense of purpose in life and wanted to get back to his wife and child. Maarten readily assented, thrilled that his son was finally embracing family life and giving up untoward relationships with housekeepers.

Nonetheless, saying goodbye to Tatiana was wrenching, and

Nicolaas's face showed it as he walked to the Customs House to meet Dirck.

"Tough to say goodbye, eh?" Dirck commented and was taken aback when his brother's eyes turn glassy. "What do you see in Tatiana? She's certainly not your type."

"She's not, and that's why I chose her. I didn't want to be tempted. She turned out to be smart, and I learned a lot. She taught me life is purposeless, so you have to find your own reason for living. I now realize that everything—marriage, work, life—gets boring after a while. When it does, I need to mix things up. Drinking and women aren't the answer. I need to create my own excitement, my own meaning in life. I'm still working on that, but you get the idea."

"Ja, I do," Dirck said, and thanked his lucky stars that Nicolaas was traveling on their father's ship, and father would be the one to have to endure more of Tatiana's words of wisdom.

The ships set sail during a break in the foul weather that had persisted throughout much of the summer and then hugged the Polish coastline for safety. In the run toward the Oresund, the sky grew ominous, the wind kicked up, white caps formed on the mounting swells, and the smell of rain was in the air. This was normally the time Nicolaas went below to ride out the coming storm, but curiosity got the best of him. How was such a small crew going to handle those new sails? He had to see for himself and, if necessary, lend a hand. He lifted his stump, amused by his little pun.

Thinking he had time before the storm turned nasty, Nicolaas became engrossed in the sight of men climbing the ratlines and trying to reef the new sails while lines rap-rap-rapped. In no time, waves were washing across the deck.

"NICOLAAS, GET BELOW!" Maarten bellowed.

"JA!" Nicolaas unwrapped his arms from the mast, tested his footing, and made a dash for the cabin. He reached it, just as a wave crashed over the bow and raced toward him. Hanging onto the cabin door latch for dear life, he braced himself. The torrent slammed into his body and carried him, flailing in its midst, toward the gunwale. The water cascaded into the sea, with him calling out, "*Help! HELLLLLP!*"

"MAN OVERBOARD!" a seaman shouted.

Maarten looked to where he had last seen Nicolaas and rushed to the gunwale. He frantically searched the angry sea. Foaming water washed the deck and knocked him down.

"CAP'N! DO YOU SEE HIM?" a seaman yelled.

Maarten scrambled to his feet and blinked the water from his eyes ... searching ... searching.

"SEE HIM?"

"Oh God, *Neeee!*"

A memorial service was held for Nicolaas at Nieuwe Kerk on what would have been his twenty-eighth birthday. Minister Arminius officiated, and Amsterdammers from all walks of life attended, from government officials and business associates to waitresses and seamen. Everyone seemed to agree that a little sunshine had gone out of their lives, and a common refrain was that his mischievous humor and infectious laugh could light up a room.

Rolfe wore the beaver hat his father had given him. Griet was inconsolable, believing she would never again find a man as fun and *unpredicable* as Nicolaas.

Maarten, Dirck and Catrijn were reeling. Two lives had been lost in less than two years: first Betje, and now Nicolaas.

A few days after the funeral, Pastor Arminius paid Maarten a visit and found him looking haggard, as though he had not slept in awhile. Together, the two sat in the front room, with Maarten saying nothing.

"Maarten, I know there is little anyone can say to diminish your pain, but I hope you will take comfort in knowing that those who live righteous lives will find a place in heaven."

Maarten's brow furrowed more deeply, not only because of concern that Nicolaas's numerous improprieties might keep him out of heaven, but also because Arminius seemed to have changed his opinion about who gets into heaven.

"Pastor, did you say I should take comfort that the righteous go to heaven? Before, you and Plancius seemed to say that God chose long ago which people would go to heaven or hell, and a person's righteous behavior could not change it."

"I have thought much about what I told you and have come to believe that free will plays a part in whether a person goes to heaven, such as your wife choosing to sacrifice her own life to save a child. Other clergy, including Petrus Plancius, argue that people mistakenly believe they are using free will, when in fact God is guiding them. Theologians will probably debate this matter for years to come, but that should not be a concern for you, and it won't change God's command that we must live virtuous lives."

Maarten forced a smile of appreciation because the pastor had been so earnest in explaining that good works earn a place in heaven, something that had been obvious to him right along.

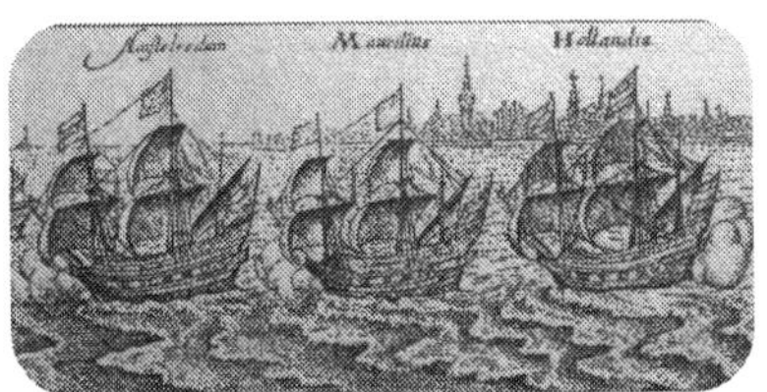

Ships of the Far Lands Company

CHAPTER 9

New Horizons – 1593-1597

Having just returned from sea, Dirck headed for home carrying a sack over his shoulder. His path took him past Griet's house, where she was sitting on the front bench taking in the late autumn sun, while Rolfe, wearing his beaver hat, was digging in the dirt with a stick.

Rolfe saw Dirck coming and ran to him.

"*Uncle Dirck!*"

Dirck dropped his sack, scooped up Rolfe, and tossed him into the air.

"I missed you!" Rolfe said between giggles. He noticed the sack. "Did you bring me something?"

"Hmm, let me see." Dirck fumbled in his sack—"Maybe."—and pulled out a wooden object with a bulbous top, pointy bottom, and string wrapped round.

"What is it?"

"A top." Dirck placed the toy on the ground, pulled the string, and launched it.

"Wow!" Rolfe watched with fascination and yelped, "Whoa!" when the top hit a stone, ricocheted, and took off down the street. He chased after it.

Dirck sat down next to Griet. "How're you doing?"

She gave a shrug to say so-so and shifted closer to him. "And you?"

"I'm fine," Dirck said, though sadness still lingered in his voice. "The voyage went well, no problems. But it seemed long, and I'm glad to be home."

Griet gave him a look that said she understood. "Have you seen your father yet?" When he shook his head no, she commented, "He's been spending time with widow Letje ter Williger. Seems happy."

"Good for him."

"The widow reminds me of your mother, superstitious and a good cook."

"That doesn't surprise me. Men tend to like a particular type of woman, and I guess Mother and Letje are his type."

"It seems so," Griet said and thought: He's letting me know I'm his type—sexy like Maria, gorgeous like Kaatje—well, maybe not *as* beautiful as Kaatje, but I have *much* bigger breasts, and I've caught Dirck staring at them.

Rolfe came running back, wanting his uncle to make the top go again.

After teaching him how to spin it, Dirck said he had to leave to visit his father and afterward deliver a present to godchild Jaane.

Rolfe grabbed his leg and hung on. "Nee, don't go!"

Dirck laughed, ruffled his hair and pulled away. "Have to go." Recalling that Nicolaas had clung to him when he left to rebuild dikes in Alkmaar, he marveled again at the similarities between the two—same cute face, mop of golden red hair ... mischievous grin—and concluded that Rolfe's going to be a handful to raise.

After Dirck had gone, Griet turned her face to the sun again and closed her eyes. Rolfe resumed digging, using the pointy end of the top.

"Hey there, little fellow. What have you got?"

"A top!"

Griet's eyes opened and squinted at the man silhouetted against the sun.

"You're Nicolaas's widow, aren't you?" the man said. When

Griet said yes, he added, "I'm Rijp Dekker, a business associate. Too bad what happened to him."

Griet tilted her head in thanks and remembered hearing Rijp Dekker's name in conversations between Nicolaas and his father. They seemed to have differing opinions of the man.

Rijp sat down next to her, leaned over to inspect the top, asked the boy his name, and helped Rolfe rewind the string.

What does this old guy want? Griet thought, not liking his undue friendliness toward her and her son. She raised the shawl around her shoulders. A gust of wind swept in, picking up some of the dirt Rolfe had been digging in and swirling it into a little whirlwind.

"Ow," Griet said, her eye fluttering. She tossed her head to the left and right, trying to get the speck of dirt out.

"Something in your eye?" Rijp brought his finger to just below her eye. "Here, let me get it."

"Nee!" Griet jerked away. She would never stick her own finger into her eye, let alone allow a stranger do it. Her eye fluttered uncontrollably. "Oow."

Rijp put his thumb on her cheek and index finger above the eye and pried it open. With a touch of his handkerchief, he removed the particle, she squirming all the while. "Now, that wasn't so bad, was it?"

"Uh, I ..." Griet's teary eye blinked several times. "I guess not." She dabbed at the corner. "Thanks."

"Don't mention it." With a sly grin, Rijp said, "Now, stick out your tongue."

"What?"

"Stick out your tongue."

She looked at him, skeptical, and did as told.

He kissed it and promptly rose to his feet. With a gallant sweep of his hat, he bowed gracefully. "Adieu."

What? That was weird, she thought. Then the word *unpredicable* came to mind. Griet watched him swagger off, dapper, and looking as though he owned the world. Like a moth to fire, she was inexplicably attracted to the odd and *unpredicable* Rijp Dekker.

With fluyts proving to be the workhorse of their northern trade, Maarten and Dirck had ordered one for the Livorno route with modifications to carry more cannons. Dirck stopped in Hoorn to check on it during his return trip from La Rochelle and noticed a man inspecting his fluyt, whose appearance indicated he was not a sea captain.

"Are you interested in ships?" Dirck asked.

"I've spent a fair bit of time on them from time to time," the man said, "but never saw one like this. What is it?"

"A fluyt. They're very efficient for our Baltic trade, but this one's for the Mediterranean. Pieter Jansz Liorne invented it. You probably know he owns this shipyard. Actually my father and I are partners with him." Dirck stuck out his hand. "I'm Dirck van der Voort, from Amsterdam."

"Jan Huijgen van Linschoten, from Enkhuizen." They shook hands. "I'm writing a book about the spice trade in the East Indies and go to Amsterdam periodically to consult with Petrus Plancius about my maps. Perhaps we can get together for a drink next time. I'd like to learn about these fluyts."

"Sure, and I'd like to hear more about your book. I know Plancius and sometimes buy maps from him. He's a good cartographer. But I'm curious about you. How did a Dutchman learn so much about that part of the world?"

"By chance really. In '76, I went to Spain to live with my older brother William and work for the merchant he was employed by. Four years later, I moved to Lisbon for a better job. The company had problems, and my brother helped me secure another position as secretary to the new Archbishop of Goa—Goa is Portugal's colony in India. I worked there until the archbishop died. Then on the way back to Portugal our ship was attacked by an English pirate, and I was shipwrecked in the Azores for two years. Finally made it back to Enkhuizen in '92."

"That's quite a story."

"There're lots of other stories similar to mine, and for the past year I've been collecting them. Dirck 'China' Gerritsz, for example, has a very interesting one; he's from Enkhuizen too."

Dirck had never heard of Gerritsz or anyone else who had been to the East Indies and was intrigued. "I want to hear more, so please look me up when you come to Amsterdam. We're on Nieuwendijk Straat. You can't miss our sign: Van der Voort & Sons."

Griet stood with one arm wrapped around her waist and a finger tapping her cheek, contemplating what to buy at the fishmonger's stand.

"Take the herring."

Griet's head whipped around. "Oh, Heer Dekker. You startled me."

"Rijp. Call me Rijp." He pointed to the herring. "They're the best ... tried 'em yesterday."

"Oh, uh, thanks," Griet said without connecting with his penetrating eyes; they unnerved her. After purchasing several herrings, she walked away and Rijp was at her side.

"Where's little Rolfe?" he asked.

"He's with Nicolaas's Aunt Margaretha, at the Begijnhof for lessons with his cousin."

"You gotta be careful with Margaretha. She'll knock the spunk out of your little Rolfe and make him a scaredy kid, always afraid of doing something wrong. I know—'cause I've had my run-ins with her."

Griet was too flabbergasted to respond. No one had ever criticized selfless Aunt Margaretha before, at least not in her presence.

"Wanna go get a drink? I own a tavern on Haringpakkers Steeg, and I'm thirsty." He touched Griet's elbow to steer her in the direction of Warmoesstraat, intending to take the long route to avoid passing by Maarten's house. He did not want to risk being seen with Nicolaas's widow, because it might jeopardize his chances of convincing Maarten to take his goods on consignment aboard his fluyts, which had the lowest shipping rates in Amsterdam.

"Why did you do that the last time I saw you—kiss my tongue?" Griet asked.

"I wanted to," Rijp said with a shrug. "Why? Didn't you like it?"

"Well, uh. No one ever did that before. I, uh ..."

Rijp let the conversation die. She's young, he told himself, go easy. She's probably never had a *real* man before. He looked at her again. Seeing a slight smile on her lips, he changed his opinion: maybe she's not so innocent either. This is gonna be interesting.

At the door of the pub, Griet noticed there were only men inside. "I don't think I should. I better go home."

"Fine, I'm not very thirsty after all." Rijp touched her elbow again. "I need to collect rent from a tenant anyway, and it's on the way to your house."

The tenant was a painter, and he whisked Rijp into the back room for a private conversation. Alone in the front room, Griet tried not to eavesdrop while inspecting the paintings. There was a half-finished portrait on the easel, a completed one leaning against the wall, and paintings of the usual biblical scenes: a weary Mary astride a donkey in Bethlehem, Jesus brought down from the cross ... martyred saints dripping in blood. In her opinion, they were much better than the family portraits done by Konrad and Catrijn's artist.

The men's hushed conversation degenerated into a heated argument, which ended with Rijp bellowing: "If you don't like it, you can get the fuck out!"

The painter burst from the back room, agitated. Rijp emerged smiling, as though nothing had happened. Griet looked askance at Rijp, thinking she had never seen anyone go from extreme anger one minute to sweetness the next. It was unsettling.

The painter realized Griet was standing next to his best picture. "I see you're a connoisseur of paintings," he said with a forced smile. "Perhaps you and your husband would like me to paint a portrait of you."

"I'm a widow."

"Forgive me," he said with penitent eyes, "I am oh so sorry." Now he was hitting his stride and moving into salesman mode.

"Any children?" When Griet nodded yes, he said, "Perhaps a painting of you and the child, Madonna and child, so to speak?"

"Would we be hugging and laughing? And could we wear our beaver hats?"

Rijp snickered.

"Well ... that's highly unusual." Seeing Griet's interest wane, the painter added, "But, of course, we could try. I must exercise my integrity as a painter. But, of course, we could try."

"I'll have to think about it. Thank you."

Damn! Rijp thought to himself. Griet's got spunk!

Worried about her financial future, Griet paid a visit to Maarten. Leaves were flying when she knocked on his door.

Pieter answered and motioned her to come in quickly. "Feels like it's going to be another early winter, and a mighty cold one," he said. When a swirl of leaves followed in Griet's wake, he swatted them out with his foot before closing the door.

"Afraid so ... brrr." Griet rolled back her hood. "Maarten isn't home?"

"Nee, but he'll be back soon." Pieter reached for his jerkin and beret. "I have to go out now. You won't have long to wait."

Griet's eyes roamed the desks, which she had paid little attention to previously. There were quill pens, shavings from a recently sharpened quill, ink stains, and ledgers. She opened one and leafed through it. It was full of numbers and words, which she could not comprehend. The door opened.

"Griet!" Maarten said as he removed his overcoat and beret with a small brim and flaps, which he had started wearing again in cold weather. "How are you? How's *Rolfe*?" He said Rolfe in the same deep voice Nicolaas always used; it was his and Griet's little shared memory of Nicolaas now. He patted her arm and motioned her to take a seat.

"We're both good. Rolfe's at Aunt Margaretha's with Jaane." Griet cleared her throat nervously and sat down opposite Maarten.

Maarten's eyebrow cocked.

Griet unwrapped her cape. "Whenever I need money, I just come to you or Pieter and you give it to me—just like you said you would."

"Uh-huh."

"Where does that money come from? Nicolaas isn't here to work anymore. I'm not working." She looked him in the eye. "I don't want charity."

Though tickled by Griet's indignation, Maarten suppressed a smile and responded in a businesslike manner. "Well, Nicolaas owned part of Van der Voort & Sons, along with Dirck, Pieter and me. And you and Rolfe now own Nicolaas's share. When there are profits, you get Nicolaas's share of them. They're not charity."

"So profits are free? Nobody has to work for them?" This was the first time she had heard of people earning something by not working. Having been a housecleaner and maid, she knew all about toiling for a living.

"Nee, profits aren't free. Nicolaas and all of us labored over the years to earn the profits, and most of those profits were reinvested in our business to create long-term value. Just because Nicolaas isn't with us anymore, it doesn't mean his hard work disappeared, as though it had no value to Van der Voort & Sons. So you get profits based on Nicolaas's past labors, as I explained to you shortly after Nicolaas died, and the value of that is now your and Rolfe's investment. You two are investors."

"So ... unless all the ships sink and you and Dirck and Pieter stop working, the business keeps going and gives profits to me and Rolfe? Because we're *in-vest-ors?*"

"That's pretty much it. But don't ever mention sinking ships in front of Pieter—he's superstitious, just like my wife was."

Griet couldn't tell whether he was serious or joking. She cleared her throat again. "I'm happy to get the profits, but I'd feel better if I worked for them. Can you give me a job?"

"What do you want to do?"

"Uh, I can learn. Help with ... uh, something."

"Maybe you should think about it. Talk to Pieter. See what type of work he does. Nicolaas started there."

"All right."

"I'll be happy to give you a job, but I want you to promise to continue to improve yourself… in reading and arithmetic. It'll make you a more valuable worker."

"I will," Griet said and brushed aside a curl that had sneaked out from the tangle of blond hair concealed under her cap. "Oh, and there's something else," she added with trepidation. "I'd like to have a portrait painted of me and Rolfe, smiling and having fun. And with our beaver hats on, as a reminder of our life with Nicolaas."

Beaver hats! Maarten chuckled silently. "Go ahead, but make sure the price is fair. The painter might try to cheat a woman, so ask Konrad what he paid for our paintings, and then negotiate with the painter if his price seems high. Anything else?"

"Nope." She had considered mentioning she wanted to take painting lessons but decided not to push her luck, because no one had ever been as nice to her as her father-in-law.

"Think about what you want to do, and we'll give you a job."

"Thanks." Griet gave him a big kiss on the forehead and asked impishly, "By the way, who's going to do Nicolaas's job in Gdansk?"

"Me for a while, then an agent." He kidded back, "So don't get any ideas."

"I won't." With a giddy grin, she left to pick up Rolfe.

At the Begijnhof, Rolfe greeted her with, "Look at Jaane, Mom! Look!"

Jaane's bright blue eyes smiled through her new spectacles.

"You see better now, Jaane?"

"Ja," Jaane said, and pushed the spectacles higher on her tiny nose. Rolfe tugged at her, and the two ran outside to play.

"I never understood," Margaretha said, "why Jaane frowned so much. It was poor vision all along. Now that sweet little face never stops smiling."

"Nice." Griet ran her finger along the edge of the table, sat down opposite Margaretha and said without lifting her eyes, "Aunt Margaretha, uh, do you think you can help me improve my talking?

I say some words wrong, like *unpredicable*. I could use help with reading. Numbers too. I want to be a better *examle*, *ex-am-pull* for Rolfe." Her eyes met Margaretha's.

"Of course. I'd be pleased to. We can start tomorrow, if you like."

Griet's eyes scrunched with excitement. "Ja, I'd like that."

The three-and-a-half-year-olds ran back into the house, and Griet started to get up.

Margaretha touched her hand and looked into her eyes. "I saw Rijp Dekker sitting with you in front of your house last week. It's none of my business, but I want you to know ... Rijp is nothing like Nicolaas." She was particularly concerned because Rijp's wife had died recently, and he was undoubtedly on the prowl.

"Oh ... uh, ja." Griet rose and called Rolfe over. Together they went out the door, with Rolfe furiously waving goodbye to Jaane and Aunt Margaretha.

"So Rolfe," Griet said, as they walked hand-in-hand down the street, "you really like Jaane's *spec-a-culls*, huh?" His head went up and down exaggeratedly. "Well, some kids might not like 'em much." She was thinking of the common belief that spectacles indicated a weak mind. "If any kid ever says something mean to Jaane, you punch him. Understand?"

"Ja!" Rolfe scowled and pummeled an imaginary mean kid with his fist.

"Good. Jaane's smart, and we love her. But kids can be mean."

Rolfe continued to punch, while Griet thought of what she could do to toughen up her reserved little goddaughter.

Dirck was disembarking at the Damrak, having spent the day getting his new fluyt ready to sail to Livorno, when he saw Petrus Plancius waving to him. Plancius met him at the dock.

"Jan van Linschoten will be here in a few days," Plancius said, "and I'm eager for all three of us to get together. He told me about your chance meeting in Hoorn, and perhaps he mentioned that he and I are organizing a sailing venture over the North Pole to China for next summer with navigator Willem Barents. We're raising money for it now."

"He didn't mention it, but, sure, I'd like to get together. Just let me know when he arrives, and I'll organize supper at my house. I'll invite Jacques and Konrad, and Catrijn too. I told them about Linschoten's new book, and they're eager to meet him." He omitted his father, knowing that anything to do with Plancius and sailing over the North Pole ranked on par with King Philip II for him. Dirck, though, did not mind Plancius as much now, because his Sunday sermons were becoming more interesting. No longer overly pious, they seemed more like lessons in cartography and astronomy with only a little piety sprinkled in.

"Splendid. I'll bring a sketch of our Arctic sailing route with me."

On the day of the supper, Dirck moved the big table and chairs from the kitchen into the front room to provide a more comfortable environment for talking. His cook was already at work in the kitchen.

Konrad and Catrijn arrived punctually, and Plancius and Linschoten followed close behind. Jacques sent his apologies. For him, life now centered on a very pregnant Maria, the silk business, Livorno trade, and the fluyt shipyard, which he had recently become involved in. China and the East Indies were merely a remote and irrelevant diversion.

After introducing Jan Huijgen van Linschoten to everyone, Plancius eagerly launched into explaining the venture, which was to discover the elusive route over the North Pole that leads to China and the East Indies. He himself was putting up part of the money, and Linschoten would be sailing on Willem Barents's ship. He added, "All the cartographers in Europe confirm the route exists," and pulled out a drawing.

"Before we look at that," Konrad said, "I'd like to ask a question. Twenty or more years ago, England sent several fleets to find the Polar route; Frobisher led one of them. Before that, France sent Verrazano and Cartier. All failed. Why do you think your venture will succeed?"

"Captain Barents will have a new, more accurate map from Gerardus Mercator. English explorers Martin Frobisher and John Davis both used Mercator's maps on their voyages and later shared their observations with him, which Mercator used to update his map."

Plancius smoothed out his sketch of the Arctic, which depicted the North Pole at the center of a large circle, labeled 60th latitude north. "This sketch is the gist of Mercator's new map. To get you oriented, here's Greenland," he said with a finger point. "It's exactly where Frobisher and Davis located it on their maps." Plancius's finger circled four blobs. "Mercator has determined there are four islands surrounding the North Pole."

Linschoten added, "Mercator knows the approximate size and shape of the islands, except for this one." His finger tapped on the blob closest to Norway. "He doesn't have an accurate southern coastline for the island, but he knows pygmies live there—little people, only four feet tall."

"Astonishing," Catrijn remarked.

"And this is even more amazing," Plancius said. "Water from all the oceans of the world flows between those four islands toward the North Pole where it's sucked into a giant whirlpool—"

"Are you saying the North Pole is actually a giant whirlpool?"

"Exactly. All the world's water goes into the whirlpool ... into the bowels of the earth ... and resurfaces to form rivers across the globe. It's a continuous flow." The room fell silent. Plancius glanced knowingly at Linschoten, for they too had been speechless when Mercator's map had first been explained to them. "Only God could have created such a masterful plan."

"And the important thing," Linschoten said, "is that those islands are surrounded by open sea in summer, so it'll be easy to sail across the Arctic to the channel leading to Asia. Not only will it be much faster than the southern route around Africa, it'll also be safer, without Portuguese competitors, Spanish ships, or English pirates to contend with."

"We'll need some time to think about your thought-provoking

drawing," Dirck said and turned to Linschoten. "In the meantime, we'd all like to hear about your East Indies manuscript."

"And what you know about the Portuguese monopoly," Konrad said.

"The Portuguese monopoly on spices in the East Indies? Portugal doesn't have one. They want you to believe they have an exclusive monopoly there, the same as they have in Europe—but they don't!"

Silence again.

"Spices grow in many different places. Some on the mainland. Others on islands. Each with a different ruler," Linschoten explained. "The Portuguese have negotiated trading rights with the rulers of the most important spice-producing areas. But they're not the *only* traders—just one of many. The Chinese and Muslims trade everywhere. So do the Persians and Indian kingdoms." Linschoten looked Dirck in the eye and then Konrad. "If a Dutchman can get to the East Indies, he can trade like anyone else. The trick is to get there safely and to know where to find the spices. That's where my book comes in."

"Do you have it with you?"

"Part of it." Linschoten lifted a sheaf of papers from his leather folder and handed it to Dirck. "These chapters describe the spices and where they grow: pepper in India, cinnamon in Ceylon ... ginger, cloves. There are other chapters, which I'm still working on, that deal with animals, plants, and gems found in each place."

Dirck leafed through the handwritten pages and passed them to Konrad.

"Very interesting," Catrijn said, looking over Konrad's shoulder.

"Do you mind if we read these and return them to you tomorrow?" Konrad asked. "We'll take good care of them."

Linschoten nodded agreement, somewhat reluctantly. "Dirck, I'll stop by tomorrow to pick them up."

"Does your manuscript tell how to navigate around the spice islands?" Dirck asked. "The Portuguese may not have a monopoly on the spice trade, but they *do* have a monopoly on navigating those waters—which I think is even more important."

"I made a copy of the rutter of pilot Vincente Rodrigues of Lagos when I worked for the Portuguese. That rutter has been used by every Portuguese captain since 1575."

Dirck's eyes bulged. "You have a rutter—*their* rutter?"

Linschoten gave an unequivocal nod yes, knowing how valuable a rutter was to a sea captain. "And it contains all the nautical details you'd expect in a good rutter and would need for safe passage: descriptions of coastlines, water currents and depths ... sandbars ... how best to approach ports, and obstacles to avoid. Everything."

"Whew, I'd like to see that."

"I can't give the rutter to you now, because I'm using it for my descriptions of the ports of call in the spice-growing areas. But I'll be glad to show it to you later."

The next day, a bleary-eyed Konrad returned the manuscript to Dirck.

"You look terrible," Dirck commented when he answered the door.

"Catrijn and I stayed up last night reading it, and just finished." He stepped inside. "Do you have a minute to talk?"

"Sure." The two sat down at Dirck's desk.

"What do you think of this plan of Barents to sail across the Arctic? Plancius said they want investors. Are you interested?"

Dirck's shrug and raised brow indicated he was undecided. "How about you?"

"I might, just to be involved, in case it's successful. But ... actually, I'm skeptical of the North Pole whirlpool. When I traveled in the Alps, villagers told me those streams and rivers were filled by snow melting high in the mountains. No one ever mentioned an underground river bursting forth, as Plancius described. Those villagers may have been repeating old wives' tales, but they made sense to me. So, if I have doubts about the accuracy of Mercator's whirlpool, perhaps—oh, I don't know. I guess I'm just skeptical, especially since the English tried the route and concluded it didn't exist."

"My father and his old sea captain friends say it doesn't exist either. I'd put more weight on their opinions than on a mapmaker like Plancius who has worked at a desk all his life." Dirck offered

Konrad an apple from the bowl on the table and helped himself to one. While they ate, each continued to think.

Dirck wiped a dribble from his chin and said, "Nee, I've decided against investing. It's just an exploratory trip. I'd rather put my money into a voyage that has potential to earn profits, like sending ships on the southern route, which we know *is* feasible. If Linschoten's rutter is as good as I expect, I'd help organize a fleet—even command it! What an adventure."

Konrad laughed. "Too much adventure for me." Turning serious, he said, "If Linschoten's rutter *is* indeed the key to the southern route, there's no time to waste. Once his book is published, merchants in every Dutch city will want to send a fleet."

Dirck had returned from his third trip to Livorno in early 1594 and was at his desk transferring the latest notes from his Waghenaer map to his rutter, when he remembered a question he wanted to ask his father.

"Father, Lodewyk mentioned that King Philip is declaring bankruptcy. Is it true?"

"That's what I hear," Maarten said with a smug grin. "It seems the problem started with his campaign against the French Huguenot king, Henry, which must of cost him a considerable sum. After that, he didn't pay his army and it mutinied. Then, of course, when Parma died and his replacements were all incompetent—that didn't help either."

"You think we're safe for a while?"

"Well. I never like to get too optimistic, but I *do* think we're pretty secure. Not because of the bankruptcy. King Philip's done that before—in the '50s, '60s, and in '75—and it didn't stop his wars. It's because of our army. Oldenbarnevelt says it's efficient, disciplined, well-paid, *and* the best in Europe. Much of the credit goes to the princes, Maurice and William Henry. They've modernized and standardized weaponry and drill soldiers to fire in volleys. And set up supply depots all along our southern border, so our army can be resupplied easily if an attack comes."

"Pretty impressive," Dirck said, "and so are our admiralties. I saw one of their new four-masted ships in La Rochelle. It had *two* gun decks."

"Another reason for optimism."

Dirck rose to refill his mug, and Maarten returned to his list of things to do. The first item—check on when the new fluyt will be ready for a trial run—brought a smile to his face, for he always enjoyed breaking in a new ship. This one was going to be especially challenging because of its design: it will have a hole in the hull for loading extra long logs, which must be sealed up before sailing. He moved onto the next item, crew for the new fluyt, and sighed. Finding experienced sailors was a chronic problem, and he knew he must start today to visit taverns favored by better seamen to get word out that he was hiring. Identifying a captain was of no concern, because one of Rykaard's sons was ready to be promoted from first mate to captain.

Maarten leaned back, scratching his ear and pondering how to make the fluyt-building operation more efficient. Shipbuilder Pieter Jansz Liorne was doing his best, but there was just too much demand for him to keep up. It was a blessing and a curse. He jotted down an idea: look into the possibility of using windmills to power the saws. And he also wrote a reminder to get back to the merchants clamoring for space on his already full ships to take advantage of his low shipping rates. His thoughts drifted to the city council and whether to take Uncle Nostrand's advice to seek an alderman position. He began cracking his knuckles. The sound made Dirck glance up, and Maarten remembered something.

"Oh Dirck, I forgot to mention Reinier Pauw dropped by and said he and a couple of other city councilors are considering sending a fleet to the East Indies. Wanted to know if we're interested. I told him you were, but I'd have to hear more before deciding. He asked me to let him know when you returned home, so we can all meet. He's heard about Linschoten."

Dirck put down his quill and wiped the ink from his fingers.

"You're not really interested, are you? Not even in the southern route?"

"Nee, we have a nice business going here, and I'm earning more money than I'll ever need. With Nicolaas gone and my work on the City Council and the continuing problems with the shipyard, I'm too busy to get involved with a new venture. Especially a risky one that probably won't make money for years, if ever."

"I think the spice trade will be lucrative, in time, and a great adventure. I wouldn't even mind commanding the fleet."

"An adventure? Sailing to Livorno is an adventure, but *this*—sailing halfway round the world, in unknown waters, and with the threat of primitive people and scurvy—it's practically suicide." Maarten's head was turning side to side. "You can forget that idea. I've already lost one son and don't want to lose you too. None of those men, not Reinier Pauw or the others, is going to risk his or his son's life on this. Money, ja. Lives, nee."

On the weekend, a meeting was held at Maarten Spil's wine tavern on Warmoesstraat with eleven men in attendance. Some expressed a preference for the northern route, hoping Barents would find it when sailing to the Arctic in summer. Others favored the southern one. All agreed, though, the decision about the route could be made later and the more pressing need was to confirm that it was indeed feasible to challenge Portugal's monopoly. Reinier Pauw said he would ask his cousin to verify Linschoten's reports about the monopoly when the cousin went to Portugal in a few months, and other men offered to solicit verifications from their sources in Spain and Portugal. Dirck agreed to get Linschoten's Portuguese rutter and report back after studying it. A few men volunteered to think about the number of ships to send and other logistics.

In late October 1594, details of the venture came together. Several sources confirmed that Portugal does not have a spice monopoly in the East Indies, just non-exclusive rights to trade. The elusive northern route had been shown to be infeasible after Barents' ships encountered impenetrable ice fields and were forced to turn back. After having examined Linschoten's rutter in detail, Dirck reported that Dutch captains should be able to rely on it to safely navigate the southern route. The cost, financing and logistics were carefully considered and agreed upon, and a departure date via the southern route was set for March 1595, a full year before Linschoten's book was to be published.

Hearing rumors about the daring enterprise, Konrad, Catrijn, Margaretha, and Jacques dropped by Maarten's house to find out whether they were true and, if so, could they invest. They found Van der Voort & Sons' owners busy at their desks, including apprentice Griet, who greeted them with a contented smile.

Dirck willingly shared the plan. "Ten merchants, including me, will form a business called Far Lands Company and serve as its board of directors. Reinier Pauw is one of them and so is Dirck van Os."

Konrad nodded approvingly, for he admired fellow Antwerper Van Os's business acumen and ability to bring ventures to fruition.

Dirck continued, "The directors will put up much of the 300,000 guilders needed, and the rest will come from investors like yourselves." His eyes went to Jacques, Konrad, Catrijn and to Margaretha. "My father has already decided to invest."

Pieter raised his hand. "I want to invest too."

"Me too," Griet said, hoping to be taken seriously.

"I'd be happy to recommend all of you as investors, if you're still interested after hearing the details: Two-thirds of the money will be spent on the ships, crew, and goods to sell in the East Indies. The other third will be taken as gold and silver coins to pay for spices. For the directors' work in organizing the venture, we'll receive 1% of the cost of outfitting the ships plus 1% of the profits. Seem fair?"

"Seems fair," Konrad said, and the others nodded their agreement.

"This idea of forming a *company* is something new," Dirck said. "The company—not individual merchants—will own the ships and goods. And directors and investors will own percentages of the company. At the end of the voyage, the company will be dissolved, the ships and spices sold, and profits distributed. If all or some of us agree to send another fleet, we'll form another company. Sound good?"

Nods all around.

"I should add," Maarten said, "both the City Council and Holland's government have agreed to help, thanks to the efforts of Heer Nostrand and Advocate Oldenbarnevelt. They're giving the company a hundred guns and other weapons, free of charge. And Prince Maurice is granting the company the right to claim land for the Dutch Republic."

"Will you be going with the fleet, Dirck?" Konrad inquired.

"Nee, I can't be away for such a long time … already have trouble keeping up with the Gdansk, La Rochelle and Livorno sailings. In fact, I'm skipping Livorno this winter, and Rykaard will lead the convoy for me, so I can finish my work on the Far Lands Company."

Everyone left, after requesting to be counted as investors.

Griet departed shortly thereafter and, not far from home, saw Rijp.

"Hey, Griet, imagine seeing you here. How you doing?" Rijp said and started walking alongside. "I hear you're working for your father-in-law now. Do you like it?"

"I'm learning a lot *and* earning my keep."

"That's good." He changed the subject. "I noticed Dirck's been meeting at Maarten Spil's tavern with a group of merchants. They say they're planning to send a fleet to the East Indies."

Griet surveyed his face. "Why do you ask?"

"No particular reason. Just interested in knowing what's happening in my city." He smiled. "Are they accepting investors?"

Griet gave him a saucy grin. "I'm one." She liked the sound of the sophisticated word, investor, being applied to her.

Rijp's eyebrow raised, and Griet took it to mean he was impressed.

It was a frigid January evening when Konrad delivered his and Jacques's final investment installments to Reinier Pauw's home. Most people had the good sense to stay home on such a bitter night, but Konrad wanted to meet the deadline. He had intended to do so during daylight hours, but a series of events had conspired against him, including a machine breaking down and Catrijn and Jaane both taking sick.

Now trudging home on a footpath along a canal, Konrad treaded carefully. Having dropped his ceramic lantern, smashing it to bits, he was having trouble identifying icy patches, much less the edge of the canal on this moonless night. All was quiet on the street, except for an occasional loud voice from behind a shuttered window. Konrad squinted at the path ahead ... a slight shimmer of ice. He avoided it and proceeded on in the darkness, looking ahead for another light-emitting window to show him the way. "Oops!" he slipped, but caught himself.

Past another faintly-lit house, he lost his footing again—"Oops!"—slid sideways, legs spread wide for balance. "Whoa." One foot went over the edge ... "Oooh" ... his body went flying. He landed on the frozen canal. THUD! His head smacked the ice.

Konrad awoke, engulfed in a mental fog. His mind waded through it, and vision slowly returned. A faint line appeared ... the edge of the canal. I'm in the canal! His hands felt around. I'm on the ice, in the canal. He tried to get up. "Ow!" Can't move my arm ... and this ringing in my ears. He shook his head to make it stop and tried again to raise to his feet, this time on his other side. On one knee ... balancing ... balancing. Just stand up, he told himself, get up! Both feet on the ice. He shook his head again ... Hold your balance! "Oh nee." His feet went flying into the air. WHACK!

By eight o'clock, Catrijn was getting worried. At nine o'clock, she bundled Jaane into her arms, lit a lantern, and walked to Maarten's house.

Maarten sat Catrijn and Jaane down by the hearth and walked to Jacques's house to see whether Konrad had stopped there; he hadn't. Maaten went on to the Night Watch meeting place to alert Dirck, who was preparing to go out on his rounds.

Returning home, he told Catrijn, "Don't worry. Dirck and the Night Watch are looking for Konrad. He probably went into a tavern to get warm. They'll find him."

Dirck sent some of the Night Watchmen to check the taverns, and took others with him to walk the path most likely taken by Konrad. Moving gingerly with lanterns held high, they mounted the bridge over the Damrak. Dirck's feet skidded out from under him. He grasped the railing and righted himself. "Damn, it's slick!" On to Haringpakkers Steeg and Nieuwendijk, then left onto the walkway along Spuistraat. It was dark, really dark. Dirck called out, "*Konrad! Konrad Teller!*" No response. He and his men walked on, slipping and sliding.

"*Dirck!*" a Night Watchman shouted, while holding his lantern over the canal. There on the ice was a man, lying face up with legs and arms splayed wide.

Dirck dropped into the canal and knelt beside him. "Aww ... Konrad." It sickened him to see Konrad's lifeless eyes staring into eternity.

Catrijn made sure every detail of Konrad's wake and funeral were perfectly executed. The mourners were many, reflecting his extensive connections in the city he had called home for fourteen years. Only Jacques and Maria were not in attendance, for they and baby Lodewyk were still in Livorno.

After the burial, a cloud of grief hung over Catrijn, which gradually gave way to thoughts about life and death: why some are spared death until late in life, others not, and the unfairness of it all. That led to confusion and upset, and lately a new dimension—anger—had surfaced. Each morning started with the same rant: It's absurd, she would tell herself, that streets are so dark a man has to lose his life just walking home! Why can't the City Council do something about it? What are Maarten and his cronies doing at those City Council meetings anyway? The more she thought about it, the angrier she became. Too many people die for absurd reasons. My father—he tried to calm a crowd overreacting to a child throwing a shoe at a painting—and he's burned at a stake! How ridiculous is that? And Godmother thinks she's condemned to hell because of heartless Plancius! And poor little Rolfe, he defends Jaane after a kid makes fun of her spectacles, and he gets a black eye! Where is God when all this is going on? Why doesn't—

A knock came at the door. Catrijn stalked across the room and yanked it open.

"Oh ... uh, Pastor Arminius."

"May I come in?"

"Oh ... certainly. Please do." She showed him to a chair and sat down opposite, while trying to bring her emotions under control.

"I thought I'd stop by to see how you're doing. Perhaps pray with you, if you like. Or just talk." He patted her hand and watched as her angry frown lines and tightly pursed lips slowly relaxed. He thought she was going to say something but instead just blinked back a tear, so he sat silently.

"Thank you for coming. I-I've been having some problems ..."

Arminius nodded sympathetically. "I thought that might be the case when you didn't come to church on Sunday, or to the organ concert. And when your sister-in-law Griet mentioned you were having some difficulty, I decided to come."

Catrijn drew back on hearing Griet's name, remembering the last time they had been together. Griet had stopped by to offer support and to share her own experience in having lost a husband. But Catrijn was in a perturbed and angry state and let Griet know in no uncertain terms that their losses were not comparable. She had lost an intellectual giant and her compass in life. What had Griet lost? Good sex? Catrijn cringed even now just remembering Griet's response and its uncomfortable truth: "You think you're better than me, don't you? You had *the* perfect marriage. Well, you can kiss my sweet arse!"

Arminius suspected something had transpired between the two sisters-in-law, judging from Catrijn's reaction, and she was still grappling with it. "God has a great capacity to forgive, but we have far more difficulty forgiving ourselves."

Catrijn was not about to forgive herself or discuss the matter with Pastor Arminius. The remedy was going to be a humble and humiliating apology to Griet.

A knock came at the door, and Catrijn rose to answer it.

Dirck was standing there, holding up one of his sacks. "I just wanted to deliver this for Jaane," he said and then noticed the pastor, "but I see you have a guest." After acknowledging Arminius with a touch to his hat brim, he took a step back.

"Nee, please stay," Arminius said and came to the door to shake hands. "I was about to go anyway, and being with family is more important." To Catrijn, he said, "We'll talk again, soon."

Dirck could see that Catrijn was out of sorts when the two sat down and she said nothing. So he put the small sack on the table and pulled out a pinwheel. "I hope Jaane likes this."

"Oh, it's lovely. She'll like it. She adores anything you give her." Catrijn blew on the pinwheel and a colorful pattern emerged. "Such pretty colors. Thanks." She looked at the other larger sack he had brought. "What's in that one? Something for me?" The question put a smile on her face, for it felt good to say something cheeky instead of angry for a change.

"Maybe it is, and maybe it isn't," he said with a mischievous grin and brought the sack to the table. "Actually, this is something for *me*, but I thought you'd enjoy seeing it." He untied the cord, and the sack fell open, revealing a sphere. "This is a celestial globe made by Mercator. I bought it in La Rochelle." He placed his elbows on the table and balanced the globe in his hands. "It's missing its stand, and I need to have a replacement made."

"That's odd," Catrijn commented. "Where's the land and sea?"

"It's a *celestial* globe, not a *terrestrial* globe."

"Hmm." Not sure what he meant, Catrijn examined its surface. "They're constellations!" she declared, delighted by her discovery and realization that the globe depicted what a person saw looking *up* at the sky—a celestial view—not looking *down* at the earth, a terrestrial view.

"Ja, there are fifty constellations. I counted them." He began turning the globe with his fingers. "I know this globe isn't very practical, but it was so intriguing I couldn't resist buying it."

"And beautiful too," Catrijn said. The two silently inspected the ethereal images floating through the heavens on the globe. There were graceful female figures like Andromeda and Cassiopeia, a muscular Hercules, the twinkling crown called Corona, and the Gemini twins ambling arm-in-arm. Stars were there too, as well as the twelve signs of the zodiac, which Betje had taught them about. Astrology had fascinated her, though scholars and not the Betjes of the world typically studied the subject.

"There's you! Capricorn." Dirck pointed at Catrijn's half-goat, half-fish zodiac sign. "A real enigma."

She slapped him on the arm friskily. Turning the globe with her hands, she searched for the image of a balance scale. "There, that's you! Libra—always balanced and logical."

Dirck studied Libra and saw Scorpio, the scorpion, with its pincers resting on Libra's scales. "Ha! And there's Nicolaas—always pestering me." The mention of Nicolaas cast a pall, and neither could force a laugh. "I sure do miss him." Dirck's hand was next to Catrijn's on the table, and his fingers reached out to give hers a little squeeze.

"Me too." She squeezed back.

Dirck was balancing on the wobbly bench in front of Griet's house, while installing a lantern and trying not to knock over Rolfe, who was on tiptoes attempting to help. Griet's house was the twelfth house on the street and, as such, was required by a new city law to have a lantern installed and candles lit every night for the welfare of all Amsterdammers. "Careful," Maarten warned and reached out to steady Rolfe.

Griet stood nearby, mulling over the heartfelt apology Catrijn had delivered yesterday. I never thought she'd admit she was wrong, especially to me. Maybe she'll start treating me more like an equal ... nee, not likely. But I *am* glad it's over. I wouldn't want to lose her friendship or the chance to learn all those fancy words and new ideas she's always coming up with. And I've got to figure out how she manages to be sophisi-*sicated* without even trying—

"What do you think, Griet?" Maarten asked.

"Oh, uh." she stepped closer to the lantern. "I think Dirck did good work."

The job done, Maarten said goodbye and went on to Jacques's home, also a twelfth house, to help install his lantern. Dirck stepped down and rubbed his cold hands together, and Rolfe jumped to the ground and mimicked him. With an impish grin, Rolfe squeezed his hands into fists and threw a punch, which set off a round of sparring.

"It's too cold out here for me," Griet said, as a shiver ran through her. "Let's go in and get warm."

In the front room, she exaggeratedly turned her gaze toward the opposite wall, and Dirck's eyes followed. "Your new portrait!" He moved closer and saw Griet and Rolfe depicted as smiling affectionately at each other and holding beaver hats, amid the usual symbols of a proper household. "Very nice."

"I knew you'd appreciate it." Griet led them into the kitchen, and the three gathered around the hearth where a pot of stew was simmering. Dirck inhaled the enticing aroma.

"Smell familiar?" she asked. "I'm making your mother's favorite recipe. Want to come tonight for supper?"

Rolfe bobbed his head up and down, telling his uncle to say yes.

"Sure I will." With a grin, he made a fist at Rolfe—"Be good"—and kissed Griet on the cheek. "Have to go back to work now. See you tonight." He did not mention he was going to swing by Catrijn's house for lunch with her and Jaane before going back to work.

Once Dirck was gone, Rolfe started hunting around for his top. Griet remembered he had left it outside and went to retrieve it.

"Hi Griet!" Rijp said as he came up the street. "Mighty cold, isn't it?"

"Ja, it is," Griet said and wrapped her arms around herself.

"Say, you've got one of those twelfth-house lanterns. Stupid idea."

"Stupid? They'll save lives."

"Sure, if people light 'em. But who's gonna do that? Candles are expensive."

"I will," Griet said indignantly, but when she glanced down the street at houses with lanterns, she realized Rijp was probably right. Old widow Voorhees was certainly too miserly to light hers, and Heer Jacobszoon was suspect too. Rijp was prescient, because it would become a problem and the city council would eventually establish a tax to pay for candles and men to light them.

Rolfe opened the door to see who his mother was talking to.

"Hey Rolfe," Rijp said, "where'd you get the black eye?"

"In a fight!"

"I hope you won."

Rolfe's head went up and down dramatically.

"He's so feisty and *unpredicTable*," Griet said.

"Ja, he is." Rijp's eyes connected with Griet's. "Mind if I come in to warm up?"

"I have to take Rolfe to the Begijnhof now. Perhaps another time."

Rijp's expression turned earnest. "You know, Griet. I like you." It was true, though he felt compelled to say it now because he had not yet found a way to be alone with her. She always kept him at a distance. It was maddening.

As Rijp walked off, Griet's eyes followed him. He's really attracted to me ... so is Dirck. A self-satisfied smile formed on her lips. I wonder which one I'll marry.

"Mom," Rolfe said, yanking on her hand. "What are you thinking about?"

"Oh, just some silly stuff," Griet said with a self-deprecating laugh. "Come on. Let's learn some useful stuff at Aunt Margaretha's."

On April 1, 1595, Maarten stopped by Catrijn's house before going to the harbor to see the ships of the Far Lands Company set sail. He wanted to tell little Jaane a story he hoped would boost her spirits, because kids kept taunting her about wearing spectacles, despite Rolfe's protective efforts. Catrijn was watching both kids while Griet was seeing the ships off.

As soon as Grandpa arrived, the kids climbed onto his lap, and he told them of the Sea Beggars capturing the town of Brill on April Fool's Day twenty-three years ago. He concluded with a recitation of the silly joke Uncle Pieter had made up about the Duke of Alva losing his *bril*, spectacles. After Jaane and Rolfe repeated the refrain, "April fool, Alva! We stole Brill. You lost your *bril!*" more than enough times, Maarten decided to leave.

At the Damrak, he met up with Pieter, Jacques and Griet, and together they watched Dirck and other directors give final instructions to the lead captains of the Far Lands Company fleet, Cornelis de Houtman and Gerrit van Beuningen. Afterward, "Good luck" and handshakes went around, and the two captains walked toward the lighter that was going to take them to the harbor where the Far Lands Company's four ships—*Mauritius, Amsterdam, Hollandia*, and *Duyfken*—were waiting with 240 men aboard. Before the two captains reached the lighter, they were quarrelling and continued to do so as it pulled away.

"What are they arguing about?" Griet asked, her anxiety showing.

"I think they don't get along," Pieter said.

"Doesn't bode well for such a long, dangerous voyage," Maarten commented.

"Will we lose our money?" That was Griet's greatest fear, for she had scrimped to make the investment. If Maarten and Pieter are already concerned, she thought, maybe becoming a big-shot investor wasn't such a good idea after all.

Dirck joined them and heard her question. "It's too early to worry about that," he replied, trying to appear confident. "They're probably just nervous and will settle down once they're underway." But experience told him it would be a problem, one way or another.

Maarten thought it best to change the subject. "Griet, you have such rosy cheeks today. You look downright cheery."

"Oh." Griet waved him off, acting embarrassed, but was in fact feeling pretty terrific because last night she had succumbed to Rijp's charms, and it was even more satisfying than with Nicolaas. She had been waiting for Dirck to make his move first, but two years without sex had finally worn down her patience. Nonetheless, she was still not counting Dirck out.

"Well," Dirck said, "maybe we should all go to Maarten Spil's tavern for a glass of wine to celebrate," and extended his arm to Griet.

Beaming at him, she linked her arm in his, feeling as though she was on top of the world. As they strolled off, she failed to notice a sullen Rijp watching from a distance.

After several glasses of wine and much laughter, other directors arrived. More wine, more toasts, and finally Maarten decided to go home for a nap. Not long after, Dirck escorted Griet home.

No sooner had Griet entered her house and begun stoking the fire, than a knock came at the door. She opened it, and Rijp walked right in. She flashed a coquettish smile.

"Why do you spend so much time with Dirck?"

"Dirck? He's my brother-in-law and Rolfe's godfather."

"Well, I don't like it—*not* one bit!"

Griet stared at him, not liking to be told what to do. On the other hand, his jealousy *was* flattering.

"Oooh ..." Rijp said, his anger rising and fists clenching. "You make me so mad!" His hand raised. "I could—" Whatever he was going to say and do, he decided not to and instead whipped around and stomped out the door, slamming it behind him.

What? Griet said to herself, bewildered and unnerved.

With the summer sun filtering through the window, Catrijn sat down with a book in hand and winked at her daughter curled up in Konrad's chair.

Jaane smiled back and resumed alternating between blowing on her pinwheel and lazily spinning the celestial globe, which Uncle Dirck had lent her after adding a base.

Catrijn closed her eyes, trying to visualize Konrad sitting

there and feel his presence. It was becoming harder and harder to do. Jaane's memory of him too was fading, even though she had tried to slow the process by keeping Konrad's belongings in place. Only recently had she come to realize the futility and selfishness of retaining his clothes and given them to Pieter to distribute to needy men. Nonetheless, she had apologized to Konrad for parting with his beautiful garments—I'm sorry, but I had to—as though he could hear from somewhere in the heavenly place he occupied. She liked to imagine him floating among the constellations, like those on the celestial globe, and occasionally bumping into her beloved father, mother, and godmother. That was how she had described it to Jaane too, in response to her questions about death.

Warmed by the thoughts, yet finding them wearing, Catrijn endeavored to meditate, as Aunt Margaretha had urged her to do since Konrad's death. Deep breath ... deep breath. Soon she was asleep and remained so while the maid came in and took Jaane away to dress her and brought her back. Finally, Catrijn awoke when Dirck arrived.

"There's my sweet goddaughter," Dirck said and lifted the bespectacled four-year-old into his arms.

Jaane planted a kiss on his cheek and waved the pinwheel until it whirled. "Aren't the colors *très jolie*?"

"*Oui*, very pretty," Dirck said, marveling again at how fluidly she moved between languages. It was her gift, along with a talent for words. Every time he saw her, she seemed to be using an impressive new word. Dirck glanced at Catrijn. "And your mother is finally awake."

"I was attempting to meditate, the way Aunt Margaretha taught me," Catrijn said and covered a yawn. "But, like always, I fell asleep instead."

"Doesn't surprise me," he said. "Your problem is you think too much and tire yourself out."

"Probably. But meditating isn't easy. Did you ever try it?"

"Nee ... well, not intentionally. But I suppose I do something similar when I'm at sea and stare at the horizon and lose track of time. Twilight is best, when the sea and sky turn silvery and the line between them blurs. It's calming, and slowly all my concerns fade away. Afterward, I feel refreshed and able to focus on more important things."

Catrijn sighed. "Exactly what meditation should be."

"For me, it's just one of those simple pleasures of being at sea."

"You're so lucky. I'd give anything to go to sea ... travel to all those exciting places."

"Ja, but it can get lonely, and sometimes I wish I could be at sea less and at home more." Dirck put Jaane down, clasped her hand, and said to Catrijn, "Ready to go?"

Their destination today was the former Convent of Poor Clares, just south of the Begijnhof, where a rehabilitation center for youthful offenders was being inaugurated. Though the City Council had approved the concept six years earlier and extensive plans had been prepared, it was only opening now because a perfect candidate had come along. He was a sixteen-year-old from a good family, who had confessed under torture to stealing from his employer, and who the magistrates believed would benefit more from rehabilitation, than from flogging.

On arriving, Jaane called out to Maria, "*Ciao!*" and while the two conversed in Italian, Catrijn and Dirck fawned over their two godchildren squirming in Jacques's arms. They then lavished attention on Jacob, the six-year-old orphan who Pieter and wife Floris had adopted. Griet showed up later with Rolfe, who insisted that Uncle Dirck hoist him onto his shoulders for a better view. Rolfe began swinging his arms to get his grandfather's attention.

Maarten, who was standing among fellow city councilors, wagged his hand at Rolfe. His eyes shifted to others in the crowd. On seeing Holland's Advocate Oldenbarnevelt, he acknowledged him with a touch to the brim of his hat. To Aunt Margaretha, he gave a warm smile after she sent a little wave his way. His eyes were drawn to pastors Plancius and Arminius, who were engaged in serious conversation, until anger flashed in Plancius's face and he brusquely pulled back. Maarten suspected it had to do with their growing dispute about free will and grumbled to himself, I wish they wouldn't argue in public. We can't afford to have divisions within Calvinism, not after so much blood was shed just to be able to worship without persecution.

At the podium, prominent men who had helped found the new rehabilitation facility waited to speak, but the man Maarten admired most was absent, Dirck Coornhert. He had written the institution's founding principles and had died recently. Coornhert had also been the chief writer for Prince William of Orange and throughout his life had tirelessly promoted religious tolerance and urged churches to put aside their dogmatic differences and come together for the common good.

The first speaker stepped forward and explained:

"The goal of this new facility is to correct and improve delinquents through work and moral teaching. Each boy will be fed an ample and varied diet, given time for vigorous exercise, and taught a useful trade. To avoid stigma, each will be brought into the facility under the cover of darkness to conceal his identity and will be released in the same way."

Maarten was thinking: Concealing their identity is an excellent idea. Lots of kids don't want to be criminals, but sometimes have no choice. Let them have a fresh start, return to society without taint, then we'll see what they're made of.

The final speaker reported, "A similar institution for women will open in the future in the former Saint Ursula Monastery. It will teach them spinning and sewing."

While the audience applauded, Griet looked around and glimpsed Rijp Dekker standing alone, lost in his thoughts and seemingly a bit angry. She studied him for a moment. I wish he wasn't so volatile, up one minute, down the next. Sometimes he scares—

"*Mom!* Look at me!" Rolfe called, while balancing precariously on Uncle Dirck's shoulders.

"Steady," Dirck warned.

In response to her son's feat, Griet's mouth formed an O in feigned amazement. To Dirck, she gave an admiring smile, while thinking: He'd make a perfect father. A good husband too, not unpredictable or particularly exciting, but completely reliable. Dirck's the one for me.

On Sunday, Maarten hosted the traditional after-church meal, and Letje ter Williger served as cook and hostess. When everyone had arrived, Maarten passed out glasses of wine and announced, "Letje and I have decided to get married." Lifting his glass, he said, "To sweet Letje. May we have many happy years together."

Competing toasts abounded, Letje served lunch, and afterward the women huddled with her to plan the wedding reception, because she had no daughters of her own to help.

On the following day, Griet dropped by Catrijn's house ostensibly to discuss the wedding and to give the kids an opportunity to play together.

Catrijn happened to be wearing a new jacket when answering the door. "What do you think?" she asked and twirled around. "This is our newest silk."

"Oh, it's exquisite," Griet said, using one of Catrijn's words she had at last mastered.

"That's exactly what I told Jacques. He's very proud of it."

Catrijn removed the jacket and stored it safely away, and the kids went into the kitchen to pester the cook. The two women sat down and talked about what foods to make for the reception, despite Letje's stubbornness in wanting to prepare everything herself. The conversation segued into speculation about Maria's pregnancy—her third!—and the results of Griet's first painting lesson—so-so. Meanwhile, Griet seemed unusually upbeat.

"You haven't stopped smiling since you arrived, Griet."

"I know, it's because—nee, I shouldn't say it." Griet shook her head. "I haven't told anyone yet. Nee, forget that I said anything."

"What? What were you going to say? Now I'm intrigued."

"I shouldn't say anything yet ... but I'm so excited. I just decided to marry Dirck."

Catrijn's jaw dropped. "Dirck?" If Griet was going to marry anyone, Catrijn thought it would be Rijp Dekker. "When?"

"Like I said, I shouldn't have told you. It's too soon. I mean, nothing's final yet." Seeing that Catrijn was upset by the news, Griet chastised herself: Why did I ever bring this up? Dirck hasn't even proposed yet. But I know he will. He finds me sexy and won't be able to keep his hands off me much longer. She looked at Catrijn and wondered, maybe I should explain what I meant: that I love him and want to marry him and know he's going to propose soon.

Catrijn had already retreated into her own thoughts.

When Catrijn said nothing more, Griet grew uncomfortable. "I should be going."

Griet departed, and Catrijn stewed. Why didn't Dirck mention this yesterday? Why would he do such a thing without telling me first? Me, of all people! After playing with her food during lunch and fretting, she asked the maid to watch Jaane while she went out.

Catrijn knocked firmly on Dirck's door.

"Catrijn," Dirck said, surprised. She strode into the house, and after he closed the door, she swung around and stood face to face with him.

"I need to talk to you," she said. "I think I owe it to you, to tell you Griet isn't worthy of you."

"What are you talking about?"

"You're going to marry Griet."

"Who told you that?"

"Griet."

"That's news to me."

"But ... she said—"

"Don't believe everything you hear. Besides, why are you always telling me who not to marry? First it was Kaatje ... too talkative, not smart enough. You've let me know, one way or another, every woman I've ever liked wasn't worthy of me." He leaned against his desk.

"Nee ... uh," Catrijn said, but it had a ring of truth.

"Why do you do that?"

Flustered, Catrijn looked at the floor. "I shouldn't have come." She started to leave.

Dirck stepped in her path and gazed deep into her eyes. "Think about it. Why do you do that?"

Once outside, Catrijn walked fast, hyperventilating and running her sweaty palms over her skirt.

Catrijn did think about what Dirck had said, while assiduously avoiding him and Griet. She too wanted answers, but everything seemed so complicated, the emotions confused. And what did Dirck think? Did he have something in mind when he asked that question?

Not really having an answer for him, she decided nonetheless to casually stop by Van der Voort & Sons at lunchtime when Dirck was likely to be alone. He was. Seeing her, he mumbled something about working on papers to take to Livorno. Mumbling was not at all like him. Before Catrijn could say anything in response, a commotion started outside involving Maarten speaking loudly. Other voices joined his, all sounding excited.

The door opened, and Maarten stepped inside, his face animated. Another city councilor was behind him. Seeing Dirck and Catrijn, Maarten said, "Oldenbarnevelt was at the City Hall and said that both the king of France *and* queen of England have formally recognized the Dutch Republic's independence from Spain."

"That's good news," Dirck said, and Catrijn, "Great news."

Neighbors came through the door, asking questions.

"Does this mean the war is over?" one queried.

A woman heard the question and said to the person behind her, "The war is over!" who said to the next person, "Maarten says it's over!"

"Nee, nee, I didn't say that!" Maarten reiterated word-for-word what he had said and added, "Even though the war isn't over, it's good news anyway because two *important* monarchs are standing up to King Philip to support us."

"King Philip will keep fighting us," the other city councilor said.

"He's right," another man added, "Philip *can't* let us leave his kingdom. If he does, other parts of the realm might try too. And ... "

While the talking went on, Maarten noticed Dirck and Catrijn were paying little attention and seemed to have something else on their minds. In fact, he recalled that Dirck had seemed preoccupied the last few days. Did they have an argument?

Dirck saw more people squeeze through the front door and realized this was not a place for a personal conversation, so he leaned over to Catrijn. "Meet me at my place, say, in half an hour? We'll have lunch."

"What about Griet? What's happening with her?" She just wanted to clear that up before agreeing to anything.

"Griet? She has nothing to do with this. Hasn't said anything to me, and I haven't said a word to her. I don't know why she told you that."

"I'll come," Catrijn said. After listening to more of the conversation swirling around the room and catching the gist of it, she slipped out the back door.

By the time Catrijn arrived at Dirck's house, he had already set out pickled fish, fresh bread and apples for lunch. With a quick "Hi" she took a seat at the table, looking ill at ease.

Dirck sat down in the opposite chair and patiently waited for her to speak.

"I've thought about it," Catrijn said, "and you're right. I have been judgmental ... about Kaatje and the others." Thinking she might have seen a smirk form on his face, she added, "But I did it for your own good."

Dirck's brows arched. "For *my* own good. Really? No other reason?"

Realizing she was approaching this all wrong, Catrijn confessed, "I know I shouldn't have done it. It's your life, and I'm sorry." Her gaze shifted to her finger with a torn nail.

"So, Miss Marriage Maker," Dirck said and crossed his arms, "who do you think *is* worthy of me?"

Catrijn saw a hint of smugness in the curve of his lips and could not tell whether he was toying with her or serious. Flustered, she looked at the finger again, and the shiny apples.

"Well?"

"Me," she said as though it was a joke but inside felt giddy, fearful, and queasy all at the same time.

Dirck got up, stood next to her, and with one hand on the table leaned over.

She stared at his chest ... raised her head, and her eyes met his.

"So you think you're the right one for me?"

She gulped and nodded yes.

Dirck bent down, cupped his hands around her face, "Me too," and kissed her tenderly.

Catrijn closed her eyes, feeling a warm rush of emotions. On the next kiss, their lips lingered.

"I've always loved you," Dirck said. "Didn't you know that?"

Catrijn's eyes blinked a yes. "I've always loved you too." Another kiss, this one full of passion.

Dirck raised her from the chair and nestled her in his arms.

"Why did it take us so long?" she asked, feeling as though she had been waiting for an eternity.

"Doesn't matter." With his lips pressing against her forehead, the two stood silently, savoring the new experience. When she looked up and kissed him, Dirck filled it with all the ardor he had saved up over the years.

"Whew." Catrijn tilted her head for another. This one was long and fervent.

Impetuously, Dirck scooped her up in his arms. Both chuckled, and she wrapped her arms around him. He nuzzled her neck and kissed it sexily, and she moaned with delight. Feeling primed and wanting privacy, he headed to the interior room where his bed was. Then it occurred to him, maybe she's not as ready as I am. She's certainly not as experienced, having had only one man, and a very gentlemanly one at that. And maybe she's still in transition somewhere between best friends and lovers. Cool down, he warned himself, go slow, see what happens. If it's not today, then tomorrow or later. We have a whole lifetime ahead of us.

As he put Catrijn down on the bench and sat down next to her, he resolved to let her signal if and when she was ready. He lifted her chin and traced the contour of her cheek and finished with a touch to her cute nose. His lips went to hers and lingered there before moving down to her neck, while his fingers were gently drifting over her arm ... and to her waist.

This is so sensuous, Catrijn thought. I'm floating ... not thinking, just feeling. I could stay here forever.

Dirck pulled her close, saw desire in her eyes, and kissed her again. Catrijn found the lush kiss incredibly arousing and sighed deeply when his hand skimmed over her hip ... to the thigh. She pulled his face closer and kissed him lustfully, ending with a little bite to the lip. She was ready.

With a flirty grin, he tugged loose the tie of her bodice. With a coquettish smile, she undid the knot of his shirt strings. As he slid her blouse off one shoulder, his lips brushed it and continued to her neck ... her breast. Their eyes met again. He raised her up and led her to the bed, and slowly his hand ran down the length of her body and slipped under her skirt ...

Daylight was fading when Catrijn reached the most delicious, exquisite crescendo ever. Slowly, she lifted her still smoldering eyes to say: That was terrific.

He kissed her ravenously, and his hips began moving in a more forceful rhythm. Her hands felt his muscles tense and skin grow hot. Soon her body was undulating with his and luxuriating in the feel of his lips on hers. His breathing grew heavier. The bed flexed and creaked. His body stiffened, face tightened almost into a grimace ... a primal moan came out. As he sank onto her, she caressed and kissed his face.

After he rolled onto his side and pulled up the covers, she lay cradled under his arm, feeling enveloped by love and marveling: That was pure ecstasy ... the shooting stars I'd always hoped for.

He lay there perfectly still, savoring her presence and his feeling of utter completeness. When she fell asleep, he mused about their sex. As I suspected, she was inexperienced beyond anything but the basics. She'd never made love nude, on top of the covers, and in broad daylight. And being sexually stimulated to heighten her pleasure before intercourse was entirely new to her, and she loved it. It was sweet that she was embarrassed slightly when we stood naked in front of each other, and I did the right thing by pointing out that we still had our stockings and garters on. The humor put her at ease. Yawn. Drowsy now, he pressed his lips to her head and closed his eyes.

Dirck walked Catrijn home, and, hearing the door open, the maid came out of the kitchen. Jaane ran to greet them, and Dirck picked her up.

"Mother, where were you?"

"I was, we were looking at, uh, maps—"

"We were at my father's house examining a new map," Dirck said, "and had lunch."

"Time just flew by," Catrijn added, without making eye contact with Dirck.

Looking skeptical, the maid asked, "Are you hungry? Jaane has already eaten."

"I'm famished," Catrijn declared.

"Nee, not me," he said, though he was. "Well, I'd better be going." Dirck put Jaane down. "Have lots to do before I go to Gdansk." When Jaane looked disappointed, he added, "I'll see you on Sunday, if not before," and departed without looking at Catrijn.

The following day, Dirck knocked on Catrijn's door when he knew she would be alone. After he stepped inside, she locked the door and put her arms around him. He restrained himself, indulging in only one passionate kiss, before taking a step back. "We need to talk."

"All right."

"It's obvious to me that we can barely control ourselves when we're together, let alone conceal our feelings from others. People will notice something's changed. I saw the look in your maid's eyes yesterday, when we struggled to answer Jaane's simple question, 'Where were you?'" He put his hands on Catrijn's shoulders. "I want our lives to be perfect together. No sneaking around, no lying, no one guessing or gossiping about us. I want us to get married as soon as possible."

"Me too."

Dirck dropped to his knee. "This is the proper way to start: Will you marry me? I love you with all my heart and promise to make you happy."

"Of course," she said dreamily, sighed, and melted into his arms when he stood and embraced her.

After the emotions settled down, Dirck said, "I don't mean to sound businesslike, but we need to decide how and when."

"You're so practical. I love that about you," she said and, with a coy upturn of the lips, added, "but oh so passionate too."

Dirck could not resist proving that with a truly sexy kiss, after which he said with a self-deprecating laugh, "Back to business," and moved them toward the table to sit down. "I have to lead the fleet on the final voyage to Gdansk, so if we start marriage banns before I go, we can have the wedding right after I return in October."

"Perfect."

"And I *won't* go to Livorno this winter. Rykaard can handle it. But I *will* go to La Rochelle in spring and later to Gdansk. *And* I'll take you with me."

"I *finally* get to see the world?" she said, visibly excited.

"Now let's decide when to tell everyone. Obviously, Father and Aunt Margaretha right away, and Jaane. We can wait 'til Sunday, after church, to let the others know."

With a nod of approval, Catrijn added, "If you don't mind, I'd like to speak with Jaane first, alone. Prepare her for the change, answer any questions. She took Konrad's death surprisingly well for a four-year-old and accepted the fact that she'd never see him again, except in heaven." She smiled. "Your globe helped with that, because I told her that Father is up there among the celestial bodies, watching over her. I'm certain Jaane will be extremely happy about us. She adores you and regards you as her second father. In fact, I plan to suggest she call you Papa in the future, rather than Uncle Dirck, to make us a *real* family."

"I'd like that."

"Oddly, I think Konrad would approve of our marriage. I suspect he knew you were his competitor and saw a yearning in me for you, first when he proposed and I hesitated, and afterward when I wanted your opinion."

"Hmm, could be," Dirck said, appearing to be thoughtful, but knew it was true, which is why he had already decided he could not live in Catrijn's house, where Konrad's memory lingered. Instead, he would buy a new one for them.

"So, should we go tell your father?" she asked.

They found Maarten working at his desk.

"We have something important to tell you, Father," Dirck said, his arm around Catrijn. "We're going to get married."

Surprised by the suddenness of the announcement, especially since the two seemed to be having an argument the previous day, Maarten rose slowly as he processed it.

"I know this is a bit of a surprise, but it was a long time coming," Dirck said.

"Took us awhile to figure it out," Catrijn added.

In Maarten's mind the past and present were merging, and he finally comprehended their relationship.

"I always knew you two had a special feeling for each other," Maarten said. "It's one of those odd things in life, when something feels right, but for some reason doesn't happen." Beaming, he put his arms around both and kissed their foreheads. "I couldn't be happier."

Catrijn and Dirck left Maarten's house after numerous toasts and arrived at Aunt Margaretha's a bit tipsy and clinging to each other.

"What's going on with you two?" Margaretha said, as she let them in and closed the door. "You look as though you're going to burst with joy ... *and* had a little too much to drink as well."

"Aunt Margaretha, you're not going to believe this, but Dirck and I are going to get married."

"It's about time," Margaretha said in her matter-of-fact way, but the tone was soft and affectionate. "It's been obvious since you were youngsters that you had a special bond. Best friends, then a mutual attraction."

"Really?" Dirck remarked. "Was it *that* evident?"

"To me it was." Margaretha knew it had also been to Betje, who was so concerned about propriety that she discouraged it at every opportunity. "Whatever happened in the past is done. The important thing is that you discovered the love you've long had for each other. And that is wonderful." She pulled Catrijn's face close to hers and kissed it lovingly, and then Dirck's. With both towering over her diminutive figure, she put her arms around their waists, and let tears of joy flow.

Catrijn and Dirck departed after more sherry, and the two agreed that he should come to Catrijn's house the next day to talk with Jaane.

When Dirck arrived, an excited Jaane came running up and said, "You're going to be my Papa!"

"That's right. Your mother and I are going to get married in two months." Jaane held up two fingers, and Dirck acknowledged it with a nod. "Then you, Mother and I will live together, as a family. The same as you and your Mother and father lived together. I will never replace your father—nobody can—but I will love you always, like he did."

"I know. I love you too."

"But you can't tell anyone else yet about the wedding. Only you, Grandpa Maarten, and Aunt Margaretha know. Can you keep a secret until Sunday, when your mother and I tell everyone else?"

To show her resolve, Jaane put a finger to her lips to seal them.

After church on Sunday the family gathered at Jacques and Maria's house. Right away, Jaane sought out Grandpa Maarten and Aunt Margaretha and pressed her finger to her lips and whispered, "Our secret."

During lunch, Maarten revealed his and Letje's plans for their upcoming wedding. "It'll be a simple family affair. Pastor Arminius will perform the ceremony, and after that we'll go to Catrijn's house for a reception that'll be similar to this casual gathering we're having today. Nothing formal or fancy, and Letje will prepare the food."

"Ahem," Letje said, "but I want to thank everyone for offering to help me cook," while smiling at Catrijn, Griet, Maria, and Floris.

"That sounds like a perfectly lovely celebration," Jacques said and raised his glass. "To your happiness!"

After everyone had drained their glasses, Jacques refilled them and raised his again. "I'd like to make a toast to my beautiful wife, Maria, who is pregnant with our third child." Maria blushed.

After the congratulations subsided, Dirck stood, picked up Jaane, and drew Catrijn to him. "I have something important to announce as well. Catrijn and I have decided to get married. The nuptials will be after I return from Gdansk."

Maarten was the first to break the stunned silence. "Congratulations!"

Others repeated, "Congratulations and best wishes!" and lifted their glasses. Then the questions started.

"I would never have guessed it," Jacques said, "you two are such good friends. When did you decide?"

"It was a long time coming ... "

Griet hung back, too numb to listen further, too embarrassed by her stupid comment to Catrijn, and wondering: Why didn't I see he was more interested in her, than me? I *know* he finds me sexy and often seemed about to make an advance ... but he never did. Flummoxed, she studied Catrijn and Dirck for clues. They're holding hands and making eyes at each other, like youngsters in love. Yet I've seen them many times talking seriously with Maarten, as though they're business partners. Dirck has a unique connection with her. One that I can't compete with. In truth, it's not the kind of relationship I want with a man.

When Catrijn looked her way, Griet panicked. What will I do if she brings up what I said? I can't tell her the truth; that would be admitting she's the winner and I'm a loser. Quick, make up something. Maybe that I was joking. That's it, I'll say I was kidding. Griet stepped forward and said:

"Congratulations you two. You're perfect for each other!"

"Thank you," Catrijn said, and Dirck added, "We think so too," and the three clinked glasses. Catrijn and Dirck said nothing about Griet's previous comment, having agreed it would accomplish nothing and only embarrass her.

Griet left early, not only to escape the awkward situation but also to get back to work on her wedding present for Maarten and Lejte, a portrait of the two of them. The previous night she had completed Maarten's image and was eager to see it in daylight and with fresh eyes. Hmm, his hair is pretty good. I did a decent job on the ruffled collar ... lots of nice detail. But not his face. The nose is too big ... mouth lopsided. Is his head too small? Something's wrong with the chair ... it seems to be floating in the air. Geez, if I have to redo Maarten, and the chair, *and* also paint Letje, I'll never finish before the wedding. I'll have to buy something else. I should go to Rijp's warehouse, he always has lots of interesting stuff. And he might be there too.

At Rijp's warehouse, Griet found that he was not there, but his employee showed her around, and she purchased a richly carved wooden box for candles.

Though Maarten and Letje's wedding was strictly a family affair, Catrijn and Dirck's marriage was a major event in Amsterdam, with every city official and Night Watchman in attendance, as well as business associates from Van der Voort & Sons' burgeoning enterprises and Catrijn and Jacques's cloth business. The Beguines and Catrijn's students were present. Rykaard and all his sons and their wives and children came from Hoorn and so did fluyt-builder Pieter Jansz Liorne. Even a Gdansk merchant traveled to be there. Pastor Arminius officiated, Maarten proudly gave away the bride, and Jacques delivered a heartfelt toast.

Throughout, Griet enthusiastically joined in the celebrations and mingled with eligible men. Soon, though, the excitement of the two weddings receded into memory, and Griet found herself alone and lonely. Dirck was not stopping by as often, his priority being to renovate the new house before winter. Afternoons with Catrijn too had pretty much come to an end with Dirck consuming more and more of her time.

To remedy her melancholy, Griet began taking the long way home from the market, enjoying the moderate weather before winter set in. During a leisurely saunter down Haringpakkers Steeg, she stopped in front of Rijp's pub and accidently dropped her basket. A man in the street stooped to help her, and she thanked him profusely and loudly.

Rijp came to the door. "Griet! Haven't seen you lately. How've you been? Wanna come in?"

"Nee, can't, not now. But I'm good. Rolfe's good." She smiled demurely.

"Beautiful day, ain't it?" Rijp said and glanced up at the cloudless sky. "You wanna go on a picnic later? You, me and Rolfe?"

"Ja. That'd be fun."

The midday sun shone brightly when the three strolled with a picnic basket in hand toward Haarlemspoort gate. Once outside the city and away from judging eyes, Rijp took Griet's hand and led her along a small canal. Dry stubbles protruded from harvested fields, and Rolfe raced through them chasing birds.

"The city's gonna expand again soon," Rijp said, "and I'm going to sell that parcel." He gestured toward a field to the north of them. "This one too." He nodded to the southwest. "And I'm gonna make a *whole* lot of money—*much* more than last time."

Rijp strode with his head high and a little further along stopped—"We're here!"—and put down the basket. "This land is mine too, and I've got *big* plans for it. I'm going to build a *huge* house right on this spot. We'll come out on weekends, the three of us. I'll get you a servant to keep up the place and cook meals. We'll have parties. It's gonna be great!"

Noticing he had said *we*, Griet beamed at him. "Sounds terrific, Rijp." She stared at the ground, trying to visualize a grand house, *her* house ... with a maid ... and an apple tree in the front yard, maybe a horse or two—she always wanted to try riding a horse. She imagined herself standing at the door, wearing a silk jacket just like Catrijn wears, and greeting guests, and them commenting on how beautiful everything was …

"Griet. Griet!" Rijp said and finally got her attention. "Are you dreamin' or something? I *said*: Do you want some cheese?"

"Oh, I guess I *was* dreaming." Griet sat down next to him, cozied up close, and took a bite of the cheese he held in his hand. "Rijp, you're really something."

Rijp reached over and pressed his lips to hers.

Rolfe arrived, demanded, "Nee kissing!" and sat down next to his mother. After a few nibbles of cheese and bread, he sprinted away.

Rijp stretched out on the ground and, with one hand propping up his head, observed Rolfe's antics with amusement. The five-year-old was wrestling with a dead stalk, and, when a good yank popped it out of the ground, he went flying backwards. Undeterred, Rolfe scrambled to his feet, dragged the stalk with much effort to the edge of a narrow canal, and started whacking at whatever was in the water.

"Your boy sure has spunk."

"Don't I know it." Griet moved closer to him and put her hand on his back.

"Come on, let's have some fun." Rijp impulsively jumped to his feet and pulled Griet up by the hand. He charged off toward Rolfe and along the way tore out two dry stalks.

"Hey, Rolfe!" Rijp said, poking the boy's shoulder. "Let's me and you have a little fishing contest. Mom, too." He jabbed his stalk into the water, pretending to spear a fish. Giggling, Rolfe jammed his in too, creating a big splash.

Griet punched hers into the water, creating an even bigger spray. Rijp threatened to throw her in, and she dropped the stalk and ran away, laughing. When he caught her and they tumbled to the ground, she declared, "Oh Rijp, you're just the *funnest* guy ever!"

"And you're the spunkiest gal I know." After a kiss, the two nuzzled and snuggled.

Rolfe threw himself on top of them. "I'm hungry!"

"All right, let's eat!" Rijp got up and grabbed the boy's hand, but soon Rolfe broke free and ran ahead. Rijp put his arm around Griet and squeezed her to him. "Griet, we should get married. How would you like that?"

Griet's eyes widened. "You're so unpredictable, Rijp!"

He glared at her. "So the answer is *nee*?"

"Nee, nee—I mean, ja. Ja, I want to marry you." She threw her arms around him, smooched him all over the face, and resumed her position nestled under his arm. "That's what I like about you, Rijp. I never know what to expect next."

Wearing his best clothes, Rijp set off for Maarten's place early Saturday morning, when he expected Maarten to be home alone. His intention was to gain Maarten's support for the marriage as well as lay the groundwork for a lasting relationship with the Van der Voorts, who held a respected place among Amsterdam's leading business and civic leaders. At the front door, he adjusted his flat-brimmed Calvinist hat, pulled the scratchy but stylish large ruffle away from his chin, and spit on his hands to tamp down the edges of his hair. With a broad smile, he knocked firmly on the door.

Maarten greeted Rijp's presence with the usual measure of distrust, but had long ago abandoned glancing up and down the street and worrying that onlookers might think they were friends.

"Maarten, good to see you." Rijp stuck out his hand to shake. "Can I come in? I got some *really* good news for you."

After shaking hands, Maarten ushered his nemesis to a seat and sat down opposite. While Rijp made a show of removing his expensive hat and gloves, Maarten stared with his eyebrow cocked, as if to say: So, what is it? What's the good news?

"I am going to get married," Rijp said with unusual decorum. "I proposed yesterday, and Griet accepted. I'm here to humbly ask for your blessing." Rijp considered it a hopeful sign that Maarten did not immediately say no.

Maarten was mulling it over. I know they've been having an illicit affair, and Aunt Margaretha has warned me that it could jeopardize my standing in the community. Marriage would solve that problem. But the thought of having that crook as my son-in-law? I don't know how I could stand it. I wouldn't be able to avoid him any longer, and he'd always be angling to make a profit from his association with me. And Griet? What would she do if I say no to the marriage? She'd keep seeing Rijp, of course.

Sensing Maarten's turmoil and fearing rejection, Rijp said:

"Maarten, we've had our differences over the years. Sometimes you thought I was an embarrassment to you. But things are different now. I do business with all those city councilors and businessmen who're in your syndicate—"

"Syndicate? What are you talking about? I don't have a syndicate and don't even know what the word means." Maarten was peeved. I haven't even given my approval, and he's already trying to wrangle his way into my business circle.

Rijp knew he had made a mistake by using a business angle to press his case. A personal approach always worked better with Maarten.

"I'm just saying, you and me shouldn't live in the past and keep fighting old battles. I've changed. We've both changed. Both respectable now ... have a place in society." Rijp added, his voice earnest, "Griet doesn't know about my early life, and I prefer to keep it that way. She knows that Nicolaas and I did some business together and got along, and you and me never saw eye to eye. She sees me as a respectable businessman who owns many properties, a pub, deals in antiques—high quality ones—and sells a lot of stuff to rich men. *And* I can provide for her."

He's right, Maarten told himself, young people and newcomers don't really know about his crooked past. Most people nowadays wouldn't have much of a problem with him being in my family. Besides, I should give Griet a chance at happiness.

"When is this wedding supposed to take place?" Maarten asked.

"So I have your blessing?"

"Blessing's too strong a word. I accept it. All right?"

"That's good with me, and I know it'll mean a great deal to Griet," Rijp said. "We'll get married as soon as the banns can be read in church. We're going to have a Calvinist ceremony." For him, one religion was as good as another, or no religion at all, but he needed to be a Calvinist for the sake of appearances.

"We'll have a small gathering with the family afterward at my house," Maarten said.

"I was thinking of something more elaborate, like Dirck and Catrijn's wedding, with all your city council friends and business colleagues."

Maarten shook his head no.

"That's all right. Griet said your *own* wedding was small and friendly. Hey, you were lucky to get Letje—a *fine* little lady."

"One last thing," Maarten warned, "Rolfe is very important to me. I don't want to see him hanging around with *your* friends or in your pub."

"Never. The little guy matters a lot to me too."

"And remember, he has a godfather, Dirck, who'll look after him," Maarten said, to which, Rijp nodded affirmatively.

The wedding occurred as planned, and Griet was happy to be able to choose her own dress this time and to be given a stunning ring—heavy gold with a diamond chip—which made everyone's eyes pop. The newlyweds settled into Rijp's house, and Griet took Maarten's advice to keep her own home and put it up for rent to give her an independent income. She continued with her career at Van der Voort & Sons and sometimes brought Rolfe to work with her, greatly pleasing Maarten.

On August 17, 1597, the town crier announced the return of the ships of the Far Lands Company, which had been gone for nearly two and a half years. Dirck gulped down the last bit of lunch, pecked Jaane on the cheek, passed his lips over his young son Kees's head and let them linger on Catrijn's lips.

At the Damrak, Dirck joined other directors to board a lighter to take them to the harbor. The *Mauritius* was already anchored, and the *Duyfken* and *Hollandia* were in the process of tying up to the Palisade. The fourth ship, *Amsterdam*, was nowhere to be seen. Dirck's eyes scanned the decks of the ships. Neither of the lead captains was in sight, but an emaciated man was waving to them from the *Mauritius*.

"Ahoy!" Reinier Pauw called to the man. "Where are Captain De Houtman and Captain Van Beuningen?"

"They're below deck, under arrest."

The directors looked at each other, alarmed.

"Where's the *Amsterdam*?"

"We had to abandon her in Asia ... not enough crew."

The directors boarded the *Mauritius*, and Dirck was disbelieving that the emaciated man they had seen was in fact the skipper. Toothless from scurvy and severely malnourished, he was almost unrecognizable. The crew, all in the same condition, listlessly converged on the directors. "How many of you are left?" Reinier Pauw asked.

"Eighty-seven."

That was a shocking number because 240 men had been sent on the ships. At the time, the number seemed more than adequate to bring all four ships home again, even accounting for the significant losses expected on such a perilous journey.

"Why were Captain De Houtman and Captain Van Beuningen arrested?"

"They made too many misjudgments and were constantly quarreling," the skipper said. "Several times the men wanted to mutiny, and finally voted to relieve them of their commands when things got really bad." He went on to explain, "For example, when negotiating to buy spices, De Houtman started arguing with the sultan of Bantam because he believed the sultan and the Portuguese were scheming against him. The sultan imprisoned him and some of the crew, and we had to pay a ransom to free them. Then De Houtman bombarded the town with cannon fire and attacked ships in the harbor, and word spread to nearby islands that we Dutchmen were dangerous. So when we went ashore on another island, after being invited to buy cloves and nutmeg, the local leader killed twelve of us."

As the Far Lands Company directors went from ship to ship, a story of horrific hardships unfolded. Casks of fish and butter spoiled as soon as the fleet reached the tropics, violent storms tore ships from their anchors, and men died in agony from scurvy. There were attacks by natives in many places, including Madagascar.

Dirck took a lighter to shore to report to the waiting investors and en route thought about what to say. I'll mention nothing about the arrest of De Houtman and Van Beuningen until we know more about the charges against them. Everyone will want to know the fate of the crew, though it's best not to give exact numbers until we confirm them. Giving a few details about their encounters is in order. The most important thing I need to stress is that three of the four ships *did* return, against all odds, and have some spices in their holds.

A rowboat passed by with Petrus Plancius aboard on its way to the ships. Plancius called out, "Dirck, was the voyage successful?"

Dirck gave a noncommittal incline of his head and said, "You'll be happy to know that Pieter Keyser completed his maps of the southern constellations for you," knowing that Plancius had trained him to record them. "Unfortunately he died, but his maps were brought back."

Plancius's face lit up, for he intended to include those constellations on his new celestial globe.

When Dirck disembarked near the Schreierstoren, the whole family was waiting.

"Did they get spices?" Griet asked anxiously. "Did we lose our investment?"

"Yes, pepper, cloves, mace, and a little nutmeg. No, you didn't lose your investment. We may cover our costs, but probably no profit. No major loss either."

That was all Griet wanted to hear—no loss—so when Dirck related more facts, she pecked Rijp on the cheek and made her way out of the gathering crowd to search for Rolfe. Seeing Margaretha, she stopped, the two exchanged congratulations for not losing their investments, and Margaretha asked about the striking blossoms embroidered on her shawl.

"I've never seen flowers quite like this before, Griet. Do you know what they're called?"

"Tulips. Rijp says the infidels grow them somewhere along the Mediterranean Sea. I just love them and hope to see a live one someday."

After Griet departed, Margaretha took Jaane's hand and moved forward to hear Dirck better. Jaane had become the spry eighty-one-year-old's constant companion after sensing her great aunt's sadness at the death of good friend Heer Nostrand.

Margaretha squeezed Jaane and herself in between Maarten and Pieter, carefully avoiding Rijp. Though she wholly believed in forgiveness and the capacity of people to redeem themselves, that did not go for Rijp. In Margaretha's opinion, it was only a matter of time before his larcenous ways resurfaced, and, when they did, Griet was undoubtedly going to suffer.

Dirck was saying, "The crew died mostly from scurvy, but some were killed in battles with natives." A question was shouted, to which he responded, "Nee, there weren't any clashes directly with the Portuguese, though they *did* instigate the islanders to raise prices and refuse to sell water and food to our fleet." In answer to a question about the extent of the Portuguese monopoly, Dirck reported, "It's been confirmed ... Portugal does not have a monopoly on spices in the East Indies, and Captain De Houtman was able to negotiate an agreement for us to buy pepper in the future." Dirck concluded with, "All in all, I'm heartened by the outcome and I support sending another fleet next year."

Maarten raised his hand slightly to get Dirck's attention and gave an appreciative smile and touch to his hat in a congratulatory salute, for he was truly impressed by the Far East Company's remarkable feat. Nevertheless, his opinion of the spice trade remained unchanged: it was an extremely risky undertaking that would never be more than an exotic sideline for Van der Voort & Sons. Their future lay in the well-established and lucrative European north-south trade, despite having had to halt Livorno sailings last winter because the famine was over and their wheat was fetching lower prices, plus a brush with the Barbary pirates had exposed the fleet's vulnerability. Trade in their now southern-most port, La Rochelle, though, continued strong and offered many unexploited opportunities. Only recently, Dirck and Jacques, a new partner in Van der Voort & Sons, had found a clever way to take advantage of the growing demand and soaring prices for French wines. They arranged to provide financing to wine makers in France in exchange for the right to buy their entire annual production at an advantageous cost per barrel.

Maarten turned away from the crowd to find a quiet spot on the quay and was approached by two mayors who exuberantly shook his hand and said he had been nominated to be an alderman. It was a relief, for he had been angling for the office, because it was the first step to becoming a mayor, a position of *real* power. As mayor, he intended to spearhead the creation of insurance to mitigate risks of operating ever larger fleets and the formation of a bank to put an end to useless coins sneaking into transactions. A mayorship would not come for several years, which would be the early 1600s, but that was fine with Maarten, because people were saying Amsterdam was going to have a golden age in the next century.

Though times were good and Maarten wanted to believe his city was entering a glorious new era, especially after enduring such hardships in the 1500s, he knew better than to get his hopes up. Setbacks happened when least expected: a key port closing to Dutch merchants or the war with Spain turning ugly again. For now, though, the rebellion was in a quiescent period, and he had a feeling it might wind down now that the Dutch Republic was recognized by some monarchs and had an impressive army. So Maarten would probably scoff if told that the revolt would go on for five more decades and become known as the Eighty Years' War, or that the latter years would engulf much of Europe and go down in the history books as the Thirty Years' War.

After reaching the far end of the quay, he sat down on a piling and took in the scene. Amid the vessels ferrying people and goods across the glistening water, he saw pastor Arminius rowing himself out to the East Indies ships to minister to the sick. He's a good man. On a lighter going toward shore was pastor Petrus Plancius, looking triumphant with an armful of maps and studiously avoiding eye contact with Arminius. Maarten wondered again how two such intelligent men could allow themselves to be drawn into a feud over who was heaven bound. He shook his head. Haven't they learned *yet* that such uncompromising religious stances never end well?

Maarten's eyes shifted back toward Amsterdam. There, among the mass of black hats and white collars, were Dirck and Catrijn conversing with directors of the Far Lands Company. He marveled again at their unique relationship that spanned love, friendship, and a sharing of worldly interests. Though Catrijn's travels with Dirck had come to an end with the birth of Kees, Maarten was confident she would be sailing again soon. A recent conversation came to mind that made Maarten chuckle. A woman said she had always thought Dirck and Catrijn were brother and sister.

At the edge of the gathering Maarten spotted Rolfe, carefree as ever and racing around chasing seagulls, and he realized that the grandkids had inherited the gentler, less savage world he and fellow Sea Beggars had dreamed of. They'll never face hunger, religious persecution, have to build a business while deep in debt ... or wait until they're fifty-three years old to finally be in the position to accept an alderman appointment. Unconsciously, he scratched his half-bitten-off ear. And hopefully they'll never have to go to war.

Seeing Rolfe balancing precariously on a piling, he shook his head. That boy's completely fearless, always looking for adventure. He'll definitely go to sea. Could even be a great sea captain, *if* he learns self-control.

Maarten observed the other kids. Jacob will probably follow in Pieter's footsteps, but then you never know. Jaane? So intelligent, yet so shy. Maybe someday she'll put that wonderful gift for languages to use, perhaps in our business. Kees? He seems smart ... so do Jacques's boys. One of them might go to university ... or aspire to a high public office, maybe be like Oldenbarnevelt—Whoa! Aren't you getting a little carried away? he said to himself, and laughed at his uncharacteristic bout of optimism.

A breeze kicked up, carrying the sweet smell of the briny sea. Maarten inhaled deeply. Possibly detecting a hint of rain in the air, he turned to check the water. It was glistening and benign. And the sky. Nothing signaled rain. Maarten reminded himself it was foolhardy to believe you could predict the weather, even more so, the future.

Epilogue

A sequel to *Amsterdam Ascendant,* "Amsterdam's World: A novel of epic voyages, fortunes, and misfortune in the Golden Age," will carry the Van der Voort saga through 1631. Though Maarten anticipates a glorious future at the dawn of the new century, inauspicious natural disasters abound and a criminal element emerges to threaten their lives and livelihood. Catrijn segues into a new role, and Griet expands her painting ambitions. Maarten angles to become a mayor, while Dirck helps launch the innovative Dutch East India Company. Burgeoning financial markets unleash speculative fervor that threatens to ruin a vulnerable family member.

Slowly, religious intolerance again festers. When it explodes into violence, Maarten suffers repercussions and struggles to shield his grandchildren. Dirck and Catrijn are drawn to exotic ports and embark on a journey fraught with danger. Rolfe sets his sights on North America and sails with Henry Hudson, while others of the younger generation hope for careers other than seafaring trade, creating opportunities and risks.

In the final book of the trilogy, Maarten makes a momentous decision, his grandchildren come into their own, and Griet indulges in the blossoming art scene, while Rolfe and his plucky wife explore the virgin forests of North America in pursuit of trade opportunities, where they encounter Indians, both friendly and hostile.

Fact or Fiction?

Because many readers understandably may not be familiar with the history of 450 years ago that underlays this novel, I offer this section to distinguish true history from fiction in the story. In crafting my tale, I conducted considerable research, endeavored to portray real events and people as I found them in history books, and strove to provide an accurate historical chronology, as pertains to my fictional characters' lives. I admit, however, to slightly altering a date or two to accommodate the story line.

FICTIONAL CHARACTERS

All members of the Van der Voort family (Maarten, Betje, Dirck, Nicolaas, and their descendants) are fictional, as well as the Hasbrouks (Papa Hasbrouk, Beguine Margaretha, Catrijn, and her descendants). So too are Pieter, Heer Nostrand, Kaatje, Rijp Dekker, Rykaard and his sons, Griet, and Konrad Teller and his relatives (nephew Jacques, cousin Lodewyk, and Maria).

Though these made-up people participate in notable historical events, their roles and details of their involvement are sheer invention.

REAL HISTORY

Dutch Revolt

The causes and evolution of the Netherlands revolt were multifaceted, and the story features only those events that are most relevant to Amsterdam and lent themselves to an action-oriented and dramatic plot. Nevertheless, the historical overview provided is generally correct. Similarly, the reasons for King Philip II's actions are complex and are only touched on. The king's intolerance of heretical

Protestants is well-known, but he was also beset with a myriad of problems inherited from his father, Holy Roman Emperor Charles V, including a vast and difficult-to-manage empire, crushing debt, as well as a costly responsibility for keeping Christendom safe from the expanding Ottoman Empire.

The revolt started in 1568 and ended in 1648 when the Dutch Republic gained its independence. It is known as the Eighty Years War.

Sea Beggars

The Sea Beggars are presented essentially as found in historical accounts. The bizarre and brutal behavior of some of their leaders is factual. Second-in-command van Treslong was a real person, as was Commander Dirckszoon, though their monologues are invented. The Sea Beggar's expulsion from Dover is true, as well as their taking of Brill.

Brill

The capture of Brill by the Sea Beggars is portrayed basically as found in historical records, including Kopplestock's role, the April Fool's Day joke, and execution of the priests. The city celebrates the event even today. Prior to the success at Brill, the revolt had achieved relatively little.

Inquisition

King Philip II did impose a Spanish-style Inquisition in the Netherlands, officially called the Council of Troubles and derisively the Council of Blood. Amsterdam was indeed called Murderdam at this time because of the Inquisition's work. Nevertheless, clandestine Protestant services reportedly were held, and some sheriffs warned worshipers when a raid was imminent. The Minor Friar Monastery, later torn down, was the seat of the Inquisitors. Despite the brutalities and deaths inflicted, the complicit monks were not killed in retaliation.

Haarlem Siege and Zuider Zee Battle

The Duke of Alva's ruthless drive through towns loyal to Prince William of Orange, his encampment outside of Amsterdam, and the siege of Haarlem are fact-based. Haarlem's heroic efforts to defend itself are straight from history, as are Prince William's deliveries of supplies and assistance by numerous means, including on sledges and boats across Lake Haarlem. Today, the lake no longer exists, having been drained in the 1800s.

The Duke of Alva's exasperation with his son Frederic's failure to defeat Haarlem is well documented, as well as his letter to King Philip II praising Haarlem's courage. The slaughter of Haarlem's residents and defenders following the city's surrender is truthful. After that, the Duke of Alva's army did refuse to move on to Alkmaar until paid. At Alkmaar, their siege failed when the city cut its dikes, a tactic used by other besieged Holland cities. The aftermath was devastating for residents, though, because two-thirds of the submerged land still lay underwater twenty years later, according to some sources.

The generalities and outcomes of the Lake Haarlem and Zuider Zee sea battles with Count Bossu's fleets occurred as described, but the specifics portrayed are pure invention.

Beguines and Their Begijnhof

Beguines were not nuns, did assist the needy, and had a tradition of mysticism. Many bought their own homes in the Begijnhof, which was not church property, and some were known as savvy investors. The Amsterdam Begijnhof exists today, and some of the buildings date to the period of the novel. The relics of the 1345 miracle were given to the Beguines for safekeeping after the Amsterdam government took over the Holy Place Church, which was mostly disused until demolished in 1910.

Amsterdam's Government and Policies

Amsterdam governed itself essentially as described. The exact circumstances that led to the Protestants entering Amsterdam on February 8, 1578, are not clearly dealt with in the historical record, and I invented the negotiations involving fictional Heer Nostrand to give a plausible explanation for it and for Protestants ultimately to be given positions in government. The Civil Guard did remove the Catholic city councilors, who were replaced by a mix of

Catholics and Protestants. For the guard's action, restrictions were later placed on them. This event ushered in an era of Protestant domination and eventually to the barring of Catholics from serving on the City Council and adoption of Calvinism as the official religion. Nevertheless, Catholics were not persecuted and continued to prosper. It is a fact that the war with Spain was a costly burden for Amsterdam, the largest city in the nascent Dutch Republic.

Immigrants from the war-ravished south and Antwerp were drawn to Amsterdam because of its openness to new businesses and relative safety. Moneyed men introduced new business practices, ideas, and fresh capital, all of which accelerated Amsterdam's economic ascendancy. In response to the influx of people, Amsterdam underwent an eastward expansion and later a westward one, much as described.

Dutch Republic

The formation of the United Provinces of the Netherlands, commonly referred to as the Dutch Republic, occurred generally as described. Prince William of Orange, his son Maurice, and nephew William Henry are portrayed as history presents them.

Advocate Johann van Oldenbarnevelt was an important historical figure who helped guide Holland and the Dutch Republic to greatness. His dialogues in the novel, however, are invented.

Maritime Trade

The Baltic grain and timber trade was in fact the mainstay of Amsterdam's economy at this time, though textiles and other manufactured products developed in the city. Trading expanded to southern ports, such as the Huguenot stronghold La Rochelle after Spanish threats diminished, and Livorno when opportunities arose. Livorno was Florence's seaport and was open to immigrants and traders regardless of their religious persuasions.

The descriptions of ships of the period are generally accurate, though the terminology is purposely nontechnical. Fluyts contributed significantly to Dutch supremacy in seaborne trade. Historians are still debating whether the fluyt was invented in the 1590s by

Pieter Jansz Liorne of Hoorn or evolved slowly through a series of innovations. Likewise, Liorne's role in building them is unclear.

Petrus Plancius and Jacobus Arminius

Pieter Platevoet, who changed his name to Petrus Plancius, was a renowned mapmaker and conservative theologian. The dramatized disputes between him and Jacobus Arminius in the story are imaginary. Their differing opinions on free will, however, are true and presage a future serious rift within Calvinism over the doctrine.

Far Lands Company

The lead up to, formation, and outcome of the Far Lands Company are basically correct, though minor discrepancies exist in historical accounts regarding the number of crew and amount of capital raised. The company had nine directors, including real persons Reinier Pauw and Dirck van Os, and they met at Maarten Spil's wine tavern on Warmoesstraat. The manuscript of Jan Huijgen van Linschoten figured prominently in the decision to send a fleet via the southern route. Linschoten, Petrus Plancius and Willem Barents did spearhead the failed expedition to find the polar route to China, which relied on Mercator maps.

Golden Age

I used this term because Americans understand what it means, but it was not used until the 1700s and now is falling into disuse among historians.

Acknowledgments

In crafting this story, I consulted a wide variety of references and list the principal ones below in case you want to learn more about a specific topic. Along the way I was fortunate to receive invaluable input from numerous individuals. Nonetheless, I wish to state that the story is entirely mine and I alone bear responsibility for any mis-interpretations of historical and maritime details contained in it.

Two experts deserve my gratitude for graciously giving of their time to answer questions and review excerpts from my manuscript. They are Jeroen van der Vliet, Head of Collections and Research at The National Maritime Museum *(Het Scheepvaartmuseum)* in Amsterdam, and Ab Hoving, ship historian and former master builder and restorer of model ships at Rijksmuseum.

Art in this book came from the sources noted in List of Illustrations. I am grateful to the son of artist Rein Poortvliet for permitting me to use his father's extraordinary drawings of daily life in 1566, which are full of humanity, pathos, and humor. I also want to thank Harold Spaninks, Curator of the Rein Poortvliet Museum, for his assistance. I applaud the Rijksmuseum for making available free, high-quality images of their art that is in the public domain, and likewise the National Gallery of Art in Washington, D.C., and the Metropolitan Museum of Art in New York City for their free, widely accessible collections.

My warm thanks go to authors, friends, and relatives, who kindly read various drafts of this novel and offered thoughtful advice and constructive criticism. They include my husband David (author D. Manning Richards), Karen Boyer, Charlie Crouch, Bill Holcombe, Sharon Korte, Reverend Jim Laughrey, Judy Laughrey, Marilyn Miscowich, Lyn Morehen, Eileen Rainey, John Ryan, Judy Searles, Stu Searles, and Gary Sheftick.

Principal Sources

ART, CULTURE & MISCELLANEOUS:

Brook, Timothy. *Vermeer's Hat, the Seventeenth Century and the Dawn of the Global World.* New York: Macmillan Bloomsbury Press, 2008.

Durant, Will and Ariel. *The Age of Reason Begins.* New York: Simon and Shuster, 1961.

Jardine, Lisa. *Going Dutch, How England Plundered Holland's Glory.* New York: Harper Collins, 2008.

Krondl, Michael. *The Taste of Conquest: The Rise and Fall of the Three Great Cities of Spice.* New York: Ballantine Books, 2007.

Kurlansky, Mark. *Salt, a World History.* USA: Penguin, 2003.

Ozment, Steven. *What Life Was Like in Europe's Golden Age: Northern Europe AD 1500-1675.* Alexandria, Virginia: Time Life Education, 1999.

Poortvliet, Rien. Translated from Dutch by Karin H. Ford. *Daily Life in Holland in the Year 1566, and the Story of My Ancestor's Treasure Chest.* New York: Harry N. Abrams, 1992.

Schama, Simon. *The Embarrassment of Riches, An Interpretation of Dutch Culture in the Golden Age.* New York: Alfred A. Knopf, Inc., 1987.

Tummers, Anna, Elmer Kolfin and Jasper Hillegers. *The Art of Laughter, Humour in Dutch Paintings in the Golden Age.* Haarlem: Frans Hals Museum, 2018.

Turner, Jack. *Spice, The History of a Temptation.* New York: Random House, 2004.

Zumthor, Paul. Translated from French by Simon Watson Taylor. *Daily Life in Rembrandt's Holland.* New York: Macmillan, 1963.

HISTORY—GENERAL AND SPECIFIC:

Barbour, Violet. *Capitalism in Amsterdam in the 17th Century.* Michigan: Ann Arbor Paperbacks, The University of Michigan Press, 1963.

Boxer, C. R. Edited by J. H. Plumb. *The Dutch Seaborne Empire: 1600-1800.* New York: Alfred A. Knopf, 1965.

Geyl, Pieter. *The Revolt of the Netherlands, 1555-1609*. London: Williams & Norgate, 1932.

Grattan, Thomas Colley. *The History of the Netherlands 50 BC – AD 1815*. Originally published in 1830 and subsequently republished and digitalized.

Haley, K.H.D. *The Dutch in the Seventeenth Century*. London: Thames and Hudson Ltd., 1972.

Hooker, Mark T. *The History of Holland*. Connecticut: Greenwood Press, 1999.

Jacobs, Els M. *In Pursuit of Pepper and Tea, The Story of the Dutch East India Company*. Amsterdam: Netherlands Maritime Museum, 1991.

Macgregor, Mary. *The Netherlands*. London: T.C. & E.C. Jack, 1907.

Mak, Geert. Translated from Dutch by Philipp Blom. *Amsterdam*. Massachusetts: Harvard University Press, 2000.

Motely, John Lathrop. *History of the Netherlands from the Death of William the Silent to the Twelve Year's Truce 1609*. 4 Volumes. New York: Harper & Bros., 1881.

Motely, John Lathrop. *The Rise of the Dutch Republic, Volume II 1574-1584*. Originally published in 1830 and republished numerous times. Available free in Kindle version.

Parker, Geoffrey. *The Dutch Revolt*. Revised edition. London: Penguin Books, 1985.

Rady, Martyn. *From Revolt to Independence: The Netherlands 1550-1650*. London: Hodder & Stoughton, 1990.

Renier, G. J. *The Dutch Nation*. London: George Allen & Unwin Ltd. for The Netherlands Government Information Bureau, 1944.

Rietbergen, P.J.A.N. *A Short History of The Netherlands*. Amersfoort: Bekking Publishers Amersfoort, 2002.

Rowen, Herbert H. *The Low Countries in Early Modern Times*. New York: Walker Publishing, 1972.

Shorto, Russell. *Amsterdam: A History of the World's Most Liberal City*. New York: Doubleday, 2013.

Vlekke, B.M. *Evolution of the Dutch Nation*. New York: Roy Publishers, 1945.

Wilson, Charles. *The Dutch Republic*. New York: World University Library, McGraw-Hill Book Company, 1968.

MAPS:

Baynton-Williams, Ashley and Miles Baynton-Williams. *New Worlds, Maps from the Age of Discovery*. London: Quercus, 2008.

Crane, Nicholas. *Mercator, the man who mapped the planet.* New York: Henry Holt and Company, LLC., 2002.

Swift, Michael. *Mapping the World.* New Jersey: Chartwell Books, Inc., 2006.

RELIGION:

Calvin, John. Translated from the Original Latin by John Allen. *Institutes of the Christian Religion.* 1536. The Project Gutenberg: EBook, Sixth American Edition, 2014.

Chadwick, Owen. *The Reformation.* New York: Penguin Books, 1964.

Cottret, Bernard. Translated from French by M. Wallace McDonald. *Calvin, a Biography.* Michigan: William B. Eerdmans Publishing Company, 2000.

Elwood, Christopher. *Calvin for Armchair Theologians.* Kentucky: Westminster John Knox Press, 2002.

Fatio, Olivier. *John Calvin and the Geneva Reformation 1536-1564.* Geneva: International Museum of the Reformation, 2009.

Graessle, Isabelle. *Reminiscences.* Geneva: International Museum of the Reformation, n.d.

Murk-Jansen, Saskia. Edited by Philip Sheldrake as part of Traditions of the Christian Spirituality Series. *Brides in the Desert: The Spirituality of the Beguines.* London: Darton, Longman + Todd, 1998.

Simons, Walter. *Cities of Ladies: Beguine Communities in the Medieval Low Countries 1200-1565.* Philadelphia, Pennsylvania: University of Pennsylvania Press, 2001.

Sunshine, Glenn S. *The Reformation for Armchair Theologians.* Kentucky: Westminster John Knox Press, 2005.

Swan, Laura. *The Wisdom of the Beguines: The Forgotten Story of a Medieval Women's Movement.* Katonah, New York: Blue Bridge, 2014.

Treasure, Geoffrey. *The Huguenots.* London: Yale University Press, 2013.

Van Heyst, Eugene. *Strength from what is hidden. The Beguinage, the chapel and the Miracle of Amsterdam.* Amsterdam: www.begijnhofamsterdam.nl, no date.

SEA VOYAGES & SHIPS:

Bontekoe, Captain Willem Ysbrantsz. Translated from the Dutch by C. B. Bodde-Hodgkinson and Pieter Geyl. *Memorable Description of the East Indian Voyage 1618-1625.* (First-hand account). London: George Routledge & Sons, LTD., 1929.

Boxer, C. R., Editor and translator from the original Portuguese. *The Tragic History of the Sea* (First-hand accounts of Portuguese shipwrecks 1552-1622). Minneapolis: University of Minnesota Press, 2001. By arrangement with Hakluyt Society, copyright 1959 and 1968.

Hawkins, John. Edited by Clements R. Markham. *The Hawkins' Voyages during the Reigns of Henry VIII, Queen Elizabeth, and James I.* (First-hand accounts of voyages from 1530 to 1607 by the Hawkins family). London: Haklyut Society, 1878.

Hawkins, Richard. Edited by C.R. Drinkwater Bethune. *The Observations of Sir Richard Hawkins, Knight, in his Voyage into the South Sea in the Year 1593.* (First-hand account). London: John Jaggard, 1622. Reprinted by Haklyut Society, 1847.

Hoving, Ab. *17th Century Dutch Merchant Ships.* Indiana: Sea Watch Books, 2014.

Linschoten, John Huyghen van. Edited by Arthur Coke Burnell and P.A. Tiele. *The Voyage of John Huyghen van Linschoten to the East Indies.* 2 volumes. Originally published in Dutch in 1598, and published in English several times. London: Hakluyt Society, 1885. Digitalized by Google.

Marshall, Michael. *Ocean Traders from the Portuguese Discoveries to the Present Day*. New York: Facts on File, Inc., 1990.

Spectre, Peter H. and David Larkin. *Wood Ship – The Art, History, and Revival of Wooden Boatbuilding*. Boston: Houghton Mifflin Harcourt Company, 1991.

Woodman, Richard. *The History of the Ship–The comprehensive story of seafaring from the earliest times to the present day*. London: Conway Maritime Press, 1997.

List of Illustrations

Book Club Discussion Guide

1. What surprised you most in the novel? What did you like best? And the least?
2. Are there any similarities between the Netherlands' rebellion against Spain and the American colonies' revolt against England?
3. Are Amsterdammers in the story in any way like Americans today?
4. Is religious intolerance today different from that exhibited in the novel?
5. Was Maarten's and Betje's marriage successful? Why or why not?
6. What motivated Dirck in life? How much was he like his father?
7. Was Catrijn in love with both Dirck and Konrad? What was she looking for in men and in marriage?
8. What attracted Griet to men and why? How was she different from Catrijn?
9. Was Nicolaas a rogue or just restless and mischievous?
10. How would you describe the culture of Dutch life and the people of Amsterdam during the late 1500s period of the novel? Are they similar to modern-day Dutch people and their culture?

If you enjoyed this first book of the Van der Voort saga, please write a review on Amazon, Goodreads, or your favorite blog or website. I will take your comments into account when writing the next two books.

About The Author

My fascination with Amsterdam and the Netherlands goes back to growing up in New York State. Dutch names were everywhere, from cities such as Batavia and Rensselaer to Vandervoort Street in my hometown. The Dutch founded New Amsterdam, which was later renamed New York City, and left behind a legacy of notable families, the Roosevelts and Vanderbilts among them. The well-known image of a little Dutch boy sticking his finger into a dike served as a symbol of resourcefulness and perseverance.

When my husband David and I decided to leave our demanding real estate development careers to write novels about great cities of the world that we love, I naturally chose Amsterdam. I knew that I wanted to start the story in the latter 1500s to answer the question: How did a small, insular city transform itself in just a quarter of a century into an international, economic powerhouse on the brink of greatness?

Because of the richness of this historical period, I knew I would be able to utilize my expertise in finance and urban development, experiences in business and world travel, and my diverse interests in history, religions, philosophy, art, mapmaking, and sailing. Most of all, I looked forward to the challenge of weaving it all into a compelling action-adventure, family saga.

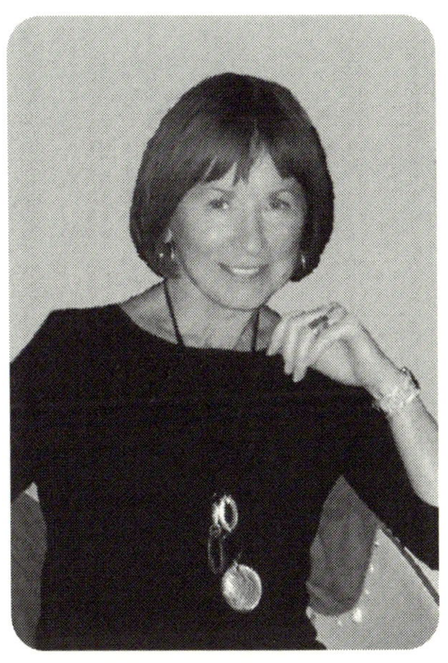

JUDITH W. RICHARDS is an American who has traveled widely, visited Amsterdam on numerous occasions, and periodically lives in France and Australia. She is married to novelist D. Manning Richards. In writing this book, Judy returned to her first love, history, the primary subject of her Bachelor of Arts degree. She also holds a Master of Business Administration in finance and spent her career in economics, finance, and as head of the commercial real estate development firm she founded in Washington, D.C. She is the author of *Fundamentals of Development Finance*, a well-regarded university textbook and guide for urban development professionals. For the latest information about her and the upcoming sequel, visit www.judithwrichards.com.

Made in the USA
Middletown, DE
22 January 2024

48256993R00222